T0386458

Studies on Hysteria Revisited

Steeped in Lacanian theory, this book is the first of its kind to present a longitudinal approach to the study of hysteria.

In these 21 seminars Dr Melman leads us from the first records of hysteria to Freud's major discovery of the principal concepts of trauma, incompatibility, repression and the unconscious. Peppered with invaluable clinical examples, the author guides readers through difficult concepts as he links hysteria to the birth of psychoanalysis itself, and demonstrates how the reader may become implicated in this discourse.

Capturing Melman's indomitable spirit, *Studies on Hysteria Revisited* will be an important read for graduate students, clinicians, and those in psychoanalytic formation.

Charles Melman is a leading French psychoanalyst and psychiatrist. Friend and collaborator of Lacan, he founded L'Association Lacanienne Internationale in Paris in 1982. He has published extensively and contributed influentially to psychoanalysis worldwide.

Helen Sheehan studied psychoanalysis in Paris where she obtained her PhD in 2000. She has contributed to psychoanalytic journals in Ireland, England and France. She works as a psychoanalyst in Dublin, and is a member of L'Association Lacanienne Internationale.

Studies on Hysteria Revisited

Charles Melman on Trauma, Incompatibility, Repression and the Unconscious

Charles Melman

Translated by
Helen Sheehan

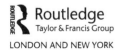

LONDON AND NEW YORK

First published 2022
by Routledge
2 Park Square, Milton Park, Abingdon, Oxon OX14 4RN

and by Routledge
605 Third Avenue, New York, NY 10158

Routledge is an imprint of the Taylor & Francis Group, an informa business

© 2022 Érès, *Nouvelles études sur l'hystérie*, Charles Melman/
Translated by Helen Sheehan

British Library Cataloguing in Publication Data
A catalogue record for this book is available from the British Library

Library of Congress Cataloging-in-Publication Data
A catalog record has been requested for this book

ISBN: 978-0-367-76632-0 (hbk)
ISBN: 978-0-367-76631-3 (pbk)
ISBN: 978-1-003-16783-9 (ebk)

DOI: 10.4324/9781003167839

Typeset in Times New Roman
by Taylor & Francis Books

Contents

Figures

Historical Context

The idea for *Studies on Hysteria Revisited* dates from 1982, when Charles Melman presented a seminar to his students and young analysts, first at the Chaslin Theatre in the Saltpêtrière Hospital (April 1982) and then in the Magnan Theatre in the same hospital (from June 1982).

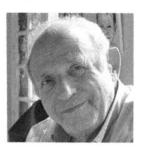

Dr Melman developed the theme of this Seminar, in the same place, during the years 1993–1994. This seminar was transcribed and edited by his analysts in formation: Jean Paul Beaumont, Claire Brunet, Marie Charlotte Cadeau, Michel Daudin, Jacqueline Légaut, Martine Le Rude, Josiane Quilichini and Denise Saint Fare Garnot. It was published by Clims in 1984. It was published again by Érès in 2010, with added corrections and re-editing, with a preface by Denise Saint Fare Garnot.

Acknowledgements

Helen Sheehan

When Dr. Melman gave me permission to translate his *Nouvelles Études Sur L'Hysterie* he accepted in advance to become the pledge of a loss already implicit in the relationship between desire and the Autre. As Lacan remarks "undoubtedly it is only too easy to see passing here the shadow of a satisfaction in being recognised."

Agreed.

There is however more at stake than this – it is that Charles Melman has liquidated his investment as the supposed subject of Knowledge thereby furrowing the possibility of a space where the discourse of the master may be eliminated. Other possibilities have been planted.

This translation was three years in the making. In October 2015 I began a monthly seminar on this book with ten colleagues. Glenn Brady, Nellie Curtin, Monica Errity, Monika Kobylarska, Eilish Griffin, Albert Llussà I Torra, Ros McCarthy, Malachi McCoy, Stephanie Metcalfe and Karolina Szafarz.

Their contributions especially our discussions during the course of these seminars assisted me greatly and for this I wish to thank them. I would also like to thank Dermot Hickey, Audrey McAleese and Michael Power for helping me to keep the work going.

Alexis O'Brien, Editor at Routledge Mental Health, quickly realised the imperative to help make Charles Melman's book available in English and just as quickly undertook to make this happen.

I wish to thank Ellie Duncan at Routledge for her kindness, enthusiasm and excellent advice.

Thanks to Pamela Bertram, Copy Editor, whose light touch editing, accuracy and close reading were of great assistance. I would also like to thank Nick Craggs, Senior Production Editor, for his care, patience and assistance in ensuring that this book is the best it can be and for making the final stages a surprisingly enjoyable experience.

This book could not have been completed without Eileen Quinn who, with a singular ability to read my writing, ensured that the signifier always found a way. Thank you Eileen.

And just when I needed it most Mary Shanahan with humour and unfailing effort helped me to meet the deadline.

Thanks to Omar Guerrero for his assistance. Thanks also to Claire Schaeffer at Érès.

Thank you to Dr. Gérard Amiel whose loyalty and enduring friendship always keeps me on track.

Thanks to Josette Zoueïn for our friendship and our work together over many years.

Nora O'Keefe, you have always been there when the going gets tough.

Anne Guaqueta, your love and support have always been vital.

This work remembers in a special way our dearest Juan Carlos Guaqueta who left us on 18 July 2021.

This book is for Garrett Sheehan.

Preface by Denise Saint Fare Garnot

To choose to publish the seminar *New Studies in Hysteria* in paperback, is to respond to the wish of Charles Melman to offer access to his preferred public audience, namely students and young analysts, to what we think is a major text of the psychoanalytic clinic.

Even though it is more accessible than the book, which was published by Clims in 1984, this text remains a tool for difficult work. Its author situates it as research linked to the time of his enunciation and open to further developments. Is he not modestly inviting his listeners to follow this research?

This is the seminar which precedes his founding of the Association Freudienne. He demonstrates his desire to transmit what he carries in him of Freud, and of Lacan with whom he closely collaborated. He brings the same ardour as Lacan in vigorously forming future analysts.

In the period which followed the dissolution of the Freudian School of Paris and the death of Jacques Lacan – a period troubled by quarrels which upset the anchors, particularly the young – the putting to work of clinical texts was the only way of helping the spirit and giving life to a new start.

The precarious nature of the organisation did not bother Charles Melman. Thanks to the confidence shown in him by Professor Duchè and our friend Professor Basquin – the Chaslin Theatre at the Saltpêtrière was invested with enthusiasm and even a certain zealousness by the audience.

At the beginning of the October term there were a considerable number of attendees. Charles Melman then acquired the Magnam Theatre, significant because it was here Lacan made his presentation of the sick. It was also here that the rest of the presentations were made when the Association Freudienne was formed in June 1982. It was led alternatively by Charles Melman and Marcel Czermak, who both renewed all that Lacan had initiated and considered as major teaching for clinical psychoanalysis.

But let us return to this publication of *New Studies in Hysteria*. "New" because it takes up again the title, and not only that of Freud's work with Breuer in 1895, but also many other of his studies including The Dora Case, Schreber, *The Traumdeutung*, and *Draft G*. All these give Charles Melman the framework for his seminars. This is a real navigation through Freud.

However, we must speak of a work of constant furrowing if we are going to use this metaphor to accentuate the Freudian foundations of hysteria which emphasise the importance of sexual desire and its repression, and will allow Charles Melman to develop Freud and Lacan's work.

In the *Letters from the Freudian School of Paris* (1973) (see the appendix), Charles Melman emphasises that with regard to hysteria, Freud did not pursue his research in the sense of his first discoveries: he was sensitive to the dimension of the word and particularly its absence, that is to say, of the eventual mutism of hysterics. This text is practically contemporaneous with the seminar *Encore* which introduces "The Four Discourses". One of the new things about these *New Studies*, ten years after *Encore*, is the dependence on precisely one of these discourses, that of the discourse on hysteria, which makes clear the expressions in the language of patients with regard to sexuality, a place which establishes the prevalence of the word on the sexual, without in any way detracting from it. This is a notable shift with regard to Freud.

In being attentive to what language conveys for women as well as for male hysterics, Charles Melman enriches his teaching by adhering to constant traits and conjectural modifications, while at the same time being sensitive to the 1980s and its influence on everybody. We may note how much he follows this evolution in his texts of clinical signs of hysteria and brings in new elements. He shows also that this neurosis is more complex than Freud thought.

There is more. It is a fact that Lacan did not do a longitudinal study on hysteria, but this book follows Lacan's teaching. Charles Melman develops the economy of hysteria, insisting on the distinction between the hysterical position and femininity, on the polymorphism of hysteria, while making a considerable contribution to male hysteria. He explains the difference between hysteria and other neurotic and psychotic pathologies.

Following Lacan, he favours the opposition between S_1 and S_2, in giving value to not only their intersubjective articulation but also to their intra subjective one.

He introduces concepts taken from Aristotle and terms with which we are not traditionally familiar, like abalility and aseity. These concepts do not seem to have been developed later. Meanwhile abalility, this dependency on the Autre which Charles Melman situates as a stage, evokes Lacan which in turn, was often taken up by Jean Bergès. "The symbolic is first" even before the mirror stage, and this is not without clinical consequences.

Charles Melman insists on underlining Lacan's teaching of the hysteric's dissatisfaction as being her specific symptom and as the motor for resistance in the treatment. Beginning with the question: "is one cured of hysteria"? he responds in a rather oblique way, because of this resistance, leaving meanwhile, a hope founded on the position of the analyst!

This book is a passionate study of the clinic of hysteria. It is extremely detailed, erudite and does not neglect essential issues discovered through a deeper and dialectical reading: This is an important work by Charles Melman, who, has given us, as with his other seminars, a fundamental psychoanalytic teaching.

Denise Saint Fare Garnot

Preface by Charles Melman

Women whose love protected my childhood, also initiated me, despite themselves, into the foundations of psychopathology.

The attention they gave me, periodically alternated with their spectacular confinements which may have misled the doctor, but did not fool those around them; he used to diagnose a suffering provoked by a demand much more intense than the attempts of the entourage to respond to it. It seemed to serve only to increase the suffering, resulting in a twofold frustration whether produced by a "yes" or "no".

How to respond? Such circumstances gave to the child witness a medical vocation, if only to make up for what allowed itself to be heard through the repetition of the symptom, that its origin might be paternal deficiency.

But this oedipal response rarely succeeded in curing hysteria, except to have erased the dramatic appeal from the list of symptoms which the hysteric makes to a father who would no longer be timorous but finally, all powerful.

Such a suppression from the D.S.M. is not without harm, because this strikes at the anthropological expression, identified since Antiquity, of a major symptom: the discordance of an organism with its environment hereby noisily attested to: nothing suits it.

Of course, this seems to have been reserved for those who line themselves up on the feminine side, because of the phallocentrism proper to diverse cultures and therefore linked in this case to the lack of the instrument which heals.

Let us note that in this eventuality, a woman evokes the insufficiency of her partner more than her own lack.

Be that as it may, the treatment through marriage of young girls and widows affected in this way has occurred since Antiquity and Freud did not think any differently. His patient, Dora, suffers because she refuses to engage. That is to say in the trust placed in an instrument which took decades to recognize that it is also poisonous: *Pharmakon.*

But Freud's genius was to decipher these symptoms as a writing, the body taken as a support and motricity as an alphabet, the writing of a wish in another place (*another scene*) but unspeakable – hysterical aphasia – and inadmissible for the conscious subject.

In the meantime, a miracle happened because the interpretation, the reading of the symptom by the therapist was enough to make it disappear, but only at the price of another miracle; a passionate love for the one who interpreted: transference.

From then on, the aim of the treatment became the question of its dissolution and the history of the psychoanalytic movement became that of resistance of students to renounce their attachment, through love or hate, to Freud.

Lacan's strength, who by the way will not escape the same kind of destiny, was to show that this denaturation of the human organism, its disharmony with the environment no matter which sex, had always been linked to its domination through the system of communication proper to our species, language.

What Freud named "unconscious" is the equivalent of what functions as instinct for the animal. Because it has to do with a knowledge unbeknownst to the bearer, guiding his thought and conduct including the sexual, despite him or without him as needs be, except that in the case of our species, this unconscious knowledge is enunciated through elements such as letters, phonemes, signifiers, phrases, but remains unarticulated because of modesty, morality, fear etc., thereby positing the word of each one of us.

And each divides and arranges in his own way, this equivalent of the instinct becoming for humankind singular, solitary, unique and creating an obstacle for any kind of generalisation which would allow a recognition and scientific understanding. Each treatment becomes in this way an individual one and bears the pain of not being able to share its effect. This goes for analysts themselves.

The only universal which brings humanity together is therefore a flaw, the object which could satisfy it lacking as a result of which humanity has only the signifier to get its teeth into and this lack becomes precious, as it is the putting into place of desire, always desire for something else, of the thing lacking.

If the Oedipus complex judges the father responsible, he is in no way guilty and his actual decline in culture does not in any way make for better days ahead.

Hysteria, because of this, is the prototype of the subjective subversion which puts the speaker in a place – "another scene" – where a destiny is decided, whether that be neurosis, psychosis, perversion or phobia. This depends on the cut to which he has consented in language and which puts into place a real – an impossible, strictly forbidden, but which from then on commands.

Charles Melman
21 July 2020

Chapter 1

Introduction

Charles Melman

We don't have any need nowadays to save either Freud or Lacan. They don't in any way need it, we should perhaps try and save ourselves. In fact, the condition by which we can escape neurosis, "do not give up on your desire", is encapsulated in the Lacanian dictum which he indicated in the *Ethics of Psychoanalysis.*[1] If this dictum brings us to something worse, have we not then got this choice only as a way of closing the question: to include a dissatisfaction which is expressed in hysterical demand or stoic resignation with regard to "this worse" which is that of psychoanalysis?

Perhaps in order to respond to this question, we have to take up again an examination of the foundations on which psychoanalysis was established, that is to say to take up once again the *Studies on Hysteria.*[2] Let us note from the outset that Freud's writings on which we continue to found ourselves, those which go from the *Project*[3] to the *Dream*[4] book are more than 100 years old and, despite the promise made by Freud in 1913 in his article on the "Unconscious",[5] he never again took up *Studies on Hysteria.* What may appear even more astonishing, is that the second topology which appeared in 1920,[6] contradicts this book. We could legitimately hope that he would have renewed his conceptions from the new economy, implied in the automatism of repetition.

Freud's students in turn, were not too eloquent on hysteria. We don't have texts or works to which we can spontaneously and immediately refer. The one and only decisive and important reference which we have to hand is the introduction made by Lacan on the discourse of the hysteric.[7] But, a question must be asked: can the discourse of the hysteric be resumed in the fact that it establishes a basis, that it gives its place to what is, properly speaking, the subjective position from where the subject expresses himself when he is able – for example, that there is no sexual rapport – in other words to say, with conviction to express his complaint, or indeed, does this algorithm resume for us the clinic of hysteria?

What we can, all the same, immediately point out, is that the discourse of the hysteric offers to the one who speaks, no matter who, a kind of *prêt-à-porter*, a ready-to-wear if he finds himself a little bare in his investment in a word. Therefore, we shouldn't be surprised if hysterical positions properly speaking, if the

DOI: 10.4324/9781003167839-1

sayings and the manifest signs of hysteria can be met within structures, in psychopathological organisations which are extremely diverse. In other words, the discourse of the hysteric presents itself at first as a possible way for everyone to contain himself in language. It is one of the major ways, quite simply, of making the social bond. And Lacan, emphasised that no matter what the structure of the patient, he will find himself being led, through the discourse of the hysteric, by the very fact of the protocol of the analytic cure.

Perhaps what we have to regret is that Lacan did not come back to the conditions which made that birth possible, that is to say, the foundation of psychoanalysis itself. It could be said with regard to this, that Lacan never wanted to approach psychoanalysis via the clinic, to establish for example, a treatise on a clinic of psychoanalysis. There is a simple reason for this: the clinic, psychoanalytic or otherwise offers itself as evidence, like a frame in which the observer finds himself privileged enough to have himself excluded. This is the principle of the establishment of all the clinics with which we deal. And precisely, in the case of hysteria, we know how he or she will freely apply themselves in giving a picture to all eventual voyeurs. Do we have to emphasise the fact that our position is different? First, for us, the subject is in the picture! In other words, the position of the observer is completely included in what he observes: he is at one and at the same time the part taken up and the part being taken up. He is himself a product of the procedure he is studying. But above all what we have to study with regards to hysteria is precisely this: in what way is the subject himself caught up in the picture? We have to be ready to conquer the resistances presenting themselves as the revelation of the most intimate of our abjection – an attempt at capturing what could amount to a certain violation.

A little remark is necessary here on the status of the clinic in the field of psychoanalysis. We can easily say that the clinic is in some way our imaginary. But, by the same token, it is fairly essential because this imaginary has a currency equal to the two other dimensions, as you are aware. You know how, in the knots for example, Lacan needed to call on this imaginary dimension to not only establish the other two but to verify them and measure their effects. For the mathematicians also, the passage through the imaginary – by the look, by the picture, by the drawing, – all of this was proved necessary. In other words, the quality of the imaginary here does not have to frighten us. If we have a meaning to give to the clinic, we will simply say that it's the study of different organisations which are the product of this fact that, there is no sexual rapport. We will not privilege one over the other and in this way, one is as good as the other.

Therefore, to conclude this introduction, there is a methodological difficulty, which is perfectly irrefutable. Studies on hysteria easily present themselves as the attempt to account for the subject by the concept. Now, what we find is that by definition, the subject is precisely that which manifests itself by escaping this concept and by denying it. That is what we call *Verneinung*.[8] This of course, means there is always a little bit of the ridiculous when we have to pretend to conclude studies on hysteria. We could be tempted by another approach and take up these studies via the way of biography, history, or the novel. We know Freud's concern when his observations are read like novels. The interest of this double impossibility which I'm emphasising about studies on hysteria is to show how this division is strictly similar to the very structure of hysteria. In what way? The subject is a product of structure, and thanks to historicisation, to the establishing of history, there is some term, some real term, some ultimate term which will finally ensure its advent.

Being is a very strict definition, which is, needless to say, not metaphysical. Being is not realised until the moment when the subject finds himself represented by a signifier which could signify himself: only then will he accomplish his being. We see this kind of division therefore between the attempt to take on board studies on hysteria via the concept itself (which always only gives an approximation, and you may remember these pages of *Encore*[9] where Lacan evokes the approximate quality to accord to these concepts) or indeed this passage via historicisation which holds the hope of an end always possible, that is to say, sends us back to a real of which, after all, we never know if it will or not be able to exhaust itself.

With regard to analysts themselves we find an opposition between clinicians – that is to say, between those who refer to the structure – and those who challenge it, to privilege instead the accent given to biography, as if reference to a clinical organisation brings along with it the germ of a decisive error. Some among us remember the quarrels which took place some years ago, which have not even today been put to rest in a satisfying way, between the partisans of structure and those of history.

Finally, in another reference, this same distinction will permit us two different modes of the apprehension of infinity: one which is founded on actual infinity, which founds itself on structure; and the other which we evoke as potential infinity and which on the contrary, animates the narrative, the historicisation. This means that when we wish to take up again studies on hysteria we don't really know if we should begin by reading books about mathematics or novels …

Our first intention in the following seminars is to take up again the concepts, those which presented themselves to Freud at the beginning, in his construction of psychoanalysis. These concepts are foundational, they are the pillars. For example, from the very first texts which support the whole edifice, we will find concepts such as *trauma* and *incompatibility*. What is an "incompatible" representation for the hysteric? What leads the hysteric to *repression* – the third concept will have for her the particularity, the singularity of veering towards that field called "somatic conversion". This repression is found in and of itself to be another essential concept because Freud called it the *unconscious*.

I hasten to say, to simplify, that I will speak of hysteria in the feminine – because that is how it was established historically – and we shall see how and why this position is so well able to respond to the feminine one. Afterwards, we shall have a seminar dealing with masculine hysteria and its particularities.

The first term I will look at this evening is *trauma*. This trauma, Freud found it in a quasi-systematic fashion, regularly, in the biography of hysterics. This will have a fairly essential role to guide us towards the place of sexuality – because these traumas are essentially of a sexual nature. This helps Freud conceive the economy of the psychical apparatus as ruled by the necessity for abreaction, which permits him to introduce a fundamental concept which is that of the *pleasure principle*. Trauma plays a harmful role by the eruption of large quantities of excitation, which cannot flow because the subject does not give them an appropriate response, whether that be a motor one, flight for example, or a sexual one: in fact, this trauma survives to an age where the subject is in a state of inadequacy to respond, a state Freud calls sexual prematuration. In the face of, this irruption, the necessary tools are not available, the subject does not have access to an appropriate verbal rejoinder. You know Freud first believed in the reality of trauma, for example in the form of violation, but he finally concluded that it is articulated around phantasy.

This question of trauma remains essential for us. Why? Because we can read there even today the way in which the subject talks about his contribution as a subject, that is to say his birth, with regard to the establishing of a real introduced by the phallic signifier, and by which the subject henceforth finds himself abolished, that is to say constituted. In other words, what trauma illustrates for us, in how it is recounted, is that this foundational act, this violent act which is in some way imposed on an "X" to make of him a subject, this inaugurates at one and the same time his place and his solitude as a subject – this act which gave him birth, gave him the light of day. We do not hesitate to say that if there is a trauma of birth, so dear to Otto Rank,[10] it is indeed this one.

We can then make a few remarks concerning this foundational act, to illustrate this inaugural trauma, this "labour". For example, if the mentally challenged person is capable of fascinating us and of being cherished by us, it's precisely because he escapes this trauma of birth and offers us the triumph of the one who manages to be here, never having had to be born. We also know how much the fantasy – we cannot speak here of phantasy, for the obsessional neurotic, is that of being kept warm and covered within the maternal uterus. We can say that this is another way of defying the separating power of the Autre. We know by what symptoms the obsessional tries to maintain this original contact, notably by this phobic contact, these obsessions of washing and indeed this other trait which for him is an abhorrence of everything with a touch of violence, because all expression of violence is considered as criminal and punishable.

We can also ask ourselves a question: from where does this scene which we call primitive get this traumatic character? The primitive scene[11] in general, as it is spoken about, gives little to see. But, it interprets the noises which it gives to hear as the very voice of this phallus which, in being presented in this way, makes the subject anxious by the fact of abolishing him, by telling him that at this moment he literally does not know where to place himself, that he has in fact lost his place. And perhaps, one can say that it is this particular mode of jouissance, pushed to anxiety, which the exhibitionist tries to capture in the look of the partner on whom he imposes himself. This initial trauma describes itself, therefore, following the scenario of a seduction which mixes the violence of the agent, with the passivity and the character, without defence, of the patient.

We can say that this character merits the name of *secondary elaboration* – as Freud introduced it, for example, with regard to the formation of dreams – and indeed, he instructs us in an essential way as to the importance of the narrative, its insertion into history. He shows us, in fact, how the construction of the narrative is only held, when it is of value, by the accident of structure which organises its agency. That is really why the truth has the structure of fiction. This can, once again make us think of the way we are forced to hear all the elaborations that we are led to produce, which are called rationalisations for example, all these elaborations which fill our exchanges whether these have to do with quarrels or so called scientific debates. Meanwhile, it is true, as I outlined earlier, that this story, this scenario, this secondary elaboration offers us pleasure, comfort, in supposing that this narrative, sufficiently faithful and sufficiently repeated, will permit us to find once again this original silence, this original mutism, this original peace. And without a doubt it was under this phantasy that Freud could construct his first therapeutic concepts, his principle of *catharsis* or even "to speak until one can say no more".[12] No matter what, it's because of this trauma that the subject will find himself accompanied everywhere, by what he can hope to leave outside, until he finds himself obsessing about rediscovering outside, the secret that he thought he had kept in his deepest inside.

With regard to this, because of this original trauma a fundamental splitting is imposed, with the introduction of the phallic reference, with the phallus[13] as referent. You know that logicians have always been interested in this question of referent. This gives us very interesting texts, but it is in any case, a question which none of them have been able to resolve. What we can take note of is that the introduction of the phallic reference takes its traumatic impact only for the little girl because it's with her that the trauma is organised, which we call the original myth of hysteria. In fact, what inaugurates the phallic signifier, is the dimension of the Autre, that is to say the sharing of speak-beings between those who have a right to be known as phallic and those, who, because they find themselves in the place of this Autre, having from then on to devote themselves to making their phallicism recognised. To say it this way, is to suggest that the narcissistic relationship is privileged upon the object relation, because it's here at the level of narcissism that suddenly, the attack will be launched. One should say that it's already hysterical to register this sharing of speak-beings as unequal and to remember this as the effect of violence, of a reduction, and as the generator of an infirmity. For the hysteric, this myth of origins will henceforth be the organiser of an existence inscribed under the sign of a demand which will never be satisfied, and a corporal assault which will be expressed just as well through illness, as a necessary malaise which translates as a feeling of dysmorphia. What matters to us, is to immediately indicate this curious paradox, which is the contradiction in which she who finds herself in this place, finds herself also engaged in a foundational contradiction with regard to castration. In fact, we are not recognised by our fellows except by representing the phallus. And, she finds herself sustained by an Autre order, which it seems, is constructed under the demand of having to renounce it, as for example the formulae of sexuation shows.[14] In these formulae, which register the feminine position, there is nothing, it seems, which sustains phallicism. She who will occupy this position about which we are talking, will find herself in this contradictory demand, on the one hand, to have herself recognised by her partner as a phallic representative and on the other hand, to sustain herself symbolically only by an order which will invite her more and more to radically exclude this phallicism. This explains the contradiction of her behaviour, in trying to get herself recognised while just as quickly being evasive and renouncing all her accomplishments, no matter what they may be. Here we could designate the typical term by which, wrongly, we call hysterical "intrigue" (because it is obvious that she is, of course, first the victim before she is the agent) and this in a twofold way: an invitation to a phallic renunciation made to the partner because she herself is sustained by this order which is precisely called this renunciation, but, of course with the fervent hope that he will resist, that he will not allow her to do this, without which of course, she would lose her way and thus, would be no longer recognisable to him.

What I'm trying to introduce this evening, is what is incompatible for the hysteric, it is exactly the kind of representation which finds itself incompatible with the order with which she is in some way trying to identify. It is not enough, as I do, to try and show this kind of disassociation for her between an imaginary, which is found to be of an order theoretically imposed on her as if it were from an outside – for example, this myth of origins of which she could not represent. On the one hand there is a xenopathic will which she will eventually find does not concern her, and on the other hand, the fact that she finds herself connected to this order, excluding everything which cannot be said. This always, of course, ensures this order is never perfectly accomplished – except at the price of sublimation, which obviously concerns love and to which we shall have to return. All this, to try and ensure that we will have even the slightest idea what this representation, called the *unverträglich*, of hysteria entails, because all these which Freud evoked in his first writings are nothing else but sexual representations. And, we will of course have to ask ourselves why these sexual representations are so incompatible for those who are in this position, and lead therefore to repression.

We need perhaps, to note the following: we are in the habit of repeating the formula "what is foreclosed in the symbolic, reappears in the real,"[15] but we have to question ourselves with regard to this. What is repressed in the symbolic, it reappears where and in what? It is very clear that we are led to think that a fundamental part of the symptomatology of hysteria finds itself dependent on place.

We have first to question ourselves about the nature of what will be repressed in this way – and this seems to be self-evident, otherwise we will not understand how the hysteric will find herself led to repression as Freud puts it, a permanent one, an activity of permanent repression – and second, with regard to the destination of what is "repressed". Perhaps, if we are able to respond to these two questions, we will be better able to understand what Freud meant by "somatic conversion".[16] The minimum is to remark that the notion of body, of soma, is somewhat enigmatic. What do we mean by body? An examination of this double trait will help us to better understand what is involved in the symptomatology of hysteria.

No matter what, we can already say this evening that we understand better what a trauma is; in so far as we are analysts, we can perhaps, say that a trauma, it's the introduction to a real where there is no father, that is to say someone who is in a position to offer what is represented by this real to semblants of masters so that they can enjoy it. The real encountered insofar as it's traumatic: it's this one. It's this real which is not occupied in that way by any father. The father here has this strict function only, to offer *jouissance* to the semblants of masters who live in this real, who represent this real. We will find, once again, a real, which tormented Freud with regard to traumatic neurosis.[17] In other words, Freud was tormented by the question of why the subject returns time and time again to a trauma which has become, in some kind of way, the cause, as if the subject is by his repetition, in fact, repeating this demand to the father. One could be tempted to say that hysterical neurosis reproduces this kind of demand, and this is undoubtedly the reason Freud found himself from the very beginning confronted with these two situations.

Such a real interests us very much as analysts, to the extent it could be said that the status of the analyst is precisely to confront a real of this kind, and this, no matter who the founding fathers are, whom he, in some kind of way, tries to imagine civilising for him this real with which he has to deal; founding fathers, who, by the same token, would authorise his work. If Lacan could say that the analyst authorises only from himself,[18] it is surely because there never was and there never is any father who could in some way civilise or prescribe the jouissance of his work.

This trauma, this notion of trauma could equally introduce us to some brief reflections on violence. Violence, we see here, is foundational and this has been wisely appreciated by philosophers well before psychoanalysts. Violence for one of them was "the mother of all things". The repugnance that we may have with everything which pertains to authority, to the imperative, this repugnance does not seem to us to be isolated from what this inaugural trauma, puts into place, mentioned earlier and insofar as the subject is, with regard to this, without defence. It cannot do much, it comes along when one is born. What we can simply say, is that analysts could have a more precise appreciation of the inevitable character of violence and, that in looking to foreclose it from the symbolic, we will obviously only find it once again where it might turn out to be even more violent or present itself from then on as being without reason.

What I would like to say before concluding this evening, is that I introduced in this lecture, two differing positions without confusing them. I referred all the time to two algorithms. One is that which emphasises S_1. The other is borrowed from the so-called formulae of sexuation insofar as it has to do with the feminine position of an Autre. And, with regard to this Autre nothing will give it a foundation, nothing will give it anything of an identification. By using in some kind of way, this two-sided approach, all I'm doing is taking up again what was a question for Freud, which still has not been resolved: Why does the feminine position find itself so willingly coinciding with the hysterical position?[19] I am happy to remark provisionally that if the feminine position is such, that it finds itself the generator of some dissatisfaction, we can understand that to be able to speak, she can only find the way in some sense a natural one, by the prêt-à-porter which I described earlier in the discourse of hysteria. You know Lacan's dictum: "It is what will fall silent if it can be articulated".[20] Feminine jouissance, it is what is not said. Therefore, this feminine position as such cannot be said. We all know the attempts and studies which are being done (which of course have to be encouraged and congratulated) to know if there is a word or a writing which could be called specifically feminine, in other words, something which could tell us immediately that it's a woman who speaks. If that were to happen, this would of course, raise the bar on *The Woman*. If, this feminine position which cannot speak as such "subjectivises" herself, in some way in the register of dissatisfaction, we can understand that she finds this expression as natural, as being self-evident – but Freud made the distinction very clearly that it's not at all the same thing – that she finds her natural expression in this prêt-à-porter, in this ready to wear, in what makes a social bond, that is to say, within the discourse of the hysteric.

Then, to begin, next week I will engage by responding to these different questions, by what is called the history of ideas about hysteria to the extent, that these first texts which we have are four thousand years old. These ideas present a character which I find absolutely admirable and exceptional: they present themselves to us today in a way that is completely unchanged. The imaginary put forward by the hysteric of four thousand years ago is more or less transmitted in an almost fossilised way, and it's a fact that has to be commented on, this inexhaustible imaginary! The question will be twofold. Did Freud in his conceptualisation of hysteria, escape from this imaginary and if so in what way? And did this possibly contribute to his first introduction to psychoanalysis? Moreover, we will try with Freud, to grasp the particularities of the symptomatology of hysteria, its specificity, which means that we are using sure and certain methods which are totally irrefutable. This will ensure that if we are in the presence of certain symptoms, even if these are atypical, strange, even extravagant, we are able, to say like we should, in a definite way that we are dealing with hysterical manifestations.

These are the two points I will deal with next week, with regard to what is called the evolution of hysterical manifestations.

20 April 1982

Notes

1 J. Lacan, *The Seminar of Jacques Lacan, Book VII: The Ethics of Psychoanalysis, 1959–1960* (ed. J-A. Miller, trans. D. Porter). London: Routledge, 1992.

2 S. Freud, *Studies on Hysteria*, Vol. II, S.E. (1893–1899). London: The Hogarth Press, 1955.

3 S. Freud, "Project for A Scientific Psychology" in *Pre-Psycho-Analytic Publications and Unpublished Drafts*, Vol. I, S.E. (1886–1899). London: The Hogarth Press, 1966.

4 S. Freud, *The Interpretation of Dreams*, Vol. IV, S.E. (1900). London: The Hogarth Press, 1953.

5 S. Freud, "The Unconscious" in *The Case of Schreber, Papers on Technique and Other Works*. Vol. XII, S.E. (1911–1913). London: The Hogarth Press, 1958.

6 S. Freud, *Beyond the Pleasure Principle, Group Psychology and Other Works*, Vol. XVIII, S.E. (1920–1922). London: The Hogarth Press, 1955.

7 J. Lacan, *The Seminar of Jacques Lacan, Book XVII: The Other Side of Psychoanalysis, 1969–1970* (trans. C. Gallagher, unedited).

8 S. Freud, "Verneinung" in *The Ego and the Id and Other Works*, Vol. XIX, S.E. (1923–1925). London: The Hogarth Press, 1961.

9 J. Lacan, *The Seminar of Jacques Lacan, Book XX: Encore, 1972–1973* (trans. C. Gallagher, unedited).

10 O. Rank, *The Trauma of Birth* (ed. E.J. Lieberman). New York: Dover Publications, 1993.

11 S. Freud, *An Infantile Neurosis and Other Works*, Vol. XVI, S.E. (1917–1918). London: The Hogarth Press, 1955.

12 Freud, "On the Psychical Mechanism of Hysterical Phenomena: Preliminary Communication" in *Studies on Hysteria*.

13 J. Lacan, "The Signification of the Phallus" in *Écrits* (personal translation).

14 J. Lacan, *The Seminar of Jacques Lacan, Book XVIII: On a Discourse that might not be a Semblance, 1970–1971* (trans. by C. Gallagher, unedited).

15 J. Lacan, "Response to Jean Hyppolite's Commentary on Freud's *Verneinung*" in *Écrits* (trans. by B. Fink). New York: W.W. Norton & Co., 2006.

16 S. Freud, "Neuro-Psychoses of Defence" in *Early Psycho-Analytic Publications*, Vol. III, S.E. (1893–1899). London: The Hogarth Press, 1962.

17 S. Freud, *Beyond the Pleasure Principle, Group Psychology and Other Works*, Vol. XVIII, S.E. (1920–1922). London: The Hogarth Press, 1955.

18 J. Lacan, *Proposal on the Psychoanalyst of the School, 1967* (trans. C. Gallagher, unedited).

19 S. Freud, "Femininity" in *New Introductory Lectures on Psycho-Analysis and Other Works*, Vol. XXII, S.E. (1932–1936). London: The Hogarth Press, 1964.

20 Lacan, *Book XX: Encore*.

Chapter 2

A history of the entity known as hysteria

Charles Melman

Six Egyptian papyrus concerning medicine have been discovered. Among those, two report on behavioural problems in women, troubles concerning anomalies in the matrix position, the uterus.

The first papyrus, well known, is called "Edwin Smith"[1] after the psychologist who found it at Thebes, 1900 years before our era, that is to say, nearly 4,000 years ago. It tells the story of a woman who loved the bed, refused to get up, refused to wash herself: another tells the story of a woman who suffered with sight problems and had soreness in her neck, a third suffered from teeth and biting problems and could not open her mouth, a fourth woman suffered from muscle problems and felt a soreness in the orbit of her eyes.

These behavioural troubles in women are attributed to two things: what is called "starvation" of the uterus and its displacement upwards. This means that the good doctor, the good therapist has a double task: the first consists in nourishing the starved organ; the second is to help it return to its place. We must take note of what is very precious for us, that this organ is treated like a living organism which is endowed with a will of its own. Therefore, treatment consisted at the time, on the one hand to ingest or breathe in fetid substances and on the other hand to do vaginal fumigations with odorous substances. Today this makes us laugh. Yet only a few years ago, hysteria was treated by giving valerian to the patient, that is to say, extracted from the same origins – *valeriana* – just like that which was given 4,000 years ago!

The second papyrus is called "Ebers"[2] after the German archaeologist who discovered it. It dates from 1600 years B.C. and it's the longest medical text we have. It has a chapter on woman troubles and takes up again all these indications so that the matrix of the woman is able to return to its place. Yet again, the same methods are used, with frictions, vaginal unctions. And, an ibis made of wax is added to the fumigations made with charcoal. Ibis, as we "don't" know represents the God that was one of the most powerful Gods of the Egyptian pantheon and specifically was a male divinity. The God Thot, the doctor of the Gods and the protector of the sick, is also the inventor of the art of writing. Finally, added to the charcoal fumigations, was the excrement of males, dried.

DOI: 10.4324/9781003167839-2

This is from where we are starting and Hippocrates, 400 years BC[3] took up all these conceptions, all these positions. These conceptions of Hippocrates as such, are there for example, in Plato. In *Timaeus*,[4] there is a paragraph which is very clear, with regard to this, where it is written that it is probable that immoral men who passed their lives in an unjust way, would, during the course of their second birth, be changed into women. Plato ends this description of the physiology of the male apparatus – (which does not interest us that much here), by saying "For man, is by nature an authoritarian and stern being, a kind of animal who does not hear reason and whose appetites, always excited, wish to dominate everything".[5]

Similarly, for women, what we call the matrix or the uterus there is, for these same reasons "an animal inside them which has the appetite for making children. And, when it happens, even despite the propitious age, this uterus stays a long time without issuing forth fruit, this animal becomes impatient and tolerates this state of affairs badly: it wanders all over the body, obstructs the airways, stops breathing, turns about in extreme anxiety and provokes all other kinds of illnesses. And this lasts a while for both sexes, alas appetite and desire do not lead them to a union, from there they can, like a tree, gather their fruits".

We understand this interpretation very well: the uterus starves because it remains sterile. We see these manifestations essentially in women of a certain age who do not have sexual relations, like widows and young girls. For these, the uterus dries up, loses weight – there is of course the theory which you will find, of dryness and humidity – it goes as far as hypochondria, looking for humidity – it interrupts the air which should descend through the abdominal cavity, and this leads to convulsions and epilepsy. There is also a whole clinic defining the extent to which this organ could reach. There is a different symptomatology as to whether or not it can reach the heart, the liver, the kidney, the head. And the treatment which Hippocrates advocated, besides these classical methods, is marriage and pregnancy. But Hippocrates also introduces, among other things, the term which specifies the relationship of these symptoms with the uterus, because it is he who introduced the adjective "hysterical" which will only become a substantive later. It is he who introduces *hustéra,* following on from *hè hustéra*, which means the uterus.

This is not without interest for us because this *hustéra* finds itself practically homophonic with *hustéros*; it is only differentiated by the accent; the mood is the same.

And *hustéros*, this means something else altogether. As an adjective, it means "what comes behind," with the idea of place. For example, to say "the train behind" we say *ta hustéra*. And, when it expresses an idea of time, *hustéros* means "what comes along afterwards". Another example, borrowed from the adjective, *hè hustéra* means "the next day" "what arrives afterwards". Or again *hustéros*: "that which arrives too late", a troop for example; *hoi hustéroi* means "those who arrive afterwards" that is to say the descendants. Finally, there is a third meaning to *ho hustéros*, which finds itself of course, metaphorised. It will be to "find itself afterwards", to "arrive too late", or to "find oneself behind". It designates also "he who comes along afterwards", who gives in to someone, he who finds himself inferior to someone, *hustéros*.

Plato's *Laws*[6] has an expression which interests us. This gives us, in Greek: "*Sôma hustéron psuchés*" (where hustéron is written with an accent, it's an adjective) which means the body is inferior to the soul, therefore it has to concede to the soul, or it is the body which is behind. In playing with the translation, one could say that "the body is hysterical to the soul", for example.

The verb which is below this, *hustereó* underlines this idea of inferiority, because it means not only to "arrive too late", "to be late", but also "to be insufficient", "to make a mistake", "to lack". For example, because *oinos* means "wine", *oínou husteréthènai*, simply means "to lack wine".

There is also *hustérèma* which directly means "lack", "penury", "indigent". And finally, I wrote something which is quite funny which is *hustérologia,* a figure of rhetoric, designating "the reversal" in the natural order of ideas, when the ideas have meaning above and below, when what is after, comes before. And *hustérolāgos* means he who plays secondary roles ...

We could think that this rapprochement is arbitrary, if we do not, we find this play on words with the Greeks (notably, Athenaeus)[7] between *hè hustéra,* the uterus and the adjective *husteros* "to be late", "to be insufficient", "to be inferior".

There is one which, for myself, I tried to give an account of the possible resonances of this word "*hè hustéra*". It's by breaking it down, as I did with *hustéras,* to try to make the homophony understandable from a Greek viewpoint. There you will recognise the word "*hus*" which is "the pig" or "the sow" depending on the article which is used to accompany it and "*téras*" which in French gives us teratology – téras which means "the fabulous beast", "the extraordinary beast"; *téras legéin* means to "tell unbelievable things", extraordinary things. And, you will see that for a Greek in this epoch, the word *hustéra* is homophonic with something like – the fantastic pig, the miraculous pig, something like this.

It has to be remarked that these conceptions of hysteria are scientific, by this I mean that they do not appeal to any supernatural cause. They try to account for manifestations of illness by anatomical and physiological changes. They also account in an imaged way, for the fact that these manifestations express unsatisfied feminine desires and the best treatment, in the final analysis, would obviously consist of course, in satisfying them.

It is very clear that these conceptions find themselves modified with the ethical changes with regard to the necessity of sexual satisfaction. In the conception of hysteria, these changes come about largely with St Augustine[8] 400 years after Jesus Christ. Illness, in a very general way, will be left as belonging to the register of sin, which the authors, in a general way in their ideas, try to denounce – that was the cause, as you know of the persecution of witches and a certain number of hysterics at this time were also made to suffer.

I don't believe that the problem is to be indulged or condemned, as works of history on the question have habitually done. It is better to understand that with a monotheistic conception this was an unforeseen, but unavoidable, conclusion. This effect imposed itself on those who found themselves involved in this issue without having to make decisions about it and therefore, was an effect of structure. All who presented with forces animating the body and escaping so-called "natural forces", expressing divine will, all those expressions which came to testify that one could escape, even contradict these natural, divine forces, such manifestations could not be logically interpreted except in the register of diabolical witchcraft. We would be wrong, in regard to this, to take the Middle Ages as a period of darkness. Everything testifies to the contrary, including what was philosophical reflection at the time, the work of scholars. They knew that the real has to do with the rational, the philosophical with the symbolic. Those among you who are interested in what philosophy was doing at that time have appreciated how much this faith in search of an intellect was nothing other than an attempt to knot the real and the symbolic. And the imaginary, also, of course. That was done, as you know, by the intermediary of a *Trinity* which was imposed at the time and which we can understand as the fruit of a long and patient work of reflection. It is still difficult (even for us, today's analysts) to understand how the three categories find themselves knotted. But it is indeed certain that one of the consequences was to give to strange powers all bodily force, all vital force, all animal force which came to contradict that which was thought of, judged as, the excitation of normal, vital forces.

And that meant that doctors were attached to this idea. It is notable, a little later, in the 16th century, that there was a certain tendency to link hysteria, in spite of this, to natural causes. We could note here well-known people such as Paracelsus[9] or Ambroise Paré.[10] There is also a very nice text of Rabelais in *The Third Book*, where we can see how the Egyptian and Hippocratic theories are maintained. Rondibilis, the doctor, expresses himself in the following way:

> Certainly, Plato does not know where to place them; as reasonable animals or brutal beasts. Because nature, has placed their bodies, in a secret and intestinal place, an animal, a member who are not men, to whom sometimes they beget certain false humours, nitrous, caustic, death dealing, – producing bitter bile, quivering with impatience (because this member is very nervous and has a lively feeling) all the body is shaken, all the senses are ravished, all feeling is destroyed, all thinking is confused. Things are such that if nature did not redden the face with a little bit of shame, you would see them as insane, chasing after a little pin more awful than the Praetides, the Mimallonides and the Thyades ever did when they feasted on their festival days, because this terrible awful

animal has a connivance with all the principal parts of the body, as is obvious from anatomy. I call this, animal, following the doctrine of the Academics as well as the Peripatetics. Because, if right movement is a sure indication of an animated thing, as Aristotle writes, and everything which is mute is called animal, then Plato is right to call this animal, recognising in him right movements of suffocation, of precipitation, of corruption, of indignation, so violent it is very often given to the woman, another meaning and movement, as if it were lipothymy, synocope, epilepsy, apoplexy and true resemblance of pale faced death.

Only you will say that little is praiseworthy regarding prudish women, those who have lived modestly and without blame and have had the virtue of arranging this frightened, deranged animal to the obedience of reason and you will be right if you assuage this quietened animal, (as assuaged as can be) by the food which nature had prepared in man, have reached the end of all their particular movements, have all their appetites assuaged, and have all their fury quietened.[11]

All this to account for the persistence with which doctors pursue interpretation, which, moreover, is not going to be so easily dismissed by them: there are always the same frustrations with the uterus as linked to a somatic manifestation.

In the 17th century, the classical era, the age of reason, doctors attempted to stop, or at least interrupt the diagnosis of witchcraft and hysteria began to be seen as having a cerebral cause. The first, an Englishman called Edward Jorden,[12] attributed hysteria to vapours which rose from the uterus and reached the brain – there is already here the introduction of the brain. A famous doctor called in Latin Carolus Piso (in French, Charles Lepois)[13] attributed a cerebral cause for hysteria and affirmed that there existed a certain masculine hysteria as well as a feminine one. There had also been earlier, a man known as Aretaeus of Cappadocia,[14] who said that hysteria was also found in men. But, it is above all an Englishman, Thomas Sydenham[15] who attributes hysteria to an illness of the spirit.

It is interesting to note that in the 18th and 19th centuries, hysteria still, nevertheless, continued to oscillate between a cerebral condition, even a mental one and a condition with genital origin. That's how, for our famous Pinel,[16] hysteria entered into the chapter of the genital neurosis of the woman. He resumed the classical Egyptian and Hippocratic interpretation, and compared uterine fury or nymphomania to what he called satyriasis in a man. Hysteria is the expression of non-controlled, libidinal feminine desires.

In 1866, which seems not that long ago, Jean Pierre Falret,[17] a doctor at the Salpêtrière, denounces the moral imperfection of these sick people whom he says "are true comediennes: they have no greater pleasure than to betray those with whom they have a rapport. Hysterics exaggerate their convulsive movements, make a travesty, exaggerate equally all the movements of their soul, all their ideas, all their acts. In one single word, the life of hysterics is made of perpetual lies: they pretend to have an air of piety and devotion and try to pass for saints while they give into, in secret, actions which are most shameful, while they make the most violent scenes, in their own homes for their husband and their children. In these violent scenes, they hold ideas which are most grotesque and sometimes obscene and they indulge in the most wild acts".

I should have mentioned earlier that for Pinel, hysteria was a genital neurosis for which treatment was still local, aiming to evacuate products which were retained by the uterus. He resumed the theory of Galen[18] which I omitted, a theory founded on a seminal retention, and treated hysterics by local manipulation before arranging what he called a sexual evacuation. He also treated them with marriage.

We therefore arrive, as we should, at Jean-Martin Charcot,[19] who in 1882, exactly 100 years ago, was named here at the Salpêtrière, professor of illnesses of the nervous system. The chair was created for him. Three years later, in 1885, Freud came to work in his clinic. What obviously thrilled Freud and what stimulated him, was that for Charcot there was nothing in hysteria which was not an expression of anatomy and the nervous system. What had been until then considered as pure comedy or bad morality was now the expression of organic disorders. On the other hand, he brought back their polymorphism and their protoform character to a strict description. And that is how the great hysterical crisis was isolated in the succession of its four stages and how the stigmatas of hysteria were catalogued. And then he put his finger on the origin of hysteria, with hypnosis, because all these ill people succeeded in being eminently hypnotisable. All these manifestations could be provoked but could also be lifted through the intermediary of hypnosis or even transferred from one part of the body to another. You know that we see Freud's term *transference*[20] appear for the first time while he was talking about his time with Charcot, to the Medical Society of Vienna, and he recounts how he was able to see Charcot passing a hysterical hemiplagia from one hemibody to another. It's on this occasion that Freud uses the term *transference*. Charcot also isolated hysterogenic zones, that is to say points of the body which could also cause excitations, provoking access, rather than stopping them. And what is even more interesting, is that he was the inventor of an apparatus, the ovarian compressor, which featured in all the good books, which was a kind of screw which helped to hold the body up, and by squeezing it to a suitable point, helped to keep the ovary in its place. We notice how, apart from these conceptions – it doesn't matter that they were incorrect – alongside this way of proceeding, which was in any case scientific, hysteria was not rejected in the same way as we saw with Falret 20 years earlier. And you will see a resurgence, with Charcot himself, of the same kind of ideas as those of the Egyptians or Hippocrates.

With regard to hypnosis, it is clear that the doctors of the time, without doubt, were themselves hypnotised by what their patients presented, because things were pushed so far that Babinski[21] who was a great neurologist, engaged in work and in publications, declared that he could cure mutism from a distance.

He had provoked mutism in a patient under hypnosis with a hypnotised patient: he had stood up and had transferred, from a distance, this cure on a patient who had been mute. If one can transfer illness from one hemibody to another, then why was it not possible to transfer this at a distance from one ill person to another? Because this could also be dispelled by hypnosis, why could one not dispel it by hypnosis at a distance? I think this is interesting for us because it shows that the circulation of hysteria is never carried out without partners. We can see how, in a certain way, doctors found themselves caught up in what is commonly known as the intrigue of hysteria, how they did not ask for more than to reply to the call of the hysteric and to supply her – today we would say of him that because of the master signifier, they were capable, from the example of the hysteric, of the greatest marvels. This would give rise to very lively conflicts in the medical milieu, in particular, in the school of Nancy with Liébault[22] and Bernheim[23] who said that this all was about suggestion – which was true – and that hysteria did not have a special affinity with hypnosis, that hypnosis was independent of hysteria. What we can today decipher in these conflicts is assuredly the way in which the doctors themselves were induced by their patients, in an attempt to give witness, to show the master signifier. The master signifier – is it not he who finds himself precisely master of the body? – they possessed it, this master signifier, and following the example of the hysteric they could demonstrate this.

A while before his death, Charcot returned to all that. We have to add that everybody says that Charcot exercised genuine hypnotism with his pupils. In 1892, he wrote the preface to a book for one of his students, Pierre Janet,[24] who had written a medical thesis with him entitled: *A Contribution to the Study of Mental Accidents in Hysterics*. With this work, Pierre Janet unknitted acute bodily illness in the hysteric transforming it to a condition of mental illness even if it had an organic basis. Charcot, therefore, wrote the preface to Pierre Janet's book, a year before his death, recognising the merit of this new research. It is in this context that Freud found himself occupied with the scientific interest in hysteria.

What is the interest for us today of this history? We must always be sensitive to the remarkable constancy of a representation, of an imaginary of the hysteric, which has found itself for 4,000 years, regularly offered up to the same reading, to the same deciphering. That is to say, that of the possession of the woman – by what? By an *X* – I will not go back to the term "animal" – which gives itself up to interpretation as the source of what would be a specifically feminine desire. An *X*, which would lead the return of symptoms to a referent which would be precisely this enigmatic signifier: original repression, cause of this desire. All this happens as if hysterical manifestations were regularly interpreted as the expressions of what would be a specifically feminine libido, having its own cause. These manifestations lend themselves to deciphering, to a reading, this imaginary imposes itself in a sort of complicity between the interpreter and the hysteric herself – who is blind and deaf and who does not know what she is saying, nor what her body is expressing – and so the spectator of this imaginary is obliged to ask who is speaking, what is happening there? This means that the question is to know, to whom does this imaginary belong?

It is usual to observe that the specific mark of a hysterical scenario is the necessity for the look of the spectator and to interrogate him by trying to disturb the small window of his phantasy. This is an important point.

Ordinarily, phantasy closes every question on the real by the putting into place of a reality, where the woman is the representative of what I would call the recommendation to enjoy what the father offers. And, it ends therefore with this conclusion: reality is validated by this kind of scheduling.

But, with hysteria it goes along as if it were caught up under a totally different look. Which one? In the hysterical scenario, in fact, it is not about the woman having to imagine herself, to represent herself for this offer of enjoyment. The hysterical scenario breaks the frame of the phantasy and forces the spectator to ask himself what this real consequently might mean for he who deals with it, at the time of this access, of this crisis, of this symptom. What could this real signify, which begins to move, to become expressive?

That is how we can see that hysterical access, in its principle of formation, resembles well what the dream realises. In this kind of token role, each element proposes itself as heavy with enigmatic signification, thereby looking for an interpretation. You know how, with regard to the Dora case,[25] Freud wanted to show the place of the dream in the analysis of symptoms. We would like to reverse that proposition: the construction, the way in which the symptoms offer themselves in hysterical access is effectively constructed in the same way as the dream. Let us remark with regard to the film which we saw last Sunday,[26] the pleasure which the silent cinema affords when the images begin to signify – this is possible only on the condition of avoiding language, or at least its articulation. That's why the hysterical scenario is so willingly silent. That's also why we encounter so often in hysteria, manifestations of aphonia or mutism, as if it had to do with an attempt at an expression of another language, a foreign language, precisely.

I will take this point up again, but I'm going to permit myself a short-circuit. A foreign language may be defined as a language, the virtue of which would be to put he who is no longer the speaker, but the "possessed", the carrier to put him in the shade of the hiatus which arises between S_1 and S_2. I would like to try immediately to validate this proposition.

In fact, what is a maternal tongue? We can give it a very precise definition: a maternal tongue, it's what you collect between S_1 and S_2, that is to say you will create a little niche as a subject, and at the same time, this will authorise you to speak as an S_1, as a master. If you don't have the right to be there, you will make it one day, a maternal tongue always leaves us this hope. On the condition that we make the effort, that we study, that we make ourselves perfect, we end up by having the right to claim it, to speak in its name. This is what the mother tongue is and it's not anything else.

What is a foreign tongue? A foreign tongue (which you can, by the way, know perfectly and speak it as well as your mother tongue) puts he who articulates it in a state where an image of himself is sent back to him as if he were in a representation. A foreign language is a tongue where the subject will never be able, in any way, and especially not in a definitive way, to express himself as a master.

Let us remark that the passage to another tongue cannot be just only the old one. It's not of the order of translation or of a radical change. Anna O.[27] expresses herself in English, because in her own tongue she has no choice, with regard to subjective positions, she has to line up one side or the other, there is no other possibility. If she speaks a foreign tongue this will say something else. But, if the hysteric engages in this expression of mimicry during her (hysterical) access it's precisely an attempt to be an expression in another tongue, which would permit her to avoid at one and the same time this distinction between S_1 and S_2, and the loss that is produced between these two signifiers.

We have seen that speculations on the cause of hysteria oscillate between a double place: the head or the body. I read for you earlier Plato's formula: *Sôma hustéron psuchés*; "the body is inferior to the soul", or again in the translation which amuses me, "the body is hysterical to the soul". If there is hysteria, is it in the head or in the body? These speculations are founded on an imaginary of bodily representation. The famous psycho-somatic history (head/body) is not nothing. As with all the imaginaries, it's very powerful, very active, has effects.

But, if we do not get our bearings from an imaginary, are we not driven to say that this opposition between head and body, it is what we will rediscover in the register of the symptom between S_1 – the place where there is the signifier which commands, where it begins – and S_2 the body in so far as it has to take orders, insofar as it has to submit to these orders?

When Freud inaugurated the concept of *somatic conversion* beginning with the schema (shown in Figure 2.1), with the division of space into four, of this drawing of the *Project* where it passes from top from bottom – with this line which separates top from bottom, the head of the body – it is clearly obvious that Freud, like us, is caught in this imaginary ego representation.

It is amazing to see just how much we, analysts, work with this concept of somatic conversion. In the same way, it's just as magical as the concepts worked with by Egyptian or Greek doctors! When we need an explanation, we say, "somatic conversion" and then we are happy! We say this more than we refer to Freud, who said it. There is, I will say, a return to this imaginary,

Schematic Picture of Sexuality

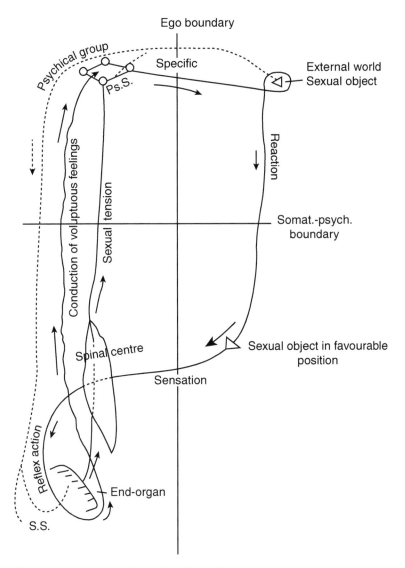

Figure 2.1 Schematic picture of sexuality. Draft G
Source: Adapted from S. Freud, *Pre-Psycho-Analytic Publications and Unpublished Drafts*, Vol. 1, p. 202.

and even a putting into place of a *cervical trait* whose imaginary effects are marked in hysteria itself. The *cervical trait* is inscribed in the representation of the hysterical body, a zone particularly sensitive and vulnerable, with a real effect of an edge. There is a whole series of symptoms which concern the effect of this imaginary partition between the head and the body. Here again, we can ask ourselves, to whom does this imaginary ego representation belong: specifically to the hysteric, or does it precisely not function in this complicity between the hysteric and the spectator?

The genesis of the Freudian conception revolves around this: the body suffers, has symptoms because something cannot be said. It is interesting to note, in Dora's analysis, Freud is persuaded about this something, concerning the expression of a desire, of a feminine desire, in particular for Mr K.

What Freud does, and this is quite decisive: is to situate the referent of desire, for the man as well as the woman, as unique. It goes for both. This is the decisive step. In other words, Freud does not enter into an interpretation which would consist in hearing the symptomatology as being the expression of a phallus which would be specific to the woman, which would, fundamentally maintain a specifically feminine libido – in which case there would be men and women because each one would have what would maintain his own libido. Henceforth, we could without any difficulty, write *The Woman*. And, at the same time, the partner would not find himself, either a semblance of a man but a real man.

We see the importance of what is at stake in this affair, in attributing to Dora a desire for Mr K. we know that Freud made a mistake. What was it in reality that interested Dora? It was Mme K., but raised to a particular dignity, because we can suppose that from then on, Dora found herself (in an imaginary way of course) the representative of a real which could have perhaps founded her own femininity. In other words, what perhaps resurged for Dora on the occasion of her becoming enamoured, was what could sustain a hysterical phantasy: the possibility to refer herself to a specific real for a woman. This specific real would be at the origin of a new language which would permit her to situate herself indeed, with regard to her partner, in a position of symmetry: To each his own! Such a representation finds itself necessarily caught up in a tacit complicity between the hysteric and he for whom this attempt is made.

This is the point at which I would like to end this evening. The next time I will take up the problem of repression.

QUESTION: Between S_1 and S_2, the subject can speak only in his mother tongue?

CHARLES MELMAN: It seems, it would appear to be only in his mother tongue.

QUESTION: What then of an analysis by an analyst whose tongue is not the same as the analyst?

CHARLES MELMAN: It's a classical question, which poses problems for interpretation. We authorise ourselves to do it. Freud did it, but it does not go without saying.

For those of you who are interested, I will recount an anecdote about the very different capacities to learn foreign tongues. Lacan was really recalcitrant with regard to this.

He knew how to learn a language. He knew how to use some foreign languages but he was incapable of articulating them correctly. He was averse to it also.

What makes a body "walk" or not? That S_2 should be good friends with S_1. What S_1 might propose to it, what might please it, does not go without saying. There is a total area here, which calls on our attention and our reflection. There are speak-beings for whom what S_2 proposes, does not please them and they find themselves very embarrassed by it. One thinks of hysterical manifestations, pithiasm, because this may be cured by suggestion, it's imitation. It's absolutely false!

We can observe a certain number of signs which bear witness to authentic bodily illnesses, which is not simply of the order of allegation or of imitation. The term "somatic conversion" has radically come to fill the gaps on that.

QUESTION: Do you make a division between a hysterical conversion which would be functional, without a lesion and the real lesion of a psychosomatic symptom?

CHARLES MELMAN: Not really. Most certainly, psychosomatic, is totally different to hysteria. With troubles of a hysterical order, we can pick up a certain number of functional modifications, not physiological, not anatomical, and one could think that these "modifications" are testimony to the biggest conversion. All this is a bit facile and we free ourselves a little too rapidly in saying that these are "modifications". It has to be explained again how this dermatographism and all these absolutely incredible things happen.

QUESTION: The psychosomatic symptom takes its exact place for the obsessional, in good management between S_1 and S_2.

CHARLES MELMAN: I'm not so sure that there is a gap between obsessional neurosis and hysteria. I think, in obsessional neurosis one can observe authentic psychosomatic manifestations.

JEAN BERGÈS: What is it that upsets the phantasy?

CHARLES MELMAN: Two things. First, the real begins to be animated. Generally, the real does not say anything special. It is for us, if I may say so, asleep, thanks to the phantasy. It is a real which loses its power to evoke. You are familiar with Lacan's seminar on "the peace of the evening".[28] In fact, this is the extreme form, this is the limited form, it's the voice of nature in what can still have an audible call. But if things suddenly begin to move, henceforth, I find myself at the same time – it's the case for the one who suffers from hallucinations – in something which is heavy with enigmatic meanings (what does that mean?) or for which I have to search. There is this procedure first of all.

The second is linked to the fact that it's not just any body, but that of the woman. Her good nature, her good standing, her politeness would mean that she is content to keep the place to which she is called, as Rabelais said, and to be the representative of what offers up to enjoyment a feminine as well as a masculine one. From the moment when she breaks this image, when she throws in the towel, this is for the spectator the phantasy, his phantasy, which finds itself disturbed and this may produce for him effects of anxiety.

We can perhaps, go a step further. The woman finds herself more willingly exposed, than her partner to the kind of oscillation between a reality which would be established, which would be fixed, of which she herself would be the guaranteed representative, and the fact that this could easily begin to move. With a question? What does this mean? What does this signify? And it's not excluded that in this hysterical access, she gives over to her partner, always in this symmetrical position, with what she in fact, finds herself so easily confronted. In other words, there is here, in a certain way, a tit for tat.

QUESTION: Could we think that there could be a semiology in connection with these oscillations at the level of corporal representations?

CHARLES MELMAN: That is another question, which concerns what is called the polymorphism or the protoform character of these cases of hysteria. Hysterics have evolved with history and we do not have the same kind of ill people nowadays which Charcot or Freud saw. Why? It is probably because the hysteric has to give an account of the truth. The manifestations of this truth are different according to the type of remarks which will come to seal this and the type of ambient remarks, of master remarks which come along to mask this truth. This may explain that hysterical manifestations can change. Meanwhile, the means of corporal expression are limited, the alphabet of it is limited. The hysterical manifestations which Freud saw or Charcot saw are not the same for a whole lot of different reasons nowadays. For example, in the American diagnostic manual,[29] in American nomenclature the term "hysteric" has disappeared. The term "conversion symptom" has replaced it. From the moment that this has a little bit of intensity, is a bit dramatic and the minute this has consequences for family life, we say immediately that this is a psychosis!

MARCEL CZERMAK: The way in which you use S_1 and S_2 from the master signifier on the one hand and from the body which should follow ... everybody knows that it's not necessarily that simple. The "body" 40 or 50 years before now, was it the same? What is a body? What is it that has to walk? This shows how little we are disengaged from being bogged down. Freud found "somatic conversion" because it was something that made one suffer, in his time. But, to consider that still as having a causative value, that's a bit limiting. To the point where someone like Daumezon,[30] not suspected of being analytically compliant, would call it "psychical conversion"!

CHARLES MELMAN: We cannot reproach Freud with anything! He used the term "somatic conversion". That was fundamental to give him an access – let us re-read the *Project*. Error always has its place, its function in discovery. We should not be either embarrassed, or blush at it or let anyone in the least be overwhelmed by it. This term "somatic conversion" was totally essential for him for the first implementation of his apparatus. It's a very simple apparatus which obeyed, and was a small group, in the mathematical sense of the term, a small group of very rudimentary permutations. This gave him the courage, which permitted him to begin to follow a scientific method, articulated according to a few ordered symbols, by allowing him a few permutations. And this is what allowed him to take on board psychoanalysis in a different way than Jung, for example, who was not less intelligent, nor less focused.

We should be careful with the French translation of *Somatisches Entgegenkommen*. *Entgegenkommen*, it's not at all "compliance" but "prevenance". Freud says that there is for the hysteric a somatic prevenance (let us write this in two words).

There is something of the body which goes in front, which offers itself up to symptomatology. In some way it's already much richer from the point of view of metaphor. It opens up a certain number of insights.

What we can expect of students, is that they will busy themselves with taking up and following on with these studies. More so, the tools which Freud has put in our hands, are not too narrow, present an interest, and permit a certain number of putting things in place.

27 April 1982

Notes

1 J.H. Breasted, *The Edwin Smith Surgical Papyrus* (translation and commentary). The Papyrus Ebers. Vol. I. University of Chicago, Oriental Institute Publications, 1930.
2 *Ancient Egyptian Medicine: The Papyrus Ebers* (trans. C.P. Bryan). London and Chicago: Ares Publishers, 1930.
3 Hippocrates, *On Ancient Medicine*. Vol. I. (trans. A.F. Adams), Vol. I. Loeb Classical Library. Cambridge, MA: Harvard University Press, 1989.
4 Plato, *Timaeus* (trans. P. Kalkavage). Hackett Classics, 1955.
5 Plato, *Timaeus*.
6 Plato, *Laws* (trans. T.L. Pangle). Chicago: University of Chicago Press, 2016.
7 Athenaeus of Naucratis, *The Learned Banqueters* (trans. D. Olson). Vol. I. Loeb Classical Library. Cambridge, MA: Harvard University Press, 2010.
8 St Augustine, *On Christian Teaching* (trans. R.P.H. Green). Oxford: Oxford University Press, 2008.
9 Paracelsus, T. von Hohenheim, *The Hermetic and Alchemical Writings.* Vols I and II (trans. A.E. Waite). Eastford, CT: Martino Fine Books, 2009.

10 A. Paré, *Oeuvres*. Lyon: Editions du Fleuve, 1962.
11 F. Rabelais, *The Life of Gargantua and Pantagruel* (trans. T. Urquhart and P.A. Motteux). New York: Penguin Random House, 1994.
12 E. Jorden, *A Briefe Discourse of a Disease called the Suffocation of the Mother*. London: 1603.
13 C. Le Pois, *Selectiorum observationum et consiliorum de praetervisis hactenus morbis affectibusque praeter naturam*, University of Lausanne. E. Typographeo. F. Hackii, 1768.
14 Aretaeus, *Consisting of Eight Books on the Causes, Symptoms, and Cure of Acute and Chronic Diseases* (1785) (trans. J. Moffat). Farmington, MI: Gale Ecco, 2018.
15 T. Sydenham, *The Works of Thomas Sydenham. M.D.* London: The Sydenham Society, 1850.
16 D. Pinel, C. Caille and L. Ravier, *Traité Médico-Philosophique sur l'aliénation mentale, ou la manie*. Paris: Richard, Caille et Ravier, an IX, 1801.
17 J.P. Falret, *Des Maladies Mentales et des Asiles d'Aliénés*. Sydney: Wentworth Press, 2018.
18 Galien, *De La Formation Des Enfans Au Ventre De La Mere Et De L'Enfantement A Sept Mois (1556)* (trans. G. Christian). Whitefish, MT: Kessinger Publishing, 2010.
19 J-M. Charcot, *Oeuvres complètes de J-M. Charcot*. Sydney: Wentworth Press, 2018.
20 S. Freud, "Hysteria" in *Pre-Psycho-Analytic Publications and Unpublished Drafts*, Vol. I, S.E (1866–1899). London: The Hogarth Press, 1966.
21 J. Babinski, *Hysteria or Pithiatism* (trans. J.D. Rollerston, ed. E. Farquhar Buzzard). London: University of London Press, 1918.
22 A.A. Liébeault, *Sleep and its Analogous States considered from the perspective of the action of the mind upon the body*. Paris: Masson, 1866.
23 H. Bernheim, *Hypnotisme, Suggestion, Psychotherapie*. Paris: Fayard, 1995.
24 P. Janet, *The Major Symptoms of Hysteria: Fifteen Lectures Given in the Medical School of Harvard University*. Whitefish, MT: Kessinger Publishing, 2007.
25 S. Freud, "Fragment of a Case of Hysteria" in *A Case of Hysteria, Three Essays on Sexuality and Other Works*, Vol. VII, S.E. (1901–1905). London: The Hogarth Press, 1953.
26 G.W. Pabst, *Secrets of a Soul*. Berlin, 1926. (A Psychoanalytic Film) viewed 24–25 April 1982, Study Days on Psychoanalytic Discourse, École Normale Supérieure, Paris.
27 S. Freud, *Studies on Hysteria*, Vol. II, S.E. (1893–1899). London: The Hogarth Press, 1955.
28 J. Lacan, *The Seminar of Jacques Lacan, Book III: The Psychoses, 1955–1956* (ed. J-A. Miller, trans. R. Grigg). London: Routledge, 1993.
29 *Diagnostic and Statistical Manual of Mental Disorders* (DSM–5), 5th edn. Washington, DC: American Psychiatric Association, 2013.
30 G. Daumezon, "Essai historique critique de l'appareil d'assistance aux maladies mentaux dans le department de la Seine depuis le début du XIX Siècle", in *L'information psychiatrique* vol. 36, 1960.

Chapter 3

Repression

Charles Melman

We are going to deal with one of the most essential concepts – repression,[1] *die Verdrängung* – which may surprise us to know that it has stayed fresh since its origins. The last time I remarked on the permanence of an interpretation lasting for 4,000 years of writing and reflection on hysteria. This was made possible, despite its polymorphism, by the stability of a representation which may be resumed like this: a woman whose animal in her would find itself dissatisfied. This permanence seems difficult to understand, to imagine, except by referring it to a fact of structure. Hysteria allowed Freud to inaugurate the concept of repression – and the unconscious because he says that one is correlative with the other – we are invited to situate repression itself as a fact of structure. How do we account for this?

Freud published this rather curious collection of texts in 1917 called *Introduction to Psychoanalysis.*[2] These are readings, which for two years during the war, was given to a very diverse public. They are interesting for us because they show well how the public could influence the formulations he adopted. In this text Freud again asks what psychical tendencies are subjected to repression, what forces impose themselves on it and what motives they obey. The response which he gives, is what undergoes repression is *die Vorstellungsrepräsentaz*, the "agent of the representative" which in French does not mean anything – but I will translate it provisionally as – the agent of the representative of a drive, whose accomplishment would be a source of displeasure. The force which imposes this repression is that of the *Ich* (which is translated in French as the "ego") and the motive of repression is of an economic order because it has to do with the pleasure principle. Displeasure would be provoked in the psychical economy if repression were accomplished.

He says a little later on, that the ill people in question, those with a transference neurosis – hysteria, obsessional neurosis, and he then adds what he called at the time, anxiety hysteria – that is to say phobia: "These patients suffer from *Versagung*, frustration, reality refusing them the satisfaction of their sexual wishes, *die Wünsche*, and the symptoms are as much substitutive satisfactions, destined to replace those which are refused in life".[3]

DOI: 10.4324/9781003167839-3

Again, in a text of the same year entitled "Repression" he says the following: "repression and the unconscious are correlative. There is no unconscious without repression".[4] It's on this occasion that he puts into place, primary repression, *die underdrängung*, primary repression, of "the agent of the representative"[5] *Vorstellungrespräsentanz* of a drive, which from then on becomes settled.

This primary repression will be a source of attraction for all the repressions to come. Freud asks a question with regard to this: do substitutive formations for this repression coincide with symptoms? Or perhaps, there is a margin, a separation between the substitutive formations linked to this repression and symptoms?[6] In this text he separates also the question of affect from that of the representative. The affect may follow a specific destiny: it could be displaced, transferred to another representative or transformed into its contrary for example, or it could be suffocated – and he cites with regard to this the words of Charcot, "The beautiful indifference" of the hysteric.[7]

To finish this recap of the Freudian position on repression, I will quote for you a very interesting sentence, which sums up very well Freud's position "In repression the ideational content, *der Vorstellungsinhalt* – I have not found a better translation – of the representative of the drive, *die Triebrepräsentanz*, escapes consciousness completely".[8] In other words, consciousness is not aware of what happens when repression occurs. It is found as a formation substitute, and at the same time as a symptom. We have an overly strong somatic innervation in cases of this type which is by nature sometimes sensory, sometimes motor and which translates either by an excitation, or by an inhibition. You can immediately see that this does not go without saying; he concludes with this "a more detailed study shows that the hyper-innervated place of the body is a part of the repressed representative of the drive itself".[9]

It is highly singular that this hyper-innervated place should be a part of the representative of the drive of the repressed signifier itself "which by a condensation, *Verdichtung*, has attracted to itself all its energy".[10] In 1915, the first idea from *Studies on Hysteria,* this mysterious leap operated by the psychical on the body is therefore conserved, and what he adds is that this body, will find itself from now on filled with a signifier, this *Triebrepräsentanz,* part of which is highly charged.[11]

So, nowadays, how are we to understand, to interpret, to read this phenomenon, which should continue to astound us, repression and its conjunction so frequent with the feminine position? What is it that is to be repressed? In the name of what and why is there repression? What is the lot of this repression? And, the final question: has it to do with a malfunctioning particular to the subject or has it to do with a fact particular to structure?

What leads us to the side of structure is that which Freud spotted very well, with his own particular divination: die *Urverdrängung.*[12] It's via primary repression, that a signifier finds itself untouched by all that could be of direct reference, of immediate reference, of a link to an object. From then on, a signifier will never be anything but representing a subject for another signifier, the signified is from now on only the equivocation for the subject produced by the procedure, and finds it sent back to him, under the form of *che vuoi?*

Insofar as we are analysts, we have the ability, a very specific one, it has to be said – to name this original signifier repressed in this way: it's the phallus. It's what fills the chain with its significance and will constitute this unique referent which meanwhile will divide speak-beings.

This primary repression, das *Urverdrängte* which means that we have from now on to do with a semblance only – and the semblant, this means something very precise, it means for example, the semblant of the woman – this primary repression has a representative which is the cause of this, which because of this the world for us will be made of representations, *Vorstellungen*. This signifier which represents primary repression has a name for Freud. We can, without too many risks, find it in what he calls the *Vorstellungsrepräsentanz*, which I translated earlier in a banal and traditional way, as "the agent of the representative" and which, I believe, should translate as "the representative because of which there are representations".

This signifier cause of representation, representing what finds itself originally repressed, I believe that we can identify it in Lacan as S_1. Let us go further. For Freud, secondary repression, repression in general, has to do with the agent of the representative of the drive. But, via a Lacanian reading we have to take a step further and say that repression does not find itself interested in just any kind of sequence, that what is implied in the procedure of repression, is in a general way S_1. Can we defend such a proposition?

What enables us to pursue things in this way, is the signifier about which the dreamer claims to be an expression. Freud notes, with surprise, that what appears there is a perfectly egotistical subject, with an ambition which nothing can stop, who is seeking essentially the expression of his power and who is witness in the dream to erotic desires which he would never admit to in a conscious state. The subject of the unconscious is therefore, a subject, who in some way, authorises himself with a signifier which precisely does not recognise any limit and who does not stop to consider anything.

We could also interest ourselves, like Freud in what he called waking or daily dreams[13] (*Tagträume* – more precisely dreams and reveries during the day). Certainly, the structure, the organisation of these daily reveries is totally different to the one of nightly dreams. We have to remark on this, it is not at all done in the same way, the scenario is constructed in a totally different manner. But Freud notices that there appears a subject which appears to be the same as the one of a nightly dream, who also authorises himself with a signifier, with a complete mastery over it. We can be a bit more precise about the day dream. The day dream is not a concrete discourse, a discourse articulated as such – I'm using here Lacanian terms you will recognise. At the same time, it is not a trans-individual discourse. In other words, it is not articulated to another, to a fellow – and you are aware, of course, the difficulty the subject has to tell his fellow about these day dreams – which would pose in an irrefutable way not only the eye but the ear of an Autre.

All sentiment held by a fellow is founded on castration, by which all the questioners make themselves known to their like. There is no other way of being a witness to him, that we come from language, that is to say that when one is a small other, one is not an animal, there is no other way but the manner in which one bars oneself in the expression that is addressed to an other. In our culture, and not in what is called our civilisation, which is founded on religion whether one wants to believe in it or imagine it, this address to a fellow implies the reciprocal renouncement of S_1. That is what we call politeness or courtesy. In the time of the gods, it did not happen like that, the way of meeting, of saluting each other, was not of the same order. In trying to follow this thread, in order to go back to the question of repression, we could say that our social relations imply this kind of lie, which has to make believe in the possibility of a co-existence of conscience and which by the same token, gives an ex-sistence to The Woman, that is to say, henceforth, puts her forward as The Woman. Let us notice that repression is not so much an individual issue, delivered up to the whims of a subject, see *Civilisation and Its Discontents*.[14] It's our culture, which demands of its participants a covering up of S_1. I did not say repression but at least this camouflage, this masking. In our culture it is incorrect to mention authority without denouncing it, under the rubric of the intolerable. One could say that the art of politics today consists precisely in knowing how to make use of this camouflage, how to let it pass. And we see how much our culture privileges neurosis.

But why, for the woman, is there a frequency not of camouflage, but of repression, of this repression of S_1, of what could be for her, the authorisation to articulate a desire? That's what Freud demanded of Dora[15] in the guise of a treatment, "why do you turn away from M.K.? In reality, it is clear that you were able to feel pleasure, why do you not consent to admit it"?

There are different ways of trying to account for repression, perhaps specific to a woman. The first is to say that if the woman is not all phallic, at the same time she is not totally taken by the phantasy of her partner, but she is divided by it – and she could have a tendency to make her partner's phantasy responsible for her division. But, if she is not totally captive of the phantasy of her partner from then on, this world of representations will partially hold for her an enigmatic and uncanny aspect: that of a signification not fully achieved, and because of this the *che vuoi?* of the Autre will always be a question for her. She is always, meanwhile, the guarantor of these semblances, these *Vorstellung* in so far as they are given for enjoyment. She cannot respond to this except by either alternately reinforcing the masquerade, which would present her as being totally phallic, that is to say completely captivated by the phantasy of her partner and a brusque renunciation, giving all the emphasis to her own existence and no longer to her representation. But this existence is from now on, deprived of representation, deprived of an ego. To say this in another way, she finds herself unwell.

In any case, when the world of representations finds this rather anxiety-laden aspect is being lived by an enigmatic signification, not completed, as if it had to do with a suffering of the Autre, on whom it will try to put a term, the subject has one way only in which to respond. It's a classical way, well known: her castration. It is as if she were there, ready to satisfy the Autre, where she will find herself rewarded with a guarantee. Her castration, that is to say the renunciation by the subject of being an expression of S_1 to authorise for herself a desire.

But, you will say, why repression and why not, for example, a dis-avowal[16] or a denegation[17] which can be perfectly well observed? What we are going to say is that repression would present itself here like a gift made by the Autre and for the Autre, the expectation, the hope of the recognition of what he would really like to deliver – a sacrifice endlessly engaged in the expectation of the procedure of this reciprocity, which is worthy of the subject, having paid in this way, to see himself finally recognised in his right to exercise his desire.

Does repression in hysteria, present itself in this way as the repetition of a sacrifice, which will never be validated, never recognised?

In any case, to make this suggestion, takes account of the clinic of alternation which I spoke about earlier, between what I would call this exalted masquerade of an all-phallic representation, which, in the name of sacrifice, could finally authorise itself with an absolute master signifier, even if only momentarily, and the depressive effects into a suffering of an unfounded ex-sistence because there is not at least One, who from that side will justify, guarantee this ex-sistence, an existence which henceforth will be unfounded, that no image will guard against in this depressive period. It was, in the preceding case, the only possible phallic reference.

This depressive consequence, what motivates it after all? This fault in engaging, the possibility of holding oneself in the presentification of an all-phallic image, this is something which intervenes in the register of frustration. There is a failure to recognise the universal character of, this all phallicism. Because, if the hysterical subject can make this quality of all phallicism recognised in the family circle or in her entourage, it is much more difficult, I would say, to impose as a fact, a civil status, capable of giving worth to this universal recognition. We could go on and on on this point by taking up all the fantasies, which could, with this daydreaming, which is organised around the status of the (movie) star, a status which would permit one to claim to be an expression of this image in a universal way, not without of course, con-siderable problems for subjectivity. We could also go on and on about these ordinary counter-phobic objects, which are necessary in such a position, that is to say the necessity of having in the hand, a child, a husband, objects, other familiar objects and occasionally, why not, a little dog.

But there is another element, which perhaps for us is even more interesting. This sacrifice alternating with depression, also repeated, also intense, no matter how exhausting, will not permit the ending of what has now become, not only frustration, but a privation of the instrument, the delivery by which the Autre will be able in some kind of way, to signal a recognition thereby acquired. It's there that we can make the problem of anatomy intervene and ask indeed if "anatomy is destiny" or not. Like some of you here, I was surprised to witness Lacan's insistence when he was making a presentation of the ill, how he never missed an opportunity, when it had to do with problems of homosexuality or of transsexuality for the man, to look for signs of an anatomical defect. He was interested not only in external anatomy but also in research in sexual chromosomes and that may appear surprising for someone, who it seems, privileged subjective determinations, put into place through our dependence with regard to language.

To be an expression of S_1, and that is why it is difficult to authorise oneself, needs the agreement of the Autre. One has to be in tune with the Autre before it will work. But, in order to be in tune with this Autre to be an expression of S_1, is it not necessary that the body responds in a satisfactory way that the body, the vector of this instrument, is able to be the witness, the body as truth, of the well-founded, of what is being affirmed here? Is it not that one of the elements of anatomy would intervene as a factor of destiny and as a cause of this depressive phase of the cycle, if it were not that of exactly: privation? That despite the sacrifice of this instrument ...

We can, with regard to this, make two clinical observations. Firstly, what is called female homosexuality, revolves around a mutual pact which wishes to imagine the presence of the instrument and purely and simply imagine it – there is not even a need for a fake for that. We are absolutely sure of this because the style of the homosexual meeting accentuates things up to the point of caricaturising the dysmorphia of male and female appearance. Those among us who may have such patients in analysis, know that this instrument functions here perfectly in a purely imaginary state and this may or may not present special difficulties.

Another clinical remark, there is a whole hysterical symptomatology which consists in demonstrating the failure of the body, at the exact moment that the subject would seem to be able to benefit from sought after recognition. At the exact moment where the subject finds himself in a society or in circumstances which would be opportune for this recognition, there are produced manifestations which betray him, which betray his truth at the level of signs, which could be extremely diverse, of a failure of the body. Why? Why, as a general rule – except in extreme cases, I've spoken about female homosexuality, but there are others – why does something like a failure of the body occur, a betrayal of the body, as if there was there some kind of prohibition, a kind of impossible?

It's an impossible of which the consequences may be fairly large. And this impossible may be raised from at least two dimensions. One is of the order of the imaginary: to be in an all-phallic representation, the hysteric is in permanent fear of a breach which would put in peril not so much herself as the phallus, of which she is the bearer of a guarantee and which must be preserved at all costs. Another prohibition, more essential, and which interests us of course, seems to be of the order of the symbolic. The feminine position comes from an order which, as such, does not authorise her to be a foil for being all phallic, unless ...

Unless we can engage in an essential activity for all of us, which is sublimation.[18] From then on, the renunciation of every private desire will find itself guaranteed, for easily understood reasons, to be validated by a social recognition, validated by the Autre, when this renunciation of every private desire finds itself authenticated, recognised in a vocation of oblativity which could be religious, social or maternal. Social recognition is really essential because in the other cases, when it's really only a private issue, it might not turn out so well. There are cases of "private saintliness" which turn around sensitive paranoia, and that is why it is not recommended in these cases, to insert them into a milieu where this saintliness could be authenticated as such. There is of course the hiding away of all addresses, of all invitations, which otherwise would constantly misrecognise her, would annoy her and would see her not as a successful sublimation, but as a failed one. There could also be success in competition with the boy, in a narcissistic challenge, in which a girl engages normally in a love with regard to her father, in this competition about knowing whom the father prefers. In these successful sublimations, it has to do with validating her, in recognition of her position as a virginal servant who would put the said phallus in some kind of way in a position to serve everybody. The phallic duty seems to be more successful in this case than the boy, who puts his own activity at the service of his father, this is well known, but who still is supposed to scrape a little bit for himself, for his own benefit, his dealings and his private adventures. He will not serve his status uniquely in the work of procreation or in the work of conjugal life.

A last question to introduce what is to follow in two weeks' time: what is the topographical destination of repression? What becomes of it? Where does it go?

I will repeat this – because we give credit to he who said it without asking in any way why? what is foreclosed in the symbolic will reappear in the real.[19] With regard to what is denied or disavowed, we know what happens to that: it subsists within the symbolic while being denied or disavowed. There, we don't have too many problems. But the repressed, where does that go? While staying in a position where it is accessible to a return of what is called conscience, it seems as if what is repressed does not go off into the real. How to understand this, except that it thereby infiltrates and orders all the signifying chain, as a symptom? How are we to understand that the signifying chain, which in primary repression finds itself laden with significance linked to the phallus, will lend itself to be filled by what is conferred, which allows me to call "parasitical" meanings which are able to infiltrate, at any stage, at any place in the said chain?

We would have to say, finally, that the hysterical scenario presents itself as a kind of symmetry, the return to a symmetry of this painful procedure which the woman has to suffer by the fact of the phantasy in which she is caught, by which she is divided. We could say that the hysterical scenario is a reply to the partner who may flatter himself to have a well-established world, a "together" world, a quiet, tranquil world where there is no reason to be astonished, where the little woman is there, as a given for enjoyment, open to jouissance, which will guarantee this reality as representative of the *Vorstellung*. A symmetrical reply which will upset the phantasy of the partner by saying "It is not as calm as you believe and the world of your representations are perhaps not as satisfying as you imagine them to be". She introduces into this world an enigmatic reality to which the phantasy of the partner exposes her. Her partner will have to try and decipher what, in some sort of way, is presented to him as an enigma. The hysterical scenario sends back to her partner what she herself, the hysteric, must tolerate: that the significations are not concluded, are not achieved, that there is a world of significations which disturb us, which interrogate us, that the question of what he wants, of his desire, of the way in which he will accomplish it, will remain open.

Perhaps, in that way, she would give vigour to her demonstration. Certainly, she is constrained by a fact of structure, to repress the signifier, the consequence of a purely mechanical type, but the latter, in this position of having been repressed, will in an imaginary way, constitute the excluded signifier which will lay claim to what the hysteric lets us hear, what she cannot articulate. Why is this not able to be articulated as such? Why does this let itself be heard? For a reason which may appear simple and complex at the same time and which has to be clarified. It's as if the signifier which she finds she has to repress is capable of functioning in a foundational position and I would say, legitimising what she has to, in this way, allow to be heard. It's as if she finds here what founds this mysterious animal, this unnamed animal – for Hans it was a horse; for the Wolf Man – we know what it was: but it could stay as an unnamed animal – with henceforth, strange new images, insofar as she will eventually have to lay claim to such an ancestor.

This is an introduction to the re-reading of *Studies on Hysteria*; to take them up again, to reflect on them, to critique them; to evaluate them by trying to allow all the questions which we have tended to leave aside, precisely because they were articulated by the Master.

To finish, I would like to make this remark. Within such a perspective, the end of analysis could be seen as the passage, the right, finally acquired through the lifting of repression, cause of neurosis and pathology, so as be able to emphasise the expression of one's desire. But what does the symptom mean? The symptom means that phallic jouissance is not everything and this has a certain number of effects, of consequences. All this will have to be of course corrected and taken up again, in particular with regard to the masculine position but for the moment, let us advance like this. We are therefore led to the idea that the lifting of neurosis goes via the condition of not having to repress, not to have to repress any more, that is to say to go straight there. Yes, this is another problem. That's true.

The other problem is that if this is a solution, it cannot be universal, because precisely the universal, there isn't one. In other words, there is no solution which will be the same for everyone. Psychoanalysis differentiates itself – Freud here is truly remarkable – from all prophetism, from all messianism, from all political action.[20] With politics of course, we lay claim to what would be good for everybody. Freud well understood that for a psychoanalyst, this is not possible. We could say that, to a certain extent, the question remains open. But, no matter what we can, all the same, conclude on this, that if a psychoanalysis could simply terminate on the fact that: "There, you go, repression has been lifted, I will not be made to yield any more, this is my desire, and that's how it is, it will be this and nothing else"! Of course, that's not bad, is it? If this did not merit all the same, this little relativisation – which seems like nothing, but which is essential, which happily Lacan introduced for us and which allows us to navigate a little better – that this master signifier is only worth arriving at the place of the semblant. This master signifier cannot take itself as a full master, as an all-over master. And, if this little addition is taken into account, by those who find themselves at the end of their analysis, who find themselves engaged in psychoanalytic work, in positions, in discussions, etc. ... this remark perhaps will help us avoid what our debates take on so frequently, as if they were fights with authority, instead of, as we would hope, for our own reflection, discussion and the possibility of taking up a dialectic. This supposes that we will never think that the signifiers to which we lay claim, even if they are of masters, are exactly that, all master signifiers, and that all we have to do is to sanctimoniously deliver ourselves up to them, to simply follow them, so that we can be in agreement with them.

This is the point on which I will finish this evening. In two weeks, we will have to test these hypotheses, especially with regard to that which we call a body.

11 May 1982

Notes

1 S. Freud, "Repression" in *On the History of the Psychoanalytic Movement, Papers on Metapsychology and Other Works*, Vol. XIV, S.E. (1914–1916). London: The Hogarth Press, 1957.

2 S. Freud, *Introductory Lectures on Psycho-Analysis*, Part III, Vol. XVI, S.E. (1916–1917). London: The Hogarth Press, 1963.

3 Freud, *Introductory Lectures*.

4 S. Freud, *On the History of the Psycho-Analytic Movement, Papers on Metapsychology and Other Works*, Vol. XIV, S.E. (1914–1916). London: The Hogarth Press, 1957.

5 Freud, *History of the Psycho-Analytic Movement*.

6 Freud, *History of the Psycho-Analytic Movement*.

7 Freud, *History of the Psycho-Analytic Movement*.

8 Freud, *History of the Psycho-Analytic Movement*.

9 Freud, *History of the Psycho-Analytic Movement*.

10 Freud, *History of the Psycho-Analytic Movement*.

11 Freud, *History of the Psycho-Analytic Movement*.

12 Freud, *History of the Psycho-Analytic Movement*.

13 S. Freud, *The Interpretation of Dreams (Second Part) and On Dreams*, Vol. V, S.E. (1900–1901). London: The Hogarth Press, 1953; S. Freud, *Jensen's "Gravida" and Other Works*, Vol. IX, S.E. (1906–1909). London: The Hogarth Press, 1959.

14 S. Freud, "Civilisation and its Discontents" in *The Future of an Illusion, Civilisation and its Discontents and Other Works*, Vol. XXI, S.E. (1927–1931). London: The Hogarth Press.

15 S. Freud, "Dora" in *A Case of Hysteria, Three Essays on Sexuality and Other Works*, Vol. VII, S.E. (1901–1905). London: The Hogarth Press, 1953.

16 S. Freud, "Fetishism" in *The Future of an Illusion*.

17 S. Freud, "Negation" in *The Ego and the Id and Other Works*, Vol. XIX, S.E. (1923–1925). London: The Hogarth Press, 1961.

18 S. Freud, "Narcissism" in *History of the Psycho-Analytic Movement*.

19 J. Lacan, *The Seminar of Jacques Lacan, Book III: The Psychoses, 1955–1956* (ed. J-A. Miller, trans. R. Grigg), London: Routledge, 1993.

20 S. Freud, "The Question of a *Weltanschauung*" in *New Introductory Lectures on Psycho-Analysis and Other Works*, Vol. XXII, S.E. (1932–1936). London: The Hogarth Press, 1964.

Chapter 4

Freud's *Studies on Hysteria*

Charles Melman

I encourage you to re-read *Studies on Hysteria*,[1] to make yourselves aware of the mystery which continues to surround this clinical entity, and try to arouse, once again, the astonishment it deserves. After all, perhaps our usage of concepts is no less magical than that of our predecessors of 4,000 years ago. Because, for us a return to magic is something really simple: it means to go back to concepts. We have seen how a concept so easily used like that of conversion was capable of posing a question for Freud himself. And because it has to do with "psycho somatic" conversion as it is called, if we could start here by asking ourselves what we mean by the words psyche and body. It is more than likely that such a question would provoke a certain embarrassment. ... This is to remind us how much we ourselves are in line with a genealogy of those who, for 4,000 years have spoken about, have written about, have studied hysteria and that we, like them, have a tendency to hand over to the magical power of the concept – perhaps because it has to do with hysteria – and to speak about psychosomatic conversion even though each one of these terms question us.

What is really going on with regard to all this? It is to know if we are capable or not of getting out of hysteria! The question does not seem today to be clear cut. Did Freud himself succeed? If we consider the reports of the cases he gave us, what we know about his entourage, even the women whom he privileged, we can think that no, we have not got out of it. It's a question which will always remain pertinent regarding the powers of our work.

What is also at stake here, is to know, once and for all, if the status of femininity should be so easily linked to hysteria.

And there is also a more general question, of an ethical order, which concerns the place we give to the subject in so far as it is about the subject of our speculations. This subject as a subject of frustration, in animating the discourse of hysteria clearly constitutes the biggest resistance to psychoanalysis and makes us question the possible end of the treatment. But the question is even more general. With this resistance of the subject as a subject of frustration, is it not also the perpetuating of the master to which we have a right? After all, it is quite easy to show and at the end of this seminar I will probably try to do this. The master's victory has to do with nothing other than this perpetuation of the subject of frustration.

DOI: 10.4324/9781003167839-4

I also think that it was sensitive, with my preceding seminars that the limit of my comment, of what I could say, was strictly regulated, commanded by what we ourselves are able to hear. This does not mean that I have a great reserve with regard to what can be articulated for an audience who are receptive. But, I think that what happens here could make us aware how much anyone's comment finds itself strictly commanded, limited, by what he is for the Autre, by what the Autre directs, imposes on him. In this inevitable game for anyone – I hope I do not plunge myself into traumatic signifiers, and I hope that I will hold on to comments which will not have a traumatic impact – we see how the exit for the subject with what is in question can never be an individual one. There is no individual salvation.

If today we resume this reading of *Studies on Hysteria*, we will see there a simple and elegant representation of its mechanism. This demonstration in its original freshness is really questioning.

We will begin with this: there are two order of things for the cause of hysteria.

Firstly: representations which are incompatible with the ego, *das Ich*. *Unverträglich*, translates as incompatible. The term would have been better translated in French as "insupportable", (intolerable in English) but the word incompatible has the advantage of making us veer towards the side of logical resonances – which is not without power to help us, so let us keep this translation. There are representations which are incompatible with the ego. The human organism is characterised by this fact that representations can occur, which have this surprising character of being incompatible with this agency, which is the *Ich*. By the same token, these incompatible representations have a traumatic impact.

But, what causes hysteria is a trauma which has remained, without a reaction. For example, as Freud says, some are inevitable, like mourning or the loss of a cherished object or again events, traumas with regard to which a reaction was not possible, through the impossibility of the social order or because the subject wished to forget about it.

With these incompatible representations, *das Ich*, the ego, will withdraw itself in a process which in *Studies on Hysteria* are not yet unique. Because there is not only repression, *die Verdrängung*, but there is a term which exists, *die Unterdrückung* to "push below", repression, and also *die Hemmung*, which will be taken up later as inhibition. There are therefore three ways to get rid of these incompatible representations: *die Verdrängung, die Hemmung and die Unterdrückung*. What is even more interesting for us is that this memory thereby pushed away, intolerable, incompatible, will find itself, through repression (we will hold on to this term of *Verdrängung*, of repression – to try and specify its mechanism), – a signifying chain will find itself being pushed away from the chain of associations. What will produce itself is what Freud called *eine Abspaltung von Vorstellungsgruppen*, a break in the groups of representations. In this way, it will form what is called a psychical group, separated from the ego. This psychical group will conduct itself, Freud tells us, like a *Fremdkörper*, like a foreign body in the psyche. But this is fairly unusual because, anatomically, if a foreign body is encysted, it surrounds itself with reactional layers. Here this *Fremdkörper* will act in a very bizarre, very unusual way. Freud tells us these elements will integrate everywhere in the elements of the normal ego. This is a rather special foreign body. Moreover, Freud says that instead of saying a foreign body, it would be better to say an infiltration. This foreign body, infiltrated everywhere, forms a second consciousness and is at the origin of motor phenomena, which, Freud tells us are partially inexplicable.

He discovered the treatment: abreaction as you know, or rather what he calls *die assoziative Denkarbeit, das Durcharabeiten*, the work of psychical association of thought. In order to be able to join the links, the foreign elements, separated from the rest of the psyche by a split, are thereby reintegrated into the general current of psychic life. In so doing, Freud says the symptom, but not the constitution is cured. Here quickly recalled is, the putting into place, which Freud traces, in a sure and elegant way in *Studies on Hysteria*.

Now, let us today re-question the different elements of this designation! What are these *unverträglich* representations? Where do we see these representations, incompatible with the ego, *The Ich*? In what do they consist? What is *unverträglich*? There are two things with regard to this: firstly, there is what Freud speaks about in the observations he brings and secondly in the way in which he categorises them. What are the incompatible representations in the observations that he brings us? Leaving aside the case of Anna O. we will take up the four observations which concern Freud and which are the basis for his theorisation.

Let us take Emmy von N., the Livonian, as he calls her. This concerns a young widow, 23 years of age, whose elderly husband has died, leaving behind two children. We could characterise all her narrative under hypnosis as *misfortune. Misfortune*, because in her memories she always has meetings with people which are disagreeable and traumatising, meetings, with animals which are very upsetting. There is here a whole zoo: toads, mice, rats, lizards etc. And also men hidden in the shadows, or men who could follow her. Finally, what characterises Emmy von N.'s text under hypnosis is that she is incessantly hitting up against, what I will call, to simplify things, unnamed beasts. If she puts her hand into a drawer, a mouse jumps out. There is always around her this something which is a source of anxiety and which I therefore call this unnamed beast.

I will remark immediately that up to now, in the observation of Emmy von N. we do not see at all what could be an incompatible representation, if it's not perhaps this endlessly traumatising, sudden appearance. We could think that this activity is inferred by what Freud is researching. Of course, we cannot put to one side the explanations which Freud has given. But, we will say this is of little importance, because, after all, it's not an exceptional situation. It could be said, this type of presence forms part of the banality of existence – the feeling that there is easily a rather mysterious presence, half hidden, half enigmatic, which risks always exposing itself, invisible, but is there all the same. It's a cinematographic theme for example, which is capable of stirring and moving everybody. It's not at all reserved for a certain category of people.

Could we advance a little on this point and attempt to interpret this presence which so easily risks manifesting itself, exposing itself, more crudely, more openly, totally and yet not seen, not perceived? Have we anything more to say on this?

We can of course say more, with the tools we have at our disposal. Let us remark that everyone is accompanied by the object of his phantasy. It is there, yet managing to remain hidden. But, because of her status, of her position, the woman perhaps finds herself particularly exposed to what – without asking anything of her, without asking her opinion – a partner well- or badly intentioned, will expose, will reveal this object. There is perhaps here a status particular to the woman, caught up in a phantasy from which she will neither be free nor in a position of mastery to decide: there could always be some person who is prepared to go further in this development, further than she herself is prepared to go. What in hysteria takes this character of an initial rape, by which Freud found himself at first fooled, perhaps it's got to do with this. This kind of situation subjectively resembles, the category of rape: that she finds herself in this way, affected by a phantasy the mastery of which is reserved for someone else, free to decide, just how far he will go and of what he is capable of revealing.

Perhaps that explains, clinically, in the style of the hysteria, a mode of retaliation with regard to the partner: no longer only an attempt at retreat and at isolation, but a turning into what could be a counter-exhibition: to play the wrong trick with the male partner which, in fact has been operated by him. And the big, hysterical crisis is perhaps the phenomenon, which has the closest possible link with this kind of attempt to turn around on the partner the truth of his own particular phantasy, of what guards over his phantasy.

This big hysterical crisis which has been so well described, including, following Charcot, clinicians who knew very early on how to distinguish it from epilepsy. What is absolutely astounding is to see how Hippocrates, 500 years before our era, knew that there was a diagnostic differential to be made. You know that this big hysterical crisis mimes a tumescence, spasmodic movements and then a detumescence. We have to say it like it is!

This symptom of Emmy von N. is interesting for us, because if what I advance is correct, we can see in what way it has to do with an incompatible representation. This would consist in a sudden appearance, in her phantasy, of a signifier which would have to remain hidden until it was time, it would have to definitively remain hidden, so that the phantasy can function. This signifier, capable of upsetting the legitimate organisation of her phantasy is always hidden there, but it always risks showing, if I may say so, the end of its nose. And, this is also capable of producing manifestations of disgust, this other symptom so frequent in hysteria.

To conclude, there is another way of questioning this trauma which Emmy von N. repeats. It is to ask if it has not got to do, after all, with a repetition which would function not in a phantasy, but as a signifier which would try and provoke a caesura: an abolition of the subject which never accomplishes itself. It's as if the trauma repeats an experience of what is expected to be foundational, foundational of a phantasy which will establish desire, give its place to the subject, but every time this trauma finds itself unable to accomplish this definitive procedure. You will see here another possibility of questioning what is involved in the repetition of this trauma.

For Lucy R. it is much more simple, it is clear. Lucy R. is a governess – we go from women of the world to governesses. She is in love with her employer who has become a widower. Her hopes to replace the deceased woman are not fulfilled and she finds herself engaged in a hysterical symptomatology, one of whose essential elements is a disagreeable odour from burnt desserts.

I have looked for other more clarifying metaphorical resonances than the burnt desserts on the occasion of this little *clash* which occurred between her boss and herself. Perhaps those of you who speak German will comment on this. No matter what, for Freud there is no doubt about what causes hysteria: Lucy R. could not talk about her desire for her boss. Therefore it forms a separate psychical group. Freud calls this an act, which has to do with an act of moral cowardice from which she could indeed have emerged, he says, by calling on a greater quantity of moral courage. In other words, if she had dared recognise her desires, she would not have been taken for a hysteric! It is interesting to note like Emmy von N., Lucy R. finds herself embarrassed by this smell of burning desserts, by this presence which does not let go of her, even if it is under another mode of sensorial presentification. There is, she says something which will not let go of her, which follows her around and goes where she goes. There is also here, this kind of presence which embarrasses her and questions her.

For little Katharina – If you remember this charming story about "fast" psychoanalysis during the course of a mountain walk – its again very easy, simple, because this dyspnoea of which she complains, is about, if we are to believe Katharina, the memory of an attempt at rape or penetration carried out on her by her parent. There again, trauma. An incompatible representation is something which will be put to one side of psychical associations. In this case, Katharina has the feeling that there is someone behind her. She is from then on, stuck to something which continues to follow her wherever she goes.

And, finally Elisabeth, this young woman, who is very sweet, very talented. Everything is simple: it has to do with a desire which she pushes away for a brother-in-law, a widower. She played the role of a boy, of son in this family. She carries herself like the eldest boy, successor to her father. Her father had told her that she could not marry. Here, she represses her desire and finds it still the cause of repression, and the constitution of a separate group and the cause also of her somatic symptom which is constituted by an astasia-abasia.

How does Freud collect all these incompatible representations? From what category does he take them? He tells us in all these cases, that it has to do with representations which provoke shame, remorse, moral suffering and also, the aversion of the ego. The ego does not like it because it is not good to have such ideas. And he has this sentence – "a representation, which accedes to the ego, finds itself intolerable and exercises on it a force of repulsion. This constitutes a defence against the dominant idea, a defence which attains its aim, the representation in question rejected outside consciousness and outside memory and not leaving, in appearance at least, any trace". In other words, the ego is conscious of it, but behaves as if it knows nothing.

Here, on this point, we have to ask ourselves; this *Ich*, what is it? What is this agency? I think we can easily reply: in refusing to see them as our own, these ideas ranged in the category of shame, of remorse, it can only be about the ego ideal. Freud tells us, it's the *Ich* which represses. In all these cases, it has to do with women, servants, governesses, who are put at the service of the family and who devote themselves to it. It all happens as if, for the love of the Autre, and for the others, fellow beings, it is necessary for them to give up on their desire. It is as if the success or the constraint operated by the ego ideal as in these cases of repression, the agency which, preserved on the first rung, commands, decides everything in order to be loved. It is as if the condition of this love for others and for the Autre, is to give up on desire and to put oneself at the service of an Other. We see how the nurse's caring vocation willingly finds its place here.

Why is this interesting for us? Because we see that, in this case, it's conscience: this is strictly confused with the imaginary. Conscience, this is what you are able to tolerate, to accept as an image of yourself, and what you repress, reject, is in some way, what finds itself incompatible, *unverträglich*, with the image, with the ego ideal. This ego ideal has to be defended, maintained no matter what the price.

What interests us even more, is the specificity of repression. That is to say the constitution of a separate psychical group, as Freud says, a *Spaltung*, a break in groups of representations. Why is this important? Because what we have to keep in mind is that this group functions as if there were, between it and the rest of these psychical representations, a radical caesura, a break, a cut, a procedure – which would have its topological support – if we continue in the same vein.

Does repression really provoke a break? What helps us to think this – you see, I will come back to that on which I finished the last time rather abruptly – concerns the place from where repression takes place. Freud describes it very well, as the henceforth indestructible conservation of the repressed, which is essential. From the moment you put it in the freezer, you can be sure that it will preserve its freshness forever, its emotional value, maintaining itself as such and not in just any way: like materials ranged in good order, at the level of a perfectly organised chain.

We can also say more: this continues without doubt like a writing. How can be sure of this? Because, we know by the psychosomatic manifestations produced, that it's not the hypothetical signified which is thereby conserved, but the signifier, indifferent to the signified which it lugs around. For example, to take the well-known story of the *glance at the nose*, this German-speaking patient, whose fetishism was linked to the *glanz*, to the "shine", when he became an English speaker, the *glance* became "a glance" "a glance of the eye" on the nose, the signifier remaining unchanged at the level of pure writing. When he changed language, his symptom moved around with the signification. What is important for us is that what is conserved functions well as a material element and I could give you other symptomatic examples which show that the final support is indeed the letter. The return of a repressed signifier can be made simply by a letter which represents it. This supposes that there is in the unconscious an alphabet, the signifying chain reduced to its strictest material support.

We are sure what this cut is about, and what goes to this side is, from now on, devoted to conservation. What interests us, is that this foreign body, this *Fremdkörper* will become the place of a second conscience. The double personality of the hysteric is this: another place for her from where it commands, from where it could command. To take the example of Anna O., there is her legal, official, social, aspiring, intelligent, devoted personality and then there is the other. For her this has a nycthemeral rhythm, but the alternation can be made in a much looser way.

We also notice how this separated place becomes the source of a second conscience which, Freud tells us, has an intelligence which is in no way inferior to the other. This goes against Breuer and Janet who said it was linked to a certain psychical weakness, psycho-asthenic, stupidity etc. But this intelligence is just as much damned as the other. We have seen that this foreign body infiltrates from this place all the elements of a normal ego. There are rejected bits from this place in all the productions of daily life. It's a place which commands in an extremely decisive way, so that all the elements of a normal ego are infiltrated by it!

What interests us also, is that this infiltration is heard. We are really dealing with symptomatology: from this second place, this second conscience, all that infiltrates the normal elements of the ego and offer themselves to deciphering. And here, a very important question: why are there not voices, heard by the ear, able to be articulated by what is heard from this second place? In other words, why does the hysteric not talk from this second place? We can interpret without a doubt that what is heard is the expression of a desire for recognition in this second place. This second place, of suffering and looking to be recognised, because nothing as we know, can exist without recognition by the other, by our fellows and by the same token the Autre.

But we can even here go a little bit further. If she speaks instead of letting herself be heard through her symptoms, from then on, whether she wishes it or not, she swallows a phallic reference – and this is inevitable – because it has to do with her giving value to and recognising this X which possesses her, what I called earlier this unnamed beast. She cannot do anything else with her symptom except offer an interpretation of this enigmatic alphabet. Freud speaks about hieroglyphics, that is the metaphor he uses, with regard to Lucy. Because, in what language, is it articulated, that which possesses her like this?

What we see, is that this separate psychical group operates as if it were a real. When this split, this caesura happens, from this *Abspaltung*, everything happens as if there were a cut and as if there was, from here, is what I would call a neo-real, the place of an enigmatic Autre from where it is formulated for her, and about which she is not the voice, but with her body, is the book, the written word. This signifier, from this place, this neo-real, will possess her and will act in a very particular way. It possesses her – we can say it like this, this is what indeed is characteristic of the symptom – it possesses her entirely, without the slightest bit of the proper distance which the subject keeps with regard to the signifier and, of the relativisation which he makes of it, as with a semblant. It has to be acknowledged that the relation of the subject to the signifier is plugged, plugged because there is a place of the subject and from then on this signifier with which he is dealing is not all phallic. He does not bring everything along with him, no matter what kind of subject he is. There is this distance, which means that the subject is not totally brought along by the butt of the nose. There is this kind of cut which is the only dimension of what is called his "freedom" which means that he is not, with regard to the signifier like a traveller, embarking onto a carriage without no other way out. What helps with this remedy involves a position which is that of the subject. But this position is capable, in totally physiological circumstances, to do away with itself. A totally banal example, he is prey to, taken along by his desire. What characterises this desire at this very moment, is the abolition of his position as subject, by the fact that he is taken, henceforth, by a chain which he uses to recover from carrying out his desire. He is then swept along by the movement of the signifier which commands him.

What can be pointed out – it is one of the incidences, why not say it, of the erotics of hysterical symptomatology – is that the hysteric presents herself with regard to the signifier which possesses her, in this position where she is entirely carried away by it and without her having any recourse to a possible position as subject. She is completely devoted to it, driven by it. It's the same position which may be found experimentally produced by hypnosis, which plays on this artificial possibility of provoking the extinction of the subject, and, from then on, gives him up effectively to the whim of a signifying chain, which could lead him to commit to a certain degree admittedly –and this is also – very interesting, this leads him to commit a certain number of actions, with, as you know, delayed effects.

What is to be noted in all these observations and which, as far as I am concerned, are not separate from what I call this pseudo-cut and this neo-real, it's the place taken by mourning. It is worthy of note that in the five observations, if we count Anna O. among them, in every one of these cases there was a central mourning, where it can be read, in following this thread, the attempt to give value to a cut. A mourning which is at every time lived, on condition of making it work – because there is a "work of mourning" of which it will, one day, have to be said what it represents – with enough intensity and duration, of devotion, of sacrifice, as if it were possible for the subject to put in place a father, a dead father, the only one who ex-sists and whom the subject could finally claim as filiation. These mournings hold, obviously, an essential place here.

So, what really allows us to decide that it has to do with a neo-real only? It is as if everything happens here, as if it were a cut, as if the repressed elements found themselves commanded by this second subject, this second conscience, a second identity, a second membership, a body, a second imaginary, a symptomatology, etc. What permits us to say, in a way, something which is I believe, difficult to refute? It is what Freud tells us with regard to his therapeutic victory. What is given to description, to interpretation, once it is recognised, when it is decrypted, it is abolished, it falls. When value is given to the purely metaphorical contribution of the hysterical symptom, which Breuer mocks, saying "Really there are symptoms which are made, so flimsy, so ridiculous so absurd, so comical", whereas Freud immediately gives all importance to the constitution of these symptoms. From the minute you give this symptomatology an interpretation of what constitutes it, that is to say a metaphor, at the same time you are making this signifier, registered on the body, in what I will permit myself to call the phallic rank. Because when it is raised to the register of metaphor, it is raised from the power of the phallus, of phallic significance. That is to say, that at this same time this second place, which looks to be recognised as such, finds itself recognised, while at the same time, abolished, by interpretation.

For example, Elisabeth, who had this symptom of astasia-abasia, her big issue, was that she took into account from then on, she was destined for solitude, in German, *das Alleinstehen*, to "hold oneself alone". And, precisely, she did not want to hold herself alone. Her symptom was that she could not hold herself alone anymore. "*Allein Stehen*". When she was put on her two feet, she could neither advance nor fall. And it's of course this interpretation given by Freud of this *Alleinstehen* – that she could not, would not, would not resign herself to hold herself up alone, to stand up – this led to the sedation of this symptom and provokes this pleasure for Freud, who tells us in finishing his observation, that he saw her dance in the arms of a soldier at a soirée.

That this has to do with elements which cede in this way to interpretation, goes along with what I've said. We are not concerned, contrary to appearances, with what constitutes what could be called a truly second conscience, we are only concerned with a neo-real, which is a pseudo-real.

The problem, and with this I will finish this evening, is that we know that interpretation can lose the symptom but it may also not lose it. I see that, I have large agreement among you! Freud finishes his *Studies on Hysteria* by saying: It's got to do with knowing if the hysteric will accept to turn her hysterical misery into ordinary unhappiness. It's obviously a rather masochistic proposition. That's the real question! Is it not after all such a good thing to go and exchange for what, is in fact, a more vulgar, a more hysterical misery for commonplace unhappiness?

So, I will finish in this way with what I began. There is an attachment of the subject to what he thinks is his character, his trait of being exceptional, that is to say this fact that he ex-sists. To be in a position of ex-sistence, it is enough to be in a place which does not exhaust phallic significance, it is enough that each subject lives as if he were totally exceptional, totally unique. All our communities, no matter who they are, are composed of so many creatures who are unique. That's how it is!

Why? There is a sliding we can locate. Let us begin always with the feminine position, to finally rejoin the subjective position which is much more general. For a woman, every man is phallic – it's this in their eyes, which creates a necessary injustice, a fundamental one – that will make this little sliding operate, which from then on, will lead her to imagine that he is all phallic. (There is yet another reason which permits her to imagine this, but let us go on). But, this man, this so-called, all-phallic man is not universal, and the proof is that there are only men.

We see how we can put this supposition in place: what supports being exsistant, to escape from this so-called, all-phallic, can only come from an X, which, from an imaginary viewpoint, finds itself – picking up again, the properties, the phallic virtues and which could really be totalising. It's from this side that a procedure of membership could be tried, permitting a universalisation. An X could be totalising and henceforth, of course totalitarian. We don't need to have any illusions, here the absolute wish of the subject is this: to have a master who would finally be an accomplished totalitarian. It is thought that the wish of the subject is freedom? That's a joke! I think that all our experiences could demonstrate this to you: freedom is the place where one can find oneself in solitude and from where one can express one's suffering. And all the demands which we can see are made by the subject, are such from which we can neither expect nor hope any liberating virtue. This, of course, may upset us.

Those who are sensitive to this kind of question may point out why psychoanalytic discourse brings us a kind of response here, on which the discourse of the hysteric cannot in any case conclude. Because the subject, the $, holds this character of being exceptional. But it is also what follows this childhood dream, this certainty of having somewhere a real father – not the puppet to whom we are accustomed – with the denunciation of this world as being made of appearances, only of shadows, the subject resigns himself in being maintained only by a semblant. From this, we can see why a Freudian interpretation is not the final say for a treatment of hysteria. But, also to verify why our existences proceed so willingly to wait for a real world, for an exit from the cavern.

This is what I will end with this evening.

QUESTION: This passion of the subject for totalitarianism, how do we articulate it with the death drive?

CHARLES MELMAN: It is very much linked to the death drive. And it can be demonstrated that there is in the clinic of hysteria an attempt to present death as a dominant agency, an agency which resolves the problem of totalitarianism. What I mean is that the absolute Master can find himself represented by hysteria. We could register this within the framework of a clinic of suicide, of which we would be wrong to think that the minute it appears within a hysterical context we should be at ease. Not at all! What is at stake is precisely a serious attempt to rejoin a place of a truth accomplished, which would no longer be the domain of shadows and appearances.

MARCEL CZERMAK: There is something which embarrasses me. Definitely, repression can be thought of only as a cut because, if it were not like that how do we account for the fact that an intervention, an inopportune or too opportune an intervention can lead to an acting out, even to, strictly speaking, an hallucination? What we normally call the real, should it not be put under the rubric of what you call the neo-real? Voices speak in the real, in the case of a psychosis, the voices say something of the subject, that is to say, indicate the place he finds himself. If, by different ways, we manage to make him assume this place, at the same time, the hallucination falls – this is also a fact of experience. And yet, this real which we usually say is ejected, it speaks, that is to say that it's the given of the symbolic. By the same token, I would rather say that this real about which we speak, with many difficulties, is always a neo-real. Because, if we would like to speak of the real, we cannot say anything, if it's not under the form of certain logical procedures and under the form of little letters. At the level of what we usually call observations, this neo-real is the only thing we can grasp.

There is a very specific difficulty in what concerns, in a general way, the problem of the real and the question of the hysteric which is distinctly the structure where an inopportune or too opportune an intervention could unleash phenomena close to psychosis. I remember Lacan being very embarrassed, with regard to the question of acting out. He used to say, "I make of acting out the equivalent of a psychotic phenomenon." This is a strange formulation, isn't it? An equivalent! There is here also a kind of embarrassment of formulation.

CHARLES MELMAN: Indeed. I appreciate what you are saying because it illustrates well our difficulty. Dominique Simonney intervened with regard to a formulation which said that the repressed signifiers went off into the real. I think that today I made it more precise. It can be repressed, it can be sacrificed (repression has also this sacrificial dimension), it can be renounced, it's not for all this, that one can constitute in the Autre a founding place. On the other hand, our clinic shows that the powers of interpretation exist in spite of everything and that all that is capable, in a certain number of cases, of dissipating, as if one was blowing on it.

I think we have to leave this debate open, not to arrive at a decision about it this evening. To respond to your question, I do not think we can use the term neo-real in psychosis. What we are dealing with is the real, full stop, to the extent that a pause, something of the order of a radical cut separates us with consequences which are not changeable, no matter the plastic arrangements with which we try to deliver ourselves. From the moment there is a cut, the feature is transformed. It is not the same thing at all as a pseudo-cut, a line which in some way is looking for itself as a cut, but which would only be a pleat, to stay in geometrical imagery. Of course, as you say we are in the presence, of the symbolic in the real. But the cut in psychosis is totally rebellious to what could be an elucidation, a dissipation through interpretation, because in fact it begins with an excess of interpretation.

What we are dealing with is a battery, something which in the last analysis, brings us to a materiality, to the brute materiality of the signifying chain. What the hysteric holds as a phantasy for us, hysterical or not, is that the real gives itself up to a perfect decrypting and by being fairly strong we will get to a complete decrypting. But we know what supports the real – not the neo-real but the real – which sense itself does not support, to take up again the excellent Lacanian formula, only *ab-sense*, we do not have a final, an ultimate sense. In other words, the final metaphor through which we are capable of acting as an interpreter is itself only the final defence, which uncorks the *dé-sens* (no sense) as Lacan describes it, that is to say, because of the fact that there is nothing else.

With regard to the effect of an interpretation, we understand it very well when it makes the mistake of aiming in too many ways, from the moment we disturb the phantasy, we are in the register of trauma and this could have, as you say, effects of acting out and other effects, effects of reorganising etc.

But at the point at where we are in this elaboration, I would like to keep the notion of neo-, of pseudo-real. This *Abspaltung von Vorstellungsgruppen* would be the effect no longer of a cut, but simply that of a line which is trying to become recognised as a cut. For the moment, I will give as a proof the fact that this could enter into the order in a magical way. In other words, we pull the curtain and the line and off we go! This is not the case at all with the real with which we are dealing.

The next time I will engage in a very audacious way – as usual! – with what there is *of* the body.

25 May 1982.

Note

1 Reference is made throughout this chapter to S. Freud, *Studies on Hysteria*, Vol. II (1893–1895), S.E. London: The Hogarth Press, 1955.

Chapter 5

The language of the body

Charles Melman

To speak about the body presents a challenge, because a successful pre-sentification leads to leaving the word only with silence, the mutism of the subject; because whether it has to do with miracles or with diabolical things, it's in an articulated way like a language with which this body expresses itself. That is why, when we wish to speak about the body, the successful thing would be to let this genitive take its value from a subjective genitive and to make us speak about *of* the body. The inconvenient thing that this kind of success hits up against is that to speak about *of* the body is by its nature without any dialectic because it is content to repeat habitually the organisation of the drive.[1] Also, we have no other recourse, despite this internal fault, than to try and speak about the body. This has an advantage, that is, in speaking about the body much more is said about he who takes the risk of speaking about it, because in a very legitimate way what will be heard will be the way in which he is trying to unravel it, to be composed with regard to it, to find peace for himself with it.

The way in which we speak about the body has always to do with an attempt to make it so that it will leave us alone, that we can hold on to our nirvana. You know the formula, *Oedipus at Colonus*, many times taken up by Lacan, "*mè phunaï*" – "oh, that I would not have been born"![2] Everything that we find concerning the body is organised in an inevitable way in wisdom, in oriental wisdom, beginning with Greece, which was our Orient for us. These are all kinds of exercises, and firstly cynical wisdom, so that we won't be the slave of a slave, because *sôma* in its metaphorical usage also means "slave" which testifies well to the position we try to take with regard to this "*sôma*", with regard to the body. All wisdom in this way seeks not to be the slave of a slave, even the slave of the dead, because *sôma* designates, in a less precise way "the corpse". In Greek there is a particular word to speak about the living body, *démas*, which we use very little. In any case, science has transmitted *sôma*. We find it in *The Gorgias*:[3] to *sôma estin émin sèma. Sôma-sèma, sèma* which is the sign, but which designates also metaphorically "the coffin", the body insofar as it is our tomb. That is why we have to make sure that our work on the body in general are only topics that the subject can give on the pain of existing.

DOI: 10.4324/9781003167839-5

All these comments have to do with the way in which we try to get by –
how we unpack things, – for example, to stay immobile or like the cynics
privilege masturbation – to make sure that it does not weigh too much. Does
Freud treat it differently? You are certainly aware of the text where Freud
talks explicitly about the body in a very interesting and illustrative way, in the
Project and in a letter, manuscript G.[4] where there is a marvellous foundational schema, because he puts into place the Freudian topology, a simple
one, happy to divide space into four:

The Central Nervous System	Object Reality
Body	Object: Put in a favourable position for sexual satisfaction

Figure 5.1 Draft G

This is a flat space R^2 in four sections, this cross with which Freud divides
space – like the four discourses! The left space is constituted by the head at
the top and the body at the bottom: the head is the central nervous system,
the body below is separated by the horizontal trait; and then the right space
with, on top, the object taken in reality, and underneath, this object put in a
favourable position for sexual satisfaction.

This is a schema which deserves our attention and those among you who
would like to do nice, good work, even a beautiful article if that amuses you, you
can see how the second topology is already included in this schema, that is to say
how the bipartition into the id, the ego, the superego, is already present there.

We can also begin with this schema to register the progress which Lacan
made in giving us the Borromean knot.[5] It's something which is able to eluci-
date itself with the substitution at the central crossing. Firstly, the passage from
R^2, a space with two dimensions, to R^3, three dimensions, which implies the
cut operated by the subject in this flat plan R^2, a cut which can be presentified
by the hole which is there at the centre, at the place of crossing. And, then,
instead of these two rights which are supposed to be infinite, that is to say the
circles which close in on themselves to infinity, there is in the knot a third,
which will "Borromeanise" them.

So, we can try to see retrospectively what Lacanian topology introduces
with regard to fundamental Freudian topology, which is there very simply in
this schema. Fundamental, why? Because it illustrates this: there is for Freud

a frontier between the psyche and the soma; there is a bar, there is a limit; there is a heterotopy between the psyche and the soma.

For those of you who pay attention to this problem, I will point out that this kind of limit, cut, frontier between the psyche and the soma is sufficient for us to understand that with regard to this Freud was not within the Hebrew tradition. In the Old Testament,[6] this division, this frontier between soul and body does not exist, there is no hierarchy between them and the Hebrew uses the same terms to designate the soul as well as the body. I will use a metaphor; instead of saying "a village of a hundred souls" it is said "a village of a hundred flesh" and this will be understood in the same way. There is, therefore, no distinction in Hebrew in the usage of terms such as: flesh, which is *basar*, and *ruah*, the spirit, which are used one for the other. This kind of heterotopy is not in any way of the order of necessity, it can distribute itself differently. In this kind of speculation, it is difficult to say that Freud follows a Hebrew tradition, but more a Greek, Platonic one, and in a certain way, already stamped because it is Aristotelian, then a Christian one.

I will remind you that at the time of this schema which divides space like this into four parts, Freud situates the function of space occupied by the psyche, which is to lower the tensions as we know only too well. To lower the excitations which come from where? Some come from outside, and these tensions from the outside, the psyche reacts very simply by ordering flight. Freud gives at this time the experience of the frog, which if you put a drop of acid on his legs, has a reflex to take off. In other words, for the excitations which come from the exterior, flight is the only course available. For those who come from the frame of the body, below and left, as a solution, flight is a little bit more complicated. Freud tells us that what comes from this space, from this place, are what he curiously calls the needs: hunger, thirst, respiration (let us note that there is a lapsus in a letter to Fliess, where he confuses *Lust* and *Luft*, air and pleasure, instead of *Lu*ftpumpe he writes *Lust*pumpe –),[7] and desire, of course, sexual. Here, the problem for the frame on top and on the left occupied by the psyche, is to get rid of these excitations. There is no other way but to work to satisfy them, and this, in two ways, the two principles of pleasure and reality.

- The pleasure principle, hallucinate the object capable of bringing satisfaction, but it is a satisfaction which risks failing, which is moreover very strange, because we know after all that actual satisfactions can be produced in the dream – nocturnal emissions exists – and this is a point on which we will, one day, have a chance to question ourselves about the function of the dream.
- And, then the reality principle. Firstly, we have to postpone jouissance because the object is not always at our disposition. It can have its whims and its humours and on the other hand, one has to work so that this object can be put in a favourable position, as Freud says, and thereby assure satisfaction.

What is interesting for us in the way in which Freud speaks of the body is that he specifies it in some way as a real of which we cannot rid ourselves. There is a real from which we can take flight and then there is a real which follows us everywhere, which accompanies us, which sticks to the skin and which permanently holds the threat of a tension, of an excitation which can be resolved only by the supply of some kind of work.

You see therefore, the interest of this putting into place, at the same time a spatial, topological location and also as a means of relation, between specific places, which puts us to say the least, in a quasi-paranoiac relationship, with regard to this body. It's interesting insofar as this rejoins philosophical pre-occupations concerning the account of reality: what proves that we are really in certain cases, not dealing with fantasies of our imagination, but, in fact, with reality?

This designation by Freud is homogenous with what Descartes tells us about signs,[8] the characters which allow us to say that a sensation, a perception, is really real and does not come from our imagination. It is very interesting for us, in a Lacanian position, to locate what was difficult for Descartes in his attempt to deduce, to put into place – to analyse is something else – what for him could be the criterion of reality, the reality principle, if I may express myself like this.

Descartes here gives us a trait: you can recognise that a perception is of the order of reality when it is not consented to, in other words simply, when it falls on top of you, when you do not want it. It's then you will recognise reality and you know that you are not in the domain of reverie or of imagination. This is in *The Meditations*.[9]

From this, a definition of wellbeing, can be outlined. Wellbeing, is to be comforted in the body. And you will see that this set-up will effectively direct us towards the death drive. That is why I say that the second topology is already present in this partitioning of space into four. The death drive, Freud tells us, it's what you aspire to, but we first of all have to make a little detour that is to say, pay your debt, pay before you arrive. Of course some people assume for themselves this right but this is another problem.

With this detour deemed necessary by Freud and because we are dealing with the question of the symptom, we see how an acceptable conceptualisation of normality presents itself to us. It appears as a way of resolving the tensions from the body by a phallic sanction, that is to say, in inscribing under the primacy of genitality, jouissance capable of resolving tension coming from the body.

I will point out here to you that the medical and Freudian viewpoints are conjoined in this definition of normality. Doctors have, by tradition, a difficulty in resolving the problem of normality. You know the difficulties of those who thought a little of the problem of the norm in medicine and I would ask you to read a book which has no successor, *The Normal and the Pathological* by Canguilhem.[10] You know that biological criteria are totally unsatisfactory, that biological equilibrium may be different according to cultures and conditions of life. Leriche's definition "health is life in the silence of organs"[11] has put us already a little on the road to hysteria. What does this mean? Health is what closes up the body, and the more the body closes, the more one is in health. But there are cycles where the body talks about itself, if I may express myself like this, but Leriche does not engage in this kind of consideration. In any case, we may define normality in medical thought in a way which finds itself homogenous with the Freudian point of view.

We can, with regard to this, note that Freud himself hesitated on the mode of resolution of the tension in this way provoked by the body, between on the one hand, cocaine and on the other hand, Martha.[12] When he wrote to Martha about cocaine he thought he had really found the answer. One takes a little bit of this thing and lo and behold! One is light, one is no longer hungry. He did not follow up on this but we can well understand that for this courageous boy, all alone, forlorn in Paris, this could also arrange things from the side of sexual desire. In the correspondence, there are places where you could ask, to whom is he writing, Martha or the cocaine, to whom does he give all his affection, all his tenderness? The difference between cocaine and Martha is that cocaine is obtained through donation; with cocaine, one is in the problematic of exchange, which is of a totally different order than the problematic of a relationship with a woman. The choice for Martha implies a certain number of procedures, of sacrifices. This happens for example, by the homage to be rendered to the father, which is not the case at all with cocaine. And that puts us on the way of the death drive, of course, whereas with cocaine, we may have the illusion that we escape. In any case, Freud chose, he came to terms with it.

What is important for us is the frontier which Freud established in this schema between the psyche and the body, and the definition of the body as a place which is characterised by its frontier. This frontier is not impassable he tells us, because representations, *unverträglich*, incompatible in the psyche, are *unterdrückt*, repressed, pass below to the inferior frame and are converted into somatic manifestations.

There is here the famous mystery of somatic conversion and up to this point, it remains like this. If it were not for what it's about in repression, which is a change of place of significant sequences. What interests us a little bit more, is that these significant sequences will give – with this change of place – the status which exploits the significance of a new enigmatic, pri-mordial repressed, this X about which I spoke the last time.

The establishing of this new, primordial repressed will therefore substitute for the phallic demand, a kind of primordial repression of the general system which is regulated by the unjust economy of the gift for nothing, of the sacrifice for nothing, with a return to an unequal distribution – that is the phallic economy, because it's not the same for everybody, it's an economy that could seem very wobbly. This will substitute for a phallic demand, an econ-omy regulated by an oblativity whose reciprocity would be perfectly guaran-teed and universal.

In this neo-economy, in this pseudo-economy, it's in some way the image of the breast – because we are in the register of the imaginary with this, which in some way is substituted for the phallus. This, according to what I'm advancing, will account for the oral fixation of the hysteric and for a certain addictive appetite, an undoubted appetite, which in the most banal of cases, is at the least medically treatable. It is clear that we live with this, this is part of our normality, and the pharmaceutical industry functions with this.

This is how I take up again what I introduced last time, with this concept of the neo-real, and I will account for a clinical picture by which the hysteric seems to be possessed by a body which manifests itself from inside her own body. In this way, we can account for, I think, this great manifestation which is in the imaginary: possession. And it is, moreover, in these terms that the hysteric speaks about it.

So, to the point, what is proposed to us is an apprehension of the body in the three registers which are familiar to us.

We are totally at ease in the register of the Imaginary because we follow Lacan's designation of the prevalence of the mirror stage.[13] The imaginary of the body, the egoic image is held up by – φ, it takes its value in the category of phallicism and that goes for both sexes. Because of that, we can conceive, in what way, by what failure of the economy, a breaking of the image can occur. Lacan, by the way, spoke about it in the following way: the image breaks because of a defect – which could be purely episodic, momentary – of this object which supports it. And, this introduces us to a geography of organic and hysterical symptoms which owe nothing to anatomy or physiology. I ask you to re-read Freud on the difference between organic symptoms and hysterical ones,[14] where he tells us that hysterical symptoms are distributed according to a purely imaginary geography and this distinguishes them from organic symptoms.

A question which I've spoken about before may be asked. In what way is this image not an illusion, a shadow of man, sloppily cobbled together, a simple appearance, a simple masquerade?

Why has it not got to do with a coat coiffed with a hat adorning a coat-stand?

In this register, where we are nothing allows us to make a distinction, and the philosophical difficulty has to do with the fact that this image lends itself to an erotic investment which could overrule bodily investment. As we know, there is an industry of images which function there. It is therefore neither the nature nor the quality of the libidual investment which allows us to settle this. And, indeed one has the wish to say that perhaps it's the contrary: the more it is invested the more illusory! It belongs to the register of fantasy, of the imaginary. What makes it valuable is that this image proposes itself in an economy of donation, which does not allow access to the body, because this economy implies other manifestations. It has to be said, this image has no authentification. Either we stay in what I called earlier, the image to which we don't consent, the image which embarrasses, or it's an image which cannot authenticate itself as real except at the price of symbolic recognition – this is not without interest because this does not work in the same way for both sexes.

If we leave this imaginary apprehension, we are able to envisage what it is about the apprehension of the body, as symbolic. If we take up again what Freud said – that the body is this place where demand, "needs" and desire are organised, we hardly make a giant leap in identifying this body as the place of the Autre. And to the extent that this place of the Autre finds itself organised by phantasy, it's also the place, where it is exercised without our knowing it, this knowledge about jouissance which animates us.

At the same time, the idea that actually there would be in this place a wisdom which would bring us beyond what we could say about it or know about it, an unconscious wisdom, a knowledge about jouissance which bears witness to the presence of the Clock Maker who will regulate all the clocks and of which we have to take notice, to guide us on the way of jouissance and the ways of rediscovering a little bit of peace. Perhaps this is worth under-lining, because in our sector, there is a conception of analysis which organises itself around this axis. It has to do with gathering up this unconscious knowledge about jouissance, insofar as the end of an analysis would give it it's free expression. This ends up in satisfying us what it is about (our) practice, because the practice has never been defined otherwise since the Greeks, but only as a knowledge which does not know itself: you do not know how you do it but you get on with it!

But the Greeks were complicated people because, besides the technique, what was important for them was the theory. It is important to know how the architect was the master of the mason. It was their way of metabolising these kind of problems. And it is interesting to see the same thing arising in our own milieu. Why is this not just a simple anecdote? Because it testifies that we are capable of speaking the same things the minute we enter the register of what provokes and causes speculation.

The term "phantasy", *phantasma*, is found in Thomas Aquinas.[15] It will be necessary, if the occasion allows it, to see how sensitive Lacan was as to how the Freudian speculation inevitably came along after philosophical specula-tion and how it introduced a radical subversion because it was not a spec-ulation, but a practice. Lacan took care to point out how the Freudian adventure took a place which he believed was conclusive of years of inevitable speculations.

The only regret that we can have is to see archaic points of view resurging in our own domain, such as those who value this intuitive and spontaneous practice as if it were like a conquest, a progress of analysis. We have also to point out how analysis subverts what is imagined under the rubric of theory. Those who went to Grenoble were able to hear a really interesting exposé on the way in which analysis definitely upset this bad habit into which one interminably takes this pseudo-couple of practice and theory. It is regrettable that we are still embarrassed by this kind of question, to pass one's existence endlessly turning around the same issues while the Lacanian advances permit us to go a little further.

Anyhow …

After envisaging the body in the register of the imaginary and the symbolic, how do we conceive of the body in the register of the real? It seems to me that we can conceive it, as what from the body, will mark its specificity, constituting its resistance, its compactness. An animal feels the obstacle but it is only the human being who can savour an object which is its consistency as such, its own resistance, which finds itself managed for us by the phallic order, because this consistence finds itself civilised by sides permitting access to phallic jouissance. Therefore, it seems to me, that with regard to the body envisaged in the category of the real, we can emphasise its compactness, its resistance, the privilege the speak-being has in feeling this special satisfaction. We can also emphasise what makes the density of an object and not to take this consistency as a given, as being self-evident, necessary, but feel that this consistency is held without doubt at this limit, this closure which is instituted by the phallic signifier. Is this not also why Lacan could say that phallic jouissance is outside the body while in the Autre as such, there is nothing which could make a limit – there is not at least one X which exists and would make a limit –and we therefore conceive how the jouissance of the Autre, in opposition to the phallic, can be said to be outside language?[16]

To give this a clinical connotation, perhaps we can attribute to this kind of disposition, this kind of malaise, I would say quasi-natural, of the woman in relation to her body insofar as, by structure, it is not all phallic. From where, of course, these kind of minor symptoms, of this fear of a possible discharge which would never stop. This is what brings us to this first economy I emphasised earlier: the persistence of a corporal tension which phallic jouissance could never totally appease, because with regard to this jouissance, the woman is not all.

We see here what Lacan says to us – I come back to the problem of normality – that there is only the male norm, the normal can only be the *norm mâle*.[17] But, its one defect is that it can never be universal, this is the small little snag which gives us so much trouble. Because of this, we can obviously see how from this feminine position, with regard to the body, a feeling of an insistent and abusive, intrusive, even an abnormal presence can occur, it really has to be said and which, by the same token finds itself being called a master signifier. A true one! Not the semblants with which we have to deal all the time. A real man! Not the semblants of a man! Such a set-up equally illustrates for us, under which place, under which rubric, therapeutic function will be registered.

From this, I will conclude with one word on this position where the woman finds herself thereby exposed to being rejected into abnormality with regard to the male norm. Because the question imposes itself on us: this hysterical symptom – I've already mentioned this phantasy which I situated between the hysteric and her male partner – this phantasy, is it that of the woman, or is it from her partner that she receives it, in an inverse way, the message which she wants to identify, for her to be a real man? In other words, in her symptomatology, who feels this abnormality? Is it she? Is it not from her partner that she receives this inverse message which wants her to thereby support this demand for her, to be a real man – that is to say in the structure, he who is not castrated.

It's on this kind of question that I will end tonight. Have you any questions?

QUESTION: This "new real" this "new primordial repressed", I have to say, is it really a primordial repressed?

CHARLES MELMAN: I will give you two answers: the first, is that indeed I put the emphasis on this *neo*, because it seems to me that a large part of the clinic of hysteria registers itself under this rubric and in particular, what is called, an awful term, the polymorphism of hysterical symptomatology. It will be said, it's a picture that looks like paranoia but it is not one, it is like a phobia but it's not one, it looks like a psychosis and so on. That is why, I try to keep the symbolic matrix which is capable of taking account of a very general disposition, which otherwise would drive you to dream of an "imitation" which belongs to our own phantasy. A paranoiac symptomatology is not invented and there is no need for a model for that. A phobic symptomatology is not invented. Therefore, really, I've emphasised this to prepare for what will eventually register itself under this rubric.

Now, why this *neo*? Well, I try to show that from the moment that there are certain significant sequences, this procedure, which to my mind is the repetition of this primordial repression, founder of a certain order, of the order of the normal, some signifiers will undergo a destiny which will be the same as this primordial repression, that is to say, will order the possibility of significant articulations. What from then on can be articulated, will find a neo-significance thanks to these sequences so called primitively repressed, and we will then find ourselves in front of topics which offer themselves up for decryption. Why is it that usually we have nothing to decipher? We walk around outside and what we perceive is exactly that, the trees, the little birds, the clouds – because the norme mâle (normal) prevails. We understand the significance of all that, all this speaks of the same thing: We are in a comfortable, well-ordered universe. You begin to ask yourself about a possible decrypting and from then on you find yourself in a world of signs, and you will ask yourself, signs of what? It does not speak the same tongue (to take up again this very precise term which I mentioned before). I'm trying therefore to take account of the way in which this repression will put into place a neo-significance, that of topics, of hysterical symptoms which Freud deciphered, and to his surprise noticed that having deciphered them, it resolved itself. In other words, we fall back into the norme mâle and that this is why I say *neo* – because I do not believe that there is in this a little devil in the body of the hysteric. I do not think that there is another body in her which agitates her without her knowledge, and about which she can do nothing. That is why I insist on this *neo*.

QUESTION: Can you talk about this "new signifier" which Lacan speaks about?

CHARLES MELMAN: I would like to very much, but I don't believe I'm there. In any case, it's the establishing of the problems to which the signifier with which we are dealing condemns us. In this sense, the "new signifier" is not of the order of the *neo*. The question is: is the norme mâle the last norm to which the speak-being is condemned, with all the consequences about which I can only remind you? It is possible that the speak-being has a relationship to the signifier which has to deal with this kind of constraint. The gods have helped me in speaking to you about the body in this kind of heat, in circumstances which make the body sensitive: You know you have a body. To keep well means that you go around without feeling you have a body. It's enough to have a dental cavity or a bunion on your foot to know that suddenly things change.

QUESTION: This is no longer of the order of the real?

CHARLES MELMAN: Of course, it's of the order of the real, the body reminds you of its real dimension. So what we call wellbeing, good health, it's precisely where this relationship to the real is plugged.

The next time, in a week, as I've spoken quite a lot here today, I would like that this would be more of a seminar than a conference. That is to say that you would be so kind as to prepare questions, things which embarrass you, things which are not working for you, so that we could discuss these points which are problematic for you, in what I'm saying. I'm advancing in a prudent as well as an audacious way and I need, I wish you would do this kind of work. For my part, I will prepare some remarks on what I very quickly mentioned today with regard to the Old Testament and with regard to what Thomas Aquinas had to say and also what follows with Descartes and Spinoza. I will do this at the beginning of the new term, but I would prefer if the next time if I could benefit from your comments and your questions, whether they are elaborate or naïve, it doesn't matter. So that I won't have the feeling that this is only a private elaboration which is being followed with regard to these questions. It has to do with a problem of structure and this has to be verified: as a means of verification I'm suggesting this. Therefore, it's up to you to work a little bit for the next week!

8 June 1982

Notes

1   S. Freud, "Instincts and their Vicissitudes" in *On the History of the Psycho-Analytic Movement, Papers on Metapsychology and Other Works*, Vol. XIV, S.E. (1914–1916). London: The Hogarth Press, 1957.
2   Sophocles, *The Three Theban Plays: Oedipus Rex, Oedipus at Colonus, Antigone* (trans. R. Fagles). New York: Penguin Classics, 1984.
3   Plato, *Gorgias* (trans. R. Waterfield). Oxford: Oxford University Press, 2008.
4   S. Freud, "Draft – G. Melancholia" in *Pre-Psycho-Analytic Publications and Unpublished Drafts*, Vol. I, S.E. (1886–1899). London: The Hogarth Press, 1966.
5   J. Lacan, *The Seminar of Jacques Lacan, Book XXII: R.S.I., 1974–1975* (trans. C. Gallagher, unedited).
6   *The Holy Bible*, Catholic Edition. New York: Harper Collins Publishers, 1989.
7   *The Complete Letters of Sigmund Freud to Wilhelm Fliess* (ed. and trans. J.M. Masson). Cambridge, MA and London: Harvard University Press, 1985.
8   Descartes, *Discourse On Method* (trans. D.A. Cress). Indianapolis/Cambridge: Hackett Classics, 1998.
9   Descartes, *Meditations on First Philosophy with Selections from the Objections and Replies* (trans. M. Moriarty). Oxford: Oxford University Press, 2008.
10 G. Canguilhem, *On the Normal and the Pathological* (trans. C.R. Fawcett). New York: Zone Books, 1991.
11 R. Leriche, *The Philosophy of Surgery*. Bibliothèque de Philosophie Scientifique. Paris: Flammarion 1951.
12 *Selected Letters of Sigmund Freud to Martha Bernays* (comp. A. Patel and A. Mehta). North Charleston, SC: CreateSpace Inc.
13 J. Lacan, "The Mirror Stage as Formative of the *I* Function as Revealed in Psychoanalytic Experience" in *Écrits* (personal translation).
14 S. Freud, "Points for a Comparative Study of Organic and Hysterical Motor Paralysis" in *Pre-Psycho-Analytic Publications and Unpublished Drafts*, Vol. I, S.E. (1886–1899). London: The Hogarth Press, 1966.
15 T. Aquinas, *Summa Theologica* (trans. A.J. Freddoso). South Bend, IN: St. Augustine's Press, 2010.
16 J. Lacan, *The Seminar of Jacques Lacan, Book XXI, Part 1: Les non-dupes errent, 1973–1974* (personal translation).
17 J. Lacan, *The Knowledge of the Psychoanalyst, 1971–1972* (trans. C. Gallagher, unedited).

Chapter 6

The ex-sistence of the hysteric

Charles Melman

I hope to conclude the ideas suggested to you during these first weeks.

Lacan taught within the context of the current philosophy represented in France by Jean-Paul Sartre[1] and which postulated and still does, the primacy of existence over essence. This philosophy asserts that giving a subject his freedom will allow him to decide what he will be, or what he could be in his essence. It's therefore a reversal of traditional philosophical positions we owe to existentialism.

The Lacanian elaboration affirms that it finds its support in a practice which exposes it to a daily challenge and verification. And it puts forward the view that ex-sistence does not in any way prevail over essence, because this ex-sistence is not supported and only proceeds by the loss of that essence. For psychoanalysis, there is only ex-sistence of the subject because essence fails. And, if the essence of a subject comes to be revealed by some chance or eventually by a difficult intervention, perhaps too direct from the analyst, the revelation of that essence – that is to say the signifier, which is the support of such a subject, the object of his phantasy – will produce effects on ex-sistence: it will find itself abolished and we will then encounter, on such an occasion, the phenomenon of depersonalisation, a phenomenon, not usual, not exceptional.

With regard to this, let us make a remark on insult. Insult is not virulent because of an excess. After all, the qualification could be anything and if I remind someone of the line from which he has come, the colour of his skin, his religion etc., we do not see in what, no matter what the cultural context, this could be insulting in itself. An insult is only active when it claims to expose the being of the subject. It is not the signifier which could be insulting, but the claim to subsume the being with whom one is dealing, to reduce him to this signifier. This has an effect not so much of astonishment as of annihilation, to be more precise.

The revelation of being pushes to one who is addressed to nothingness. In our daily work, to specify someone in the category of being (he's a "this", or he's a "that") which we can very easily do, it's a way of getting rid of him. And this is one of the questions which our diagnostics pose for us: In categorising him in his being, we close the question which he sparks off for us and

DOI: 10.4324/9781003167839-6

the question which he has about himself as to who he is. Meanwhile, we know that this question is fed by him from this lack which he feels in trying to be a man or a woman, because he cannot approach it except through the category of the semblant. From hence all that functions as a sexual parade for the speak-being as well as for the animal, all that is used in the category of the imaginary. This is a way that cannot be avoided to gain access to the sexual.

"I am who I am". You know this formula taken up by Lacan[2] from an exact translation of the Bible. Of course, it is only God who could sustain this ultimate enunciation, which would claim to come from a signifier that would signify itself. That is, the category of being. Therefore, it is only God who could advance such a formulation, that is to say, let us not hesitate to underline it, to support such an ignominy – an ignominy which the obsessional neurotic knows well because this truth sticks in his throat, and he has no other recourse after that, no other recourse except to try and avoid contamination, contacts, and wash his hands.

The other translation of this formula "I am he who is" is totally different because it has to do with an enunciation and not with a statement. An enunciation which is exerted at the place of the subject, a subject who bears witness at a glance at this curious affair, even to a question on what this subject is trying to fabricate. "I am he who is", ex-sists, such a one is a mortal. But "I am who is" does not exist in any way, cannot be supported by any ex-sistence. And that is why we can assuredly remember that the real father, after all, is the dead father.

All this interests us because what we notice in the symptomatology of the hysteric is that she shows herself to defy all entification, to defy all "être-fication" (This is a play on *être* and *ent* in French). She denounces the insufficiency of every diagnosis because what she feels from the signifier, as it is it's effect of cutting, she exists from the fact of this signifier. That is what she complains about. And, in this kind of defiance at all êtrefication, she calls on a signifier which would be a true master, and which will come to install itself in her being.

We say that the subject is divided. He is divided because S_1, to call it in the real, meets not only the object which would evidently be the solution of our ills, but another signifier and we know that the repetition of this encounter will henceforth celebrate the loss which proves to be active between these two signifiers. It's from this interval, from this cut, that the subject sustains himself. That is why, following Lacan, we are led to repeat that a signifier is what represents a subject for another signifier.[3]

A big question, why doesn't the hysteric satisfy herself with this function of representation? Why does she show herself to be so hostile? Why does she so willingly denounce the semblant, the masquerade? Why is she not satisfied with the identification which is proposed for her? Why does she protest so much against this kind of small instrument? Why does she put all the weight of her words on this place which is that of ex-sistence?

It seems as if we could see here again how the conjunction between a feminine position and the hysterical position is found to be favourable. Precisely, a woman sees herself symbolically refusing to found her word, to be an expression of, to authorise herself from S_1. We can recognise how the totally symbolic prohibition operates, that the woman can thereby express, give value to her speech, beginning with the master signifier – it doesn't matter what she will do with it, but it is like that. She will find herself from then on being driven to assert her word beginning with S_2, to authorise her word from S_2. Let us immediately remark, it is no less of the order of knowledge and this will permit us to outline later what relation the woman has to knowledge.

But more decisively why isn't a woman satisfied, because of the failure of S_1, to base her proposal on S_2? Because the first one finds itself refused, why not then the second? What seems essential, is that for him or her who authorise themselves from S_2, this authorisation will not be registered by any symbolic sanction. That is the problem. This authorisation will only have value if it is incessantly recognised and validated by the partner – to be more precise and not to give in to ambiguity, he who authorises from S_1. In other words, and barely more metaphorically, it seems that a woman will take her phallic value only on the condition of being recognised by a male counterpart. With this exorbitant power which is reserved for her, we see the importance which will unfold for her of the symbolic pact which will link her to this other, male, in the register of marriage, but more than that, in maternity – and this is beyond the capriciousness of this partner, of his free arbitrariness, and of his power.

What is called seduction by the hysteric, which she dispenses as if it were to do with the accomplishment of a duty, is a work. It is called seduction by the hysteric with a little nuanced pejorative, and indeed one wonders why. This seduction is nothing other than a call to recognition, a call willingly disappointed in being registered in the register of a sexual advance when, fundamentally it has to do with love.

What complicates the situation, is that one makes a mistake also in believing that one has to respond by some favourable gesture, a benevolent one. Because it has to do with love, it's a love which implies that it will not satisfy, again being careful to preserve the Autre. The hysterical position is constructed on the fact that the masquerade which she upholds cannot be worthy of a true love and from then on this demand, this call can only stay frustrated and protected as such.

Failing to sustain oneself from S_2 because of these kind of impasses, the other possibility which is offered to her is, in spite of the symbolic defection about which I've spoken earlier, is to express herself from S_1, to be a man. You know the Lacanian formula: "the hysteric is the woman who makes the man".[4] There again, we would be wrong to see there an egoistic conclusion. It's the worry to protect the Autre, a devotion, a care for the Autre. That is to say to make the man, to hold the place for the one for whom castration bears witness, after all, that he is not so much up to it, that he is never only a semblant of a man, only a semblant of a father.

Because of the fact that the woman is not all phallic, this gives her a greater freedom with regard to castration, which she notes towards her partner in the register of cowardice. She feels with regard to this much freer, much less engaged. She can say everything about it, as Lacan will say, and this refers us immediately towards a very explicit clinic of her relationship with the father. This theme was taken up in a very interesting way during the study days in Grenoble. There is here again a kind of double impossibility. Either the father is interpreted as impotent and why would he not be interpreted in this way, after all, he will prove to be incapable of validating the filiation of his daughter, because for this he is obliged to pass her to another in what is called the laws of family. Or else that father is interpreted in the register of phallicism, and this has the effect only of exacerbating the competition and the rivalry with him.

This reintroduces us to the generally contradictory character of what is demanded of the male partner from a hysterical position, or rather from what is regularly denounced in him. Either he makes castration a part of his condition and it is under the rubric of insufficiency that this is registered, or else, he shows himself to be active, and this will reignite the competition and rivalry with him.

To conclude this seminar, what we call the polymorphism of hysteria, its contradictory and incomprehensible character orders itself in a very precise way in two ways – either the frustration attached to the hysterical position is interpreted as privation, it is heard as a reduplication of what privation is, of the infirmity of the father, hence the genesis of the caring vocations (and in *Studies on Hysteria* the caring vocations present themselves at every page); – or else this frustration is interpreted as a link with an injustice in the distribution of goods, and from then on, there is an organisation of subjectivity around a grievance, around an inaugural foundational damage: maintaining an economy which illustrates itself by a demand which never ends, because it only supports the position of the subject on the condition that it is never satisfied.

To authorise oneself from knowledge, from S_2, is what would sustain the feminine position. Hence, the particularity of the relationship of the feminine position with knowledge, because we encounter – in a way that is not exceptional – the co-existence between, on the one hand, a feeling of ignorance, and on the other hand, a spontaneous and intuitive certainty in the solidity and the truth of knowledge, proper to this position. Why so much difficulty with the S_1 and the S_2 and why is this privilege accorded to this word, which works itself from the subject, from the barred subject the $? I will try to assert that, being an expression of S_2 that is to say, what is proposed as S_1 and therefore categorised as knowledge by the "good men", the "types" those who make the theory, introduces a kind of difficulty in the apprehension of the concept. So, that the support taken from S_2 permits one to validate a spontaneous and intuitive knowledge, about which we know all the pertinence.

I am taking up this little clinical point to verify the pertinence of our concepts, their procedural value, if they are able or not to orientate us in this apparently complex phenomena. We see them co-exist in a natural way where the contradiction is valid only for those who express themselves from reason. But this is a pretension of pure blah blah blah; none of us function with reason. We all function in contradiction and this is what we recognise when we are more or less normal, we let these contradictions exist without being in any way worried. Except of course, in a quarrel with a partner, to whom we will say he is contradicting himself. But that's what we do all the time!

On a previous occasion I said, with regard to the relationship to knowledge and to conceptualisation, how, even in the psychoanalytic milieu itself, we can see this hesitation between S_1 and S_2. On which side would it be better to stand? There is no side to be chosen, there is not in the least any bit wrong, but we have to make do with different positions. We have to try and get our bearings with regard to them, that is to say, not to privilege one or the other, but to put them in their place.

There is a word to be said on the question of transference,[5] because the hysterical word meets the goodwill of the entourage who, for the most part do not ask anything better than try to respond to this call, which is incessantly relaunched. But, the entourage is disappointed, they do not understand, they think that their responses, no matter how precise and exact they may be, are never satisfying. What is demanded is what is presented as a need, may articulate itself as a desire and as a desire which would remain unsatisfied. Everything happens as if we had to do here with a subject in search of a phantasy, a subject who is looking for the shell which will make her well established, by the fact of having been taken hold of by the phantasy, will establish her in her quality, her dignity as a subject.

Here, we can introduce the question of identification for the hysteric. What Freud has so remarkably shown in Group Psychology (*Massenpsychologie*),[6] in the chapter on identification, is that the hysterical position presents itself as being in search of a phantasy, into which she can come along and live, in which she can participate in search of the cause to which she can dedicate herself.

And, I will indeed say: this reintroduces the question of transference, this leads us to re-question the Lacanian formula of transference.[7] We can see the pertinence of upholding this by a subject supposed to know. I took the trouble of questioning it, this subject supposed to know, with regard to this impossible ex-sistence: because of the fact that the father is never other than a dead father, then we can be devoted to him, to make him ex-sist.

We have to re-examine what is produced from the hysterical position in analysis, that is to say the meeting with this personage, who has in general, this faculty of hearing topics in their power of metaphor, to not consent to this procedure in which the entourage gently struggles, to try and satisfy what it hears as being of the order of need. This personage reintroduces the virulence of metaphor in the utterance which is proposed to him and we know how active this virulence is in hysterical speech, really it is what should interest us. Not without provoking a scandal: that the question posed should not be heard in its reduction to the object demanded does not go without provoking hurts and storms. But what I'm keeping here as a thread, which has to be resumed, is the question of what founds the transference, which should be reopened.

The question of what I tried to reintroduce with this kind of link between $S_1 S_2$ and the $, is by what way does the $ find itself privileged in certain cases, and why, in certain cases, the conjunction risks making itself equal to the feminine position. We will see later the masculine position and we will discuss, if this is no less, than what could be presented as being of the order of hysteria.

I would like to finish on this. There is a fourth position, the position validated by Lacan as being that of the *objet a*.[8] What can we immediately say about it? What does this imply and what will we be able to recognise when a comment comes from this place? What does this produce?

Firstly, this place excludes the reference to a signifier. The object *a*, what founds it, no matter what the signifier is which comes along to represent this place for a subject, it's a hole. It seems to me that it's like this that we can hear Lacan's formula. "The psychoanalyst can authorise only from himself":[9] there is no signifier which would give him authority, he cannot be an expression of any signifier. That is why it is a difficult and precarious position to uphold, that is why there are collective eruptions among analysts and the constitution of places which are looking for a support in the reference to authors, founders, and so on.

The second remark is the following. All the other positions articulate themselves as so many kind of defences with regard to castration. After all, there is only hysterical discourse to represent the pathology of discourse. The other discourses, university, the master, these support themselves as palliatives, remedies with regard to castration. And yet, psychoanalytic discourse does not defend itself against castration, but affirms it on the contrary, as a master position. That is to say as a place from which everything is commanded for a subject, a speak-being, and not on the side of S_1, of which it is the representative, from S_2 of which it is an effect, not from $ is caught up with his efforts and his devotion.

It's a position which excludes all temperance. Temperance constitutes the foundation of our wisdom and of our good education, but this temperance is driven by the other discourses. This means that it doesn't matter that one never goes to term, because the term is purely and simply this hole. The temperance in which we swim, it's the commandment to have to defend ourselves against this ultimate revelation, to be decent enough, correct enough, to … I could here make use of a metaphor, to hide the nakedness of the mother. This can be entered, inscribed in this register.

This means that if we take the consequences of these little inscriptions which have the air of being nothing at all, when one writes *a* and when one plays with it, there is a kind of effect of which we would be wrong to believe that they can be tolerated. A certain number of you feel that with regard to Lacan's style. With *hubris*, the Greeks had a category which they assert, on feast days, Dionysian feast days, but otherwise, it was better not to be too excessive! It is something which is always in the register of scandal. Therefore, this little remark to make you sensitive to the fact that these little letters, if we take them seriously and if we try and assert them, have consequences with which we cannot legitimately approve. I think no one will believe that this is progress.

That is the question on which I will finish for tonight, that is to say the question which Lacan opened up for us, with the rigour which we know. He was someone who was totally devoted and obedient to what supports us; he explored the avenues which are ours to their last consequences. He was not content with spaces that were well managed. Is there something here that could be ranked among the rubric of progress? You know that Lacan said, not unfounded, that he did not believe too much in progress. We can, in this circumstance understand why! But the question remains for us: in this position inaugurated by analytic discourse – to command a word which no longer authorises itself from any signifier and which can give the feeling of being always unfounded – is it possible to assert progress, if we understand by this an exit from neurosis, that is to say the exit from the discourses by which we are normally hemmed in, restricting each and every one? This is a question which deserves to be put forward to conclude on these first seminars on hysteria.

As you undoubtedly know, the analytic position has been for a long time confused with the hysterical one. It was not long ago that I had to bring this kind of assertion up with one of our friends. Finally, the weight of these writings is to bear witness that it is not like that. An analysis does not have to finish on this kind of hysterical impossibility. You see that I come back to the question of the end of analysis, to the question of the pass. The worry of our generation – we can call it like that without affectation – what weighs on our shoulders, is to know if analytic discourse can or cannot constitute an exit and not be part of the circle which buckles in on itself: The four discourse, where one could think that the analytic discourse supports the others, they hold each other there, the four by the hand, and it turns around.

Is analytic discourse a possible exit for neurosis, a neurosis which is the model which founds, not only our subjective structure but also all our social relationships? There's the point – I've spoken a lot longer than I thought I would, to where I wanted to get to today.

15 June 1982

Notes

1 J-P. Sartre, *Being and Nothingness: An Essay in Phenomenological Ontology* (trans. S. Richmond). Abingdon: Routledge, 2018.

2 J. Lacan, *The Seminar of Jacques Lacan, Book XIII: The Object of Psychoanalysis, 1965–1966* (trans. C. Gallagher, unedited).

3 J. Lacan, "The Subversion of the Subject and the Dialectic of Desire" in *Écrits* (trans. by B. Fink). New York: W.W. Norton & Co., 2006.

4 J. Lacan, *The Seminar of Jacques Lacan, Book XVI: From an Other to the Other, 1968–1969* (trans. C. Gallagher, unedited).

5 S. Freud, *Introductory Lectures on Psychoanalysis.* Part III, Vol. XVI, S.E. (1916–1917). London: The Hogarth Press, 1963.

6 S. Freud, *Beyond the Pleasure Principle, Group Psychology and Other Works*, Vol. XVIII, S.E. (1920–1922). London: The Hogarth Press, 1955.

7 J. Lacan, *The Seminar of Jacques Lacan, Book VIII: Transference, 1960–1961* (trans. C. Gallagher, unedited).

8 J. Lacan, *The Seminar of Jacques Lacan, Book XVII: The Other Side of Psychoanalysis, 1969–1970* (trans. C. Gallagher, unedited).

9 J. Lacan, *The Proposition of the School* 1967 (trans. C. Gallagher, unedited).

Chapter 7

The body since Aristotle

Charles Melman

According to Aristotle, everyone has the duty to extend towards the accomplishment of his being, because every object has a spontaneous tendency to regain its natural place. I ask you to reflect on what you know about Greek physics. What is light rises up, to gain its natural place, the heavy falls and what's in the middle floats between the two. This has played a role in the idea of hysteria, this conception which proposed that hysteria be linked to the uterus, suffering from not finding its proper place: too light, it would climb and take the woman by the throat, from hence the necessity to irrigate, to fill it for example, with a pregnancy. That every object has a tendency towards its own place tells us enough about the confidence Aristotle has in the power of the symbolic, and I will also ask you to read "The Seminar on *La Lettre Volée*":[1] everything in its place. We could however think that for Aristotle this confidence is tempered by the assertion by which there is no science which is not general, there is no existence which is not particular. In other words, it seems that the power of the symbolic stops with the classification of species[2] and genus, even in the isolation of *species infirma*. According to Socrates, for example, science is not able to say anything about the individual – because it is too particular – for it to be scientific it would have to have general value.

On the contrary, the Lacanian enterprise of the Borromean knot tells us there is no science possible apart from the subject and that, moreover, things depend not on the way they are placed, but in the way in which they are knotted. The Borromean knot subverts the notion of place itself, because in the knot, it is not the place of the round which is important, but the way in which it clings.

Does Aristotle's conception appear to you a little bit anachronistic? I will reply to you that the realisation of being is still something intriguing, even among analysts. There is still an Aristotelian ideal circulating among us: analysts would have to come to what would be their being, their being-an-analyst for example. And the notion of an ownership of the place attached to a being or to a thing still merits the most bloody and the craziest of quarrels. This is to make us sensitive to the fact that, if Aristotle seems to us to be more than strange, his logic, his method of thought continues to activate the most spontaneous, the dearest movements, even the most elaborate ones among many of us.

DOI: 10.4324/9781003167839-7

If I qualify my studies on hysteria as being new, it's not because they attempt to contradict Aristotle – something which their feeble means does not permit us to do – by remembering that a science of the individual does indeed exist and that it even has the same aim as psychology. This is not either about teasing Freud by remarking that the second topology of 1920[3] assigns a new conceptualisation of hysteria, because this second topology is totally incompatible with how the idea of hysteria was constructed.

It is not so much about showing the artifice of a subjectivity which would propose itself as the acme of modernity. In fact, what is involved in hysteria is: to enjoy one's solitude faced with a world which is strange and for which one has only to wait for it to pass, but in a position secretly complicit with the Autre, which only death can rejoin. What is new in this work, is the implication, it has to be said, of a modern subjectivity, – that is to say, the discourse of the hysteric – insofar as this subjectivity leaves us only a little hope. In fact, it is primordially a call to the master – it is effectively the motivation of psychoanalytic discourse – and at the same time engages mysticism. It's something, I believe that is verified every day.

After this reminder of the circumstances which can justify a work, let us try and advance in taking up the question of the body. I will begin – with a brief detour: for the speak-being who makes an order? It is remarked that he who makes an order never authorises from himself. He refers himself obligatorily, no matter what, to he who in the Autre situates himself as the supreme commander. He who gives the orders offers himself forward regularly, as his delegate or his interpreter. And yet, analysis shows us that this position is, properly speaking, that of transference, that is to say this movement which supposes that there is a subject in the Autre and that it's the subject, who knows and at the same time, commands. This is what allows Lacan to say, that analysis is the questioning, of the transference – pardon! – the putting into act of the transference. In fact, it offers to this transference the putting into action of a possible ending. A failure to do this would only be the pure and simple exasperation of a movement of the soul which did not wait for analysis to prosper.

To the question "who commands", analysis replies by showing from where it is commanded: it commands at the level of this $ça$ and we are right in putting the Freudian Es there. That is to say that $ça$ commands from the place which marks pure loss, the hole, pure and simple, which organises the phantasy. It's from there that $ça$ commands for us; it's from there that the subject is commanded. And from the very willing confusion that proceeds between a and A, the subject from then on lives in a dependency on "he who organises" "he" who is led to organise for him the ways of his jouissance, that his to say, his world. It's therefore, from this place, this pure hole, that the signifier takes its authority. It's from there, that it exercises, if I may say, it's terror. It's from there that it makes a master signifier. It's from there it finds itself conferred with an authority for he who can or who wishes to be an expression of it and to authorise himself from it.

But it's here that things become more alive. As we can sense, the exercise of this authority depends on a complicity. It is not enough for he who is an expression of the master signifier to tap his fist on the table. It is even necessary that the real from which this authority emanates, that the real consents to give its guarantee to S_1. In other words, whether or not he wishes to do it, he will consent to do it. This is necessary, because the first one fails, the second hit with which you can reach the real, otherwise S_2, responds "yes".

But, what characterises S_2, is to say no, to say that it's not that. And the signifiers succeed to S_2 repeating the inaugural challenge: "the *essaim* of signifiers" as[4] Lacan puts it so nicely, to designate the results which accompanies S_2. If S_1 is successful, it is enough to be at S_2, it could stop there, we are there. Therefore, all those who follow the S_2, the swarm of signifiers, those have no need to be numbered, it is not necessary to call them S_3, S_4, S_5 etc, because they are just repeating the inaugural failure. It could even be said that they speak only of this failure. And it really is for this that the signifier represents the subject, it's from there exactly that the question finds itself posed, that the signifier only represents the subject for another signifier.

It could be pointed out, that this failure, of the swarm of signifiers which follow each other, speak about, constitute an introduction to the question of reality. We find that for Freud the "judgement of reality" which is already a formulation, asks a question and also another concept "index of reality", *das Realitätszeichen.*[5] What tells us that we are in reality and that we are not about to go off our rocker? Precisely, because we have to do with S_2, which succeed each other, and which tells each one of us that it's not that, this is to say all of them, say "no" to us.

And, when by some accident, some event happens which says "yes", some signifier for such a subject says "yes", this may provoke some disorders. For example, the birth of a child may be capable of provoking this psychotic episode, in general, briefly what is called a puerperal psychosis because something for this subject, which for her is personal, has brusquely come to lift this failure, this no.

This is something which could happen for the gambler. It's a pity we don't have recent works on the psychology of the gambler. You know that he waits until the good signifier appears, the real one, the one which will not say no to him, that is to say the signifier which will give him the big share. We have to ask ourselves; do we too numerate the rest of the signifiers?: We say that from S_2 the others only repeat the first failure, but perhaps, the unconscious counts the successive hits. As Lacan remarked with regard to a bone that he had seen at the museum of Saint Germain-en-Laye and the notches marked on it recording the number of killed animals, perhaps the unconscious, it puts numbers on all the signifiers which succeed each other. In any case, what interests the gambler – it's not the big share – when he gets it. The gambler is never someone who gets rich, it's not someone who has such trivial aims! Once, he has obtained the big share, he runs off, of course to give it back to the Autre, even if it is in the fear that he will lose it and even he puts a little bit into his pocket. And he engages himself in the position of waiting again on the emergence of what would be the good signifier, the good number.

So, we can remark that if the master, the real master, is someone who in general does not go mad – there are cases, all the same, where it happens – this can only be because precisely there are around him signifiers which can be heard saying "no" to him. If we have to make an epilogue on that, there was in the entourage of the kings, people whose precise social function it was to say "yes". There was one who was charged with saying the truth, it was exactly the work of the fool, he who was mad enough to put things back in their place.

The question of the body will allow us, on the course of the journey, to make other remarks … Firstly, the place where the *ça* commands, the place of power, is usually occupied by someone we know well and who it is important to name. I talked earlier about the signifier which authorises itself from this place, which takes its authority in being an expression of this place. But this place itself is occupied by the one who has the power to appear as *at-least-one*, this place is occupied, structurally by *The* Woman: she is, if one can say it, the natural representative. You know that Lacan first of all spoke about – *at-least-one* – there is at least one who escapes castration – and then afterwards in a very explicit way, he pinned it more by saying that this *at-least-one* (in the masculine mode) to escape from castration, becomes *at least one* (in the feminine mode).[6]

This is to point out that there are structural reasons for believing that the Autre is not barred. Often, this belief is attributed to the neurotic who wants to defend against castration, but there are reasons which make us think that by insisting …. because, if one is there in an unlimited domain, in an open ensemble, if we know how to give value to the demand as we should gently, politely, with authority, as you wish, what would stop us thinking that this will not end by its arrival? We have to point out also that it's the position of the woman which should make it a little clearer for us what fetishism is.[7] It is often said that fetishism allows us to think that the woman would have it. Let us re-situate things simply by saying that after all, a certain part of fetishism intervenes in the most common eroticism, the most ordinary, the most daily!

The second point on which we can remark with regard to implementation, it's the kind of knotting operated by the Name-of-the-Father[8] between this real from where the woman takes her power, where she holds herself, and the symbolic, that is to say the effect produced by the paternal signifier on the knot between the symbolic and the real. What comes back to the phallus, is to make a limit, we will have occasion to return to this. But, if the phallus closes up the series – otherwise in a constant expansion like the universe, if you wish – if it makes a limit and a prohibited one, an inaccessible limit towards which the series may tend, then the Name-of-the-Father, the paternal signifier, will confer on he who is an expression of the signifier, a new authority to enjoy and aims for that achievement to go to the end of the chain. How? Because of the intervention of the paternal signifier, the knot between the symbolic and the real is changed. The symbolic does not take its authority any more from the real but from a signifier which in some way enjoins, gives as an imperative to have to use this real in conformance with jouissance – it's that of the superego: *enjoy!* It renders this real right for jouissance and invites the subject to an achievement which would consist in going all the way.

By the same token, this paternal signifier modifies the feminine response. If, in the preceding case, she isolates herself by saying no, to remember that it was not that, to mark from her own leadership a refusal, on the other hand, in this new situation, she is invited to the masquerade, invited to respond "yes". We know that this is one of the demands of the institutions of marriage: everyone has her own, it's hers, she had been arranged for him. That is to say, that in this new case, she has to respond "yes", that in some way it is really her, but because of the fact of structure she continues to know perfectly she is not loved for herself and that she finds herself being brought back to reflecting an ideal woman, which always as you know, arouses her jealousy and for whom she will look, to catch a glimpse at least in her husband's look. This is, for example, Dora's history, without going into the "passionate" register.

Can we say that this paternal signifier assigns to the woman in order to ensure this masquerade, which would consist for her in presenting herself as the unique one, as the true one? The question is worthy of being asked. Because if it's true that the woman finds herself assigned to that role, we are led to say that hysteria is really a fact of structure and it verifies itself as being simply the effect of discourse. In other words, the hysteric in trying to be an expression of *The Woman* (with all the work which this could represent, the effort, the attention etc.) would not only accomplish from her side the achievements the father would demand of her. She would have to, at the end of this difficult situation in assuming this masquerade, respond to the achievement that this father, the paternal signifier will expect of her.

There is a little inconvenience always produced here. If the validation of this achievement, of this effort, for the woman cannot in some way be verified, except by being once again the source from where the signifier takes its authority, what guarantee does the woman have here for her success? If she does not find herself in the position of investing in the place from where the signifier would take its authority, she finds herself in this banal position of the woman who because of her, the husband takes power, who because of her, her man has signifiers which can be an expression of his authority. But, if on the other hand the woman succeeds, by the same token she finds herself subverting the power of the father who has put this effort into effect, this father who henceforth becomes the master for whom she governs. You see how this formulation illustrates itself perfectly. But, to protect this master, she is pledged to a rocking game of a phallic emergence in eclipse; to show that she can accomplish this duty, and half the way travelled, abdicate, renounce, even mutilate herself to preserve her partner. The success appears for a minute only and has to just as quickly disappear at the price of a kind of voluntary amputation.

Failing this eclipse, what is produced in the signifying chain, which I mentioned earlier, is this fault where the woman stands, this fault from where a chain of signifiers originate, endowed with all powers with regard to which the child will have some difficulty in finding the smallest place, the smallest hole where he will be able to find his lodgings. We know that this is a clinical problem, this difficulty faced with a chain in some way a generator of all hiatus, of all impossibility, a difficulty for the child to be able to arrive there to "cram" the smallest bit of room for himself. What could he abandon, give of himself, sacrifice, if only as a guarantee, to a chain which is not only an expression of himself, but which in some way proves to be completely opaque to all that could be an attempt at a gift on his part? We could bring forward a curious symptomatology, which I don't believe has been listed in the work of analysts: subjects who cannot escape their home, their domicile, in fear that they will not find on their route the little place where they can pee, where the fault of perception in space proves very difficult for them, even plunges them into anxiety. This is a symptomatology which has nothing exceptional to it.

So, all this way to put in place what the body is for us. We will take up next week the question of the hysterical symptom: why is the hysterical symptom first of all a bodily symptom? To deal with the body, we have to mention the three registers which are familiar to us: imaginary, symbolic and real, and a certain number of traits will isolate themselves for us, thanks to that distinction.

The imaginary body is evidently the one which appears to us the easiest to represent, which we apprehend the most easily, because Lacan has given us this introduction with the imago, the mirror phase and the discovery by the child of what makes the body for him.[9] That is to say, the gathering up of parts about which we know very little, little pieces, at the level at which they hold together and which make a body, thanks to this capture in the mirror. There is therefore the emergence of a totality which takes on narcissistic value by arriving at the place of *desêtre*: the child does not know what he is. To the question "what am I" responds the "It's you" then in return begins the "It's me". With regard to this image of the body, I think we can retain two traits which are seldom evoked.

The first is a clinical fact which I find striking. The image we have of our own body, we cannot auto-represent it, except in its totality, and this, no matter what the anatomical real is. This deserves our attention, this mental incapacity for us to represent our body outside its totality. There is every reason to think that this incapacity has physiological effects, analogous to those which Lacan refers in his work on the mirror phase, these physiological effects which can be observed in the animal, when the image of his fellow creature is discovered. For example, the phantom limb, when a real amputation of a limb gives way before the persistence of its mental representation, with its movements outlined as if the member were always active, always present: incapacity to think, to register this amputation. And, also another interesting neurological fact, observed in certain hemiplegias: the ill person who can at other times stay perfectly lucid, is totally incapable of knowing, of recognising that half of the body is impotent or paralysed: when asked where is his right, he raises an arm and if he is asked where is his left, he raises the same arm, but he is bound to an image of himself which remains intact. It seems as if this could not be done in another way and this illustrates for us the formative and irreducible power of this imago. If this appears for some among you as being risky, I will tell you that I had the opportunity to debate this with a brilliant neurologist, Professor Lhermitte, one of whose ancestors was interested in the image of the body, and what I am bringing forward here seemed to him to be perfectly admissible.

The second trait is not pointed out any more: at the level of the image, there is after all no sexual identification. I mean with what one identifies is not the image of a man or the image of a woman but an image full stop. And, we could say that the hiding of the genital zone – which the φ would achieve, which Lacan proposes to us in the putting into place of this image – contributes in neutralising the imago of the body with regard to sex. Which means that in what concerns the imaginary, there will not be a proper bodily trait at the level of the imago which will permit us to distinguish or to specify the other sex. It is possible to consider that the investment of the imago has by itself a feminising character. I would like to say, to simplify, that the narcissistic investment manifested as such of the imago would be a permanent trait in making itself recognised at the level of femininity – because there is no specific trait, isn't that so? Let us add that it's without doubt, it's to this narcissistic investment of the image, for the man as well as for the woman, that we can attribute a part of the bisexuality which is constitutive of everybody. At the level of the narcissistic investment of the imago, every man passes necessarily through a process marked by femininity.

What is the symbolic body? It's relatively easy to grasp. The symbolic body is supported by the chain of S_2, a chain itself vectorised by jouissance. That is the symbolic body. That is to say that the body finds itself the seat of a knowledge, a natural knowledge, or even a practical knowledge, because it is a knowledge which has no need to go to school, nor be instructed to go into action. It's a willingly given knowledge in an example, as it has been said to us, why not say it, by God Himself, by the Creator. He could have given us a knowledge which we wouldn't have to deal with, which would work on its own, a practical knowledge – which is opposed to a theoretical knowledge, which would be fabricated, invented, always a little demoniac and in some way a testament to the pretentiousness of the *speak-being*. The body is therefore in this way the receptacle of the wisdom which guides us. Henceforth, it is the representation which allows us to join microcosm and macrocosm, because it is the seat of this microcosm which is in harmony with the wisdom which regulates the world.

To give you a little example of the ever-active effects of this conception, I will remind those of you who are interested in the theories of Hughlings Jackson,[10] those inspired by the evolutionary English philosopher, Spencer.[11] These theories gave in France the organic dynamism of Henry Ey,[12] who had a large place in French psychiatric thought. The theories of Hughlings Jackson make of the body the seat of a structure progressively hierarchical, which reaches its summit at the isolation of an executive – which the stoics isolated by calling it the *hègémonikon* – the hegemonic part, in some way, of the individual, from where it commands: a structure progressively hierarchical, which reaches an executive acting for the wellbeing and the equilibrium of diverse elements of the said structure. Hughlings Jackson did not see any better model for speaking about this organisation of the body than the British parliamentary system! This idea of a physical order of the universe which would unite our microcosm is constructed under this phantasy of a reconciliation between *hègémonikon,* hegemony which commands, the S_1 and those who have to obey it. The phantasy of this natural wisdom, of this wisdom of the body, is based on the idea that there exists a natural harmony linking the executive, the leader and those who carry out the orders. The messages of these would be well received by the leader who would in return give orders – hormones, nervous influx and whatever you like – the ones most appropriate for the interest of the community. In other words, this symbolic body would realise the ideal of a reconciled society. And, I have no need to tell you how such an idea is still so powerful. We can find a thousand examples bearing witness to this kind of phantasy always at work in our societies, always very active. An example, among others – natural medicines. They are called natural, they are called gentle nowadays, it's nicer. They are based on the idea that the world around us, carries with it the instruments for a possible reconciliation. All we have to do is look for them and use them.

I think that this establishing of the body which I call symbolic will be of some interest for us to find our way in the symptomatology of hysteria, and will tend to respond to this big question: why is it in her body the hysteric produces, or in some way, makes the symptom emerge?

Finally, a last word on what the real body is. After all, the real body seems to go without saying. What to say about the real body? The real body is the way we are made, each and every one. Everybody has its own particularities, its mode, its reflexes, its growth, its coldness, its sensitivity, its reactions etc. There are as many real traits as possible which diversify the body we inhabit and it is assuredly a specification which should be made concerning the real body.

But something else deserves our interrogation. It seems as if the real body never presents itself as a homogenous area, contrary to the image of the body. The real body always marks itself as a divided body, that is to say the carrier of a limit and including, if I may say so, the exclusion of a part of this body – I will not bring forward this evening here what would be the process of such exclusion. To give a major example to which you will be immediately sensitive, I will evoke the problem of laterality. Animals do not know laterality: there is not a dog, a cat, or a flea or whatever you like which can distinguish left from right. Laterality seems to well imply something in the depth of ourselves, a separation from the part that commands and then the other, which has only to submit to it, not to be noticed, to follow on nicely. This division is observed in other cases, for example, in our postural tonus. The tonus implies a certain division between the muscular mass. There are muscles which we need in order to stand up, and those for which it doesn't matter if they are left to one side. And, then there are others which should function to permit the learning of a certain number of gestures, of actions, whether that be playing the piano, playing the tambourine, playing golf, swimming, whatever you like. And learning implies this partition between the muscles, which will have to enabled to function and those which can be left aside. In laterality, everything happens as if there was, in the very core of this body, an application of the division which I tried in a subtle way earlier, to show you the ins and outs of which you did not grasp. That is to say, there is this division of place from where it commands and the signifier which may or may not inspire itself to command. It's as if the real body finds itself indeed crossed through by this kind of division, a division which permit us in a certain way to understand the problems of laterality. Those children who do not know precisely which side commands, they do not know if it should be on the side of place or on the side of the signifier, and from where this signifier possibly takes its authority. Perhaps one could set about doing an analysis of a certain number of problems of laterality from this. ... All the more so, as the evacuated, the bad part should not talk about the bad part, and I will go as far as saying the shameful part, the part which would have to be rejected, should not talk about that either.

I think that these remarks concerning the apprehension of the body in these three registers of real, symbolic and imaginary can introduce us to an interpretation of hysterical symptomatology and therefore can allow us to better distinguish its otherwise, paradoxical richness. Why the body, for the hysteric? If one of you has any response, I would be very happy to hear it. Freud called it *das Entgegenkommen*, "pre-venance" and not "somatic compliance" as it has been translated in French. I will recall for you that in *The Project*[13] this schema has four sectors where what is incompatible in the domain of thought finds itself repressed in the body. Evacuated in the body because Freud says, for the hysteric there is something of the body which comes to the front – *Entgegenkommen*. We will have to try and see what could come to the fore; for the hysteric we will have to see what of the imago could serve us to interpret hysterical symptomatology. You know that Lacan used this from the beginning, and his mirror stage served him to account for a part of hysterical symptomatology. We will also have to account for our establishing the real of the body to try and get our bearings a little.

12 October 1982

Notes

1 J. Lacan, "Seminar on 'The Purloined Letter'" in *Écrits* (trans. B. Fink). London: W.W. Norton & Co., 2006.
2 Aristotle, *Organon* (trans. O.F. Owen). Vol. II. London: G. Bohn, 1853.
3 S. Freud, *Beyond the Pleasure Principle, Group Psychology and Other Works*, Vol. XVIII, S.E. (1920–1922). London: The Hogarth Press, 1955.
4 J. Lacan, *The Seminar of Jacques Lacan, Book XX: Encore, 1972–1973* (trans. C. Gallagher, unedited).
5 S. Freud, "Project for a Scientific Psychology" in *Pre-Psycho-Analytic Publications and Unpublished Drafts*, Vol. I, S.E. (1886–1899). London: The Hogarth Press, 1966.
6 Lacan, *Book XX: Encore.*
7 S. Freud, "Fetishism" in *The Future of an Illusion, Civilization and its Discontents and Other Works*, Vol. XXI (1927–1931). S.E. London: The Hogarth Press, 1961.
8 J. Lacan, *The Seminar of Jacques Lacan, Book XXII: Joyce and the Sinthome Part 2 (1975–1976)* (trans. C. Gallagher, unedited).
9 J. Lacan, "The Mirror Stage as Formative of the Function of the *I*, as Revealed in Psychoanalytic Experience" in *Écrits* (trans. B. Fink). London: W.W. Norton & Co., 2006.
10 J. Hughlings Jackson, *Evolution and Dissolution of the Nervous System (1881–1887)*. London: Thoemmes Continuum, 1998.
11 H. Spencer, *On Social Evolution*. Chicago: University of Chicago Press, 1975.
12 H. Ey, *Manuel de Psychiatrie*. Paris: Masson, 1960.
13 Freud, "Project for a Scientific Psychology".

Chapter 8

The hysterical symptom

Charles Melman

Hysteria – I would like to remind you of it because it seems my comments can sometimes provoke some emotion – is the mode of expression of the position of the subject, of the subjective position. With regard to this, from the minute we are endowed as a subject, we are invited one and all to explore in an intimate way what it is about this position and its diverse expressions.

We know that hysteria is a way of knotting a social bond. I mean that it comes from a discourse, that it can be the occasion of a passage through a certain type of discourse. If Lacan could allow himself to say that Socrates was a hysteric, it is not only because he was able to hold himself up on the street, alone, on one foot, his head buried in his hand and plunged into his thoughts. It's because Socrates, from a hysterical position, inaugurated the interrogation of the master. In this society of masters, sure of itself, sure of its good rights, sure of its knowledge, Socrates arrives and was the first to say, "you speak there of certain things, virtue for example. Do you know what virtue is?" – "Ah – says the other, indeed I do! Moreover, I'm virtuous." – "Well, then you will explain to me what virtue is."[1] And, the other, engages himself, obviously in a series of comments which showed, that no matter what kind of master he was, even a virtuous master, he did not know what virtue was, he could not say anything which would hold. This is the inauguration of the position of the hysteric in the history of thought. Therefore, it is certain that the position of the hysteric can be an occasion for discourse. But it can also be a way of living.

Lacan used to say that the passage to the couch brought about a hysterical discourse.[2] You will of course have read the work of analysts who ask themselves the question: how does it transpire all the same that obsessionals are able to present in a parallel way a symptomatology of a hysterical type? And Lacan specified that the passage to the couch – that is to say the establishment of a discourse addressed to the Autre from a position of suffering, of demand, of questioning, – was enough to bring about, even for an obsessional, a hysterical position. This helped him to better understand a certain number of manifestations which could be produced.

In speaking about hysteria because I'm claiming to be doing it in a new way, I'm prolonging our remarks on the impact of this subjective position.

DOI: 10.4324/9781003167839-8

There are a certain number of such positions, private or public, in our lives. And the unchanged and valorised persistence of the discourse of the hysteric constitutes, without doubt, the strongest obstacle to an appreciation of what could be a psychoanalytic discourse. Hence, an appeal, and maybe a necessity to develop what is in the position of the hysteric insofar as it is a resistance to analytic discourse. We cannot wait for the goodwill of the subject for this to change because this subjective position is surely what everyone holds most dear. Here there is a form, not of impossibility but of resistance. I will take the risk, in developing this clinic of hysteria to disturb certain people to whom I am attached, so that I can get their attention. I meet resistances among my nearest and dearest. But, if my comments in some cases may hurt, in these cases, I say it without regret and without the slightest irony. I believe that they will forget very quickly and that they will be hurt only momentarily. It seems to me that there is all the same, interest and necessity to pursue this, despite meeting these resistances in such a manifest way.

The last time, we finished on the question of why hysterical symptomatology has essentially and primordially the body as a place of expression. What separates hysteria – in a dichotomic way, that's exactly how Freud presented it – from obsessional neurosis, where the place of suffering appears as the mental process itself? We are called by these kind of questions. We cannot let go of them as easily as Freud who, I will remind you, conceived neurosis as being linked to a *unverträglich*, an incompatible representation. As in logic, there are things which cannot enter the system and therefore have to be expelled. From then on, this incompatible representation, *unverträglich*, finds itself repressed, *verdängt*, suppressed, *unterdrückt*, pushed below. And it is the topological distribution of this repression, that is to say the place from where it will pass, which accounts for the topography of the symptom. I will ask you to read a letter to Fliess,[3] *The Project*[4] and in *Studies on Hysteria*.[5] And I recalled the last time, that for Freud, it is what explains the somatic symptomatology of hysteria, corporal fixation, its "somatic compliance" its *das somatische Entgegenkommen*. In this conception, Freud obviously uses an imaginary representation of the body, because he himself divides this body into top and bottom. There will be repressions which are produced on top and which will therefore stay in psychical life, and others, underneath which will manifest themselves in the body. We can see as well, how this imaginary gives in to the idea of *unterdrückt,* that is to say the idea of what is suppressed below, is injected below. In hysteria, what is *unterdrückt* will of course go towards the below, and the body, opposed to the head, offers itself as the place in some way predestined to express in a local way the suffering of this intolerable representation, henceforth maintained.

We will try to substitute for the imaginary representation of the body an interpretation which owes more to the symbolic, because it's from here that we begin. To be more precise, an interpretation which owes more to the three categories to which we are used.

Let us begin with the following question: if what is foreclosed in the symbolic reappears in the real, where does what is repressed in the symbolic reappear? We really have to ask this elementary question. We can make use of what we know about the functioning of metaphor: a signifier falls down below, passes under the bar, thereby giving way to the substitutive signifier. And Lacan tells us it is thanks to the metaphor that an injection of the signifier into the signified is possible – if there was only metonymy we could not see why a signifier would pass under the bar – that is to say a passage of the signifier into the real.[6] And, this signifier, which is not foreclosed, which is repressed, where will it reappear? It will reappear in the symbolic, under the form which we know: in the clinic of neurosis: the lapsus, the stumbling block, the witticism, even, for example, the obsessional idea. It will be a parasite on the symbolic, where the symbolic will not be able to find itself vectorised except by phallic signification, and let us take a step further, it will be a parasite on the non-sense which supports it, the non-sense which phallic signification conceals! Where the symbolic would have to only, if I may metaphorise like this, sing the glory of life, the glory of God, there is produced this little thing. This signifier below, if it is repressed (because in the normal game of the metaphor, we imagine very well that the signifiers fallen down could come back into the usage of the word without otherwise causing a problem), if this is a "caught" signifier, to take up a Freudian term, with regard to something else there will be signifiers caught below, there will be signifiers entering the word and they will begin to speak about this signifier in this position, in the real. There will be, simply a letter. ... It is here that the game of the unconscious illuminates itself as being constructed by the letter: a single letter of this signifier is able to resurge and provoke a stumbling block in a word, which analysis permits to isolate, to distinguish as belonging to a repressed signifier. Therefore, the word instead of being happy to sing or to celebrate the glory of life, will find itself as a parasite on this repressed signifier. It is indeed in the symbolic that this repressed signifier will resurge.

To say it like this leaves us always with a question. Why the body? We do not always see why the body should be the elected place for the basis of a symptomatology.

We can still, to make things even clearer, observe what we can call the facility of experimental neurosis. It is very easy, even if one is – happily or unhappily, as you wish – not neurotic, to induce an experimental neurosis in oneself. All is needed, in any circumstance, is to make oneself consciously avoid such and such a subject out of politeness, discretion, holding back, whatever you wish. And there will be lots of chances, you know, that your word will find itself like a parasite, by what you have wished to keep below. Here is the most simple and easiest expression of an experimental neurosis and the effects produced by repression.

But, why a somatic symptomatology? What is it, an incompatible representation for the hysteric? What is this *Vorstellung*, which when it surges up in a hysterical system cannot stay there, and will find itself, automatically and unconsciously of course, rejected down to the below, *unterdrückt?*

With regard to this, during the previous months, I advanced a suggestion that what the hysteric represses, is S_1. The hysteric cannot authorise her word from the signifier S_1, which it is an expression of the phallus, to intimate to the real, to lend itself to jouissance. It's incompatible with her system. I will leave this sentence for your reflection and your critique.

We forget the following too easily: the real lends itself to jouissance, what comes from the real lends itself to jouissance for example S_2. It does not go without saying, it's not a procedure inscribed in the natural order of things and we have in the clinic, markers, precise situations, which show us what happens, when on the contrary we have to do with a real which is not put forward to offer itself to jouissance. This kind of transformation is linked to the intervention of the Name-of-the-Father, which I mentioned the last time. It has to do with a civilisation which comes from the real, or an establishment of slavery, a domestication, if you prefer. What comes from then on from the real will not present itself under a strange, disturbing, enigmatic or demanding castration. Because it is equally this kind of message which the subject receives from the real; that he has only to renounce his pretention and castrate himself.

The hysteric would find herself in the position where she could not (or instead – *he:* every time, to avoid our facility to put the hysteric in the feminine, I will take the care to specify that the masculine hysteric is not any the less interesting and I will speak about it) the hysteric cannot be an expression of this S_1, to intimate to the real to lend itself to jouissance. Why?

I will emphasise that, the inconveniences and the impossibilities are linked to the system and do not come from his choice, the reasons are structural. From the mirror stage, a sharing takes place, with one's fellow. The image of this fellow shines with a mysterious object, an object contained by this image. It is always attributed to this image of the other, to be maintained by this mysterious object which gives it its shininess – I will remind you of the very clear text of Lacan on St Augustine (the child who looks at his *amare conspectus*, the other child at the breast).[7] The meeting with the image of one's fellow implies a sharing: either him, or me. Or indeed, it's the other who has it and his image contains and takes shelter, supports itself with this treasure, or else it is me. We know that symmetry is never realisable. It is enough, for example, to check out what happens for twins. They organise themselves regularly, inevitably, in an asymmetrical mode for which we can find the matrix in this disposition of the mirror. It is one or the other, but it cannot be for both at the same time.

The first sharing with the image of the other is regulated by the structure which inevitably isolates two places, one which Lacan characterises or names as that of the agent (at the top and on the left in the four discourses)[8] and the *autre*, the small other, which is also the place of jouissance. You see I'm not straying too much by pointing out how much S_1 is called the place of jouissance! This kind of sharing between me and the small other is validated by what is used by the structure because of the separation between the place of the agent and the place of the other. It is this kind of dialectic which the philosophers found from their own speculations, for example in the dialectic of the master and the slave.[9]

Who decides this choice with regard to the place? Why will you have an inclination to occupy such or such a place? It's obviously a huge question. Some will find themselves totally at ease in the place of the ordinary *agent*, marked by S_1 by this coloration, this pretence at mastery. Others will, voluntarily or not, arrive at the place of the other, at the place which gives enjoyment, which offers enjoyment by the effect of some obscure forces. What is it that incites this choice? This choice is never free, as we may doubt – there are very few who are! – there is, all the same, a certain availability with regard to this.

I am suggesting that what leads in making the choice or in making the choice oscillate to one side rather than the other, it's the real of the body. It's probably here that anatomy could be destiny, by the presence or not of this piece of skin, whose possible erection would give witness of what could be the will of the Autre. As if the Autre would say "you see, you can, and therefore, if you can you should". What I'm advancing here accounts, in a contradictory way for a formulation of Lacan, which says that he who desires authorises only from himself.[10] This is a formulation to which we will have to return. It is undoubtedly correct if we refer to the structure, which on its own does not allow any indication to be heard, nor does it deliver any authorisation. It's perhaps only a subject, from the interpretation he gives, who makes himself socially admitted, which supposes a desire in the Autre. Because, we know, moreover, that the Autre is only a place, that the Autre does not exist and we cannot see therefore how it could deliver a prohibition or authorisation! But, in any case, let us note this position of Lacan saying, "He who desires authorises only from himself", although that we know that in the constitution of the phantasy for a subject, this is never the case. I mean to say, that a subject in the constitution of his phantasy, authorises himself to say what he has at his disposition, he authorises himself, for example, from a parental desire, or, simply from the social imagery of which he is an expression, according to whether he is a little boy or a little girl, totally different behaviours. In the cases of transsexualism, we could say that the subject authorises only for himself, but the case of transsexualism is not the rule. Generally, we obey this legitimacy we find in anatomy, but insofar as this becomes significant, finds itself in some way a vector for desire which we loan to the Autre, even the obligation it makes for us, because the superego, it's what says, "you must, you must go there, you cannot rest on your laurels, you cannot escape it; You can, therefore you must"!

So, how can we say that the hysteric represses this S_1, incompatible in her system? These, let us say *her* for what I invoke as the establishing of, that is to say, a destiny regulated by anatomy. Because of this sharing, could she not authorise herself from S_1? Why, after all could she not admit, as existing in the universe, and simply recognise that it's not up to her to authorise herself? Why does she have to repress this and simply not renounce it?

We can advance on this by saying that if she is not content to renounce it and furthermore represses it, it's because to be dependent on a place Autre, she inserts herself from henceforth in an order, the demands of which become very different: an order structured in such a way that it has to do with he who comes to this place not only to desire, but to please, not only to enjoy but to be loved. To occupy this place suggests to the subject an interpretation of the desire of the Autre which would be the duty of the creature – what the structure intimates to him – to please the Autre, to honour him. We link an essential question here: how to better guarantee being loved by the Autre than by castration? Because after all, it's never other than this, that a creature could offer in his interaction with the Autre to try and find security there. How better therefore to guarantee the love of the Autre except by castration this time taken to its term, that is to say to sublimation?[11]

It would be in this involuntary way, linked to structure, that the hysteric finds herself engaged, vis-à-vis her male partner, in a curious negative competition where it is a question of, he who sacrifices the most, he who is most castrated, will win. It's being caught up in these moods, in the jouissance of the body of the fellow human marked by this irreducible of a foundational failure – because it works only on the condition of not being that – to this jouissance of the body of the fellow, the hysteric substitutes a specular jouissance with the Autre, a specular exchange with the Autre. To enjoy the supposed look of the Autre on this likeable image which is offered to her – at the price therefore, of a castration taken to its term, that is to say to sublimation, to the renunciation of sexual jouissance – on the one hand, the hysteric finds herself taken in a series of models, I will allow myself to say, which find themselves more or less involuntarily close to those very instructive works which were written in the style of *The Imitation of Christ*.[12] Do not make me say what I do not say, I would never allow myself in any way to register the existence of Jesus Christ under the rubric of hysteria! But the model of a life as an example of renunciation and sacrifice operated for the glory of the Autre – very easily and very naturally proposes itself in this case.

What hysteria here proposes for us is a world Autre – we can write this with a small a or a big A – which means what? A world animated by Another phantasy than what supports sexual jouissance, covered and supported, by other values. This world Autre is regulated by other laws, other imperatives, other duties, and regulated by an Autre jouissance. This Autre world refers to a father, henceforth the dead or impotent father. You will know how much curiosity we will find again in the first observations of Freud concerning the father of patients he was dealing with: the dead father, impotent, even supposed unwell. I will of course come back to this point.

The order to which the hysteric refers herself is an order of which none of the signifiers authorise her desire. They all prescribe debt, love, even care: this is the reference to the moral order which the hysteric inaugurates. This is why Freud said (it was at the beginning as you are aware): "While hysterics are people who are highly moral their reputation is so angry". But of course! The moral order of hysteria implies that S_1 should not be present but removed. Because of this, we can conceive the destiny prescribed for S_1 will be that of repression, because it is here and isolated as such, so what other destiny could it undergo? Perhaps, obviously, censorship or denial. All that is at work, by the way, but the most ordinary process is repression. We will have to try and evaluate the consequences.

An objection, why not think about this repression of S_1 as a repetition equivalent to *das Urverdrängte?* Because the establishing of this system is founded on foundational repression, original (*urverdrängt*), and it is precisely the phallic signifier which finds itself thereby *unverdrängt*, why not, after all, do we not assist simply at a kind of repetition, at a renewal of this exercise, the establishing of at least One, from which the game of desire usually organises itself?

But, precisely, it's here you see the difference, it's not any more an *ur-verdrängt*, but a repression which comes after the fact, which comes in second position. In not being original, this hysterical repression has totally different consequences. It has foundational effects which are different if only for a reason of which I will immediately make you aware. If it operates as if it were originally repressed (*urverdängt*) that is to say, if it puts itself in a founding position, it will appear clearly to you that it is a new moral order which it registers as the will of the father, as the wish of the father. From then on, it's the male partner who finds himself in the position Autre. If this second repression operates as an original one, as a founding one – that is to say, if he puts, in some way, this new moral order on the side of the law, but a law totally different to the law of desire – it is the male partner who will find himself returned to the position Autre.

And I will remark to you, in passing, that if the male partner is designated as Autre, as you will guess, for the little boy to be born from a couple constituted in such a way, this will easily orientate him for a homosexual destiny. This child will not any longer have to interest himself in those who are there, in this Autre position, that is to say having to serve as support for jouissance. But, in addition, he will interest himself only in their little organ, their little organ insofar as it should not be there, that it begs a question, because this has escaped the partner the order which was prescribed, was recommended. That is to say the value and the price that it takes. It is therefore not superfluous to note how the key to male homosexuality passes without doubt, through a certain disposition of maternal hysteria. This is not a surprise. This is totally banal.

But, to stay with our aim of trying to account for the predilection of hysterical symptomatology for the body, let us rapidly make clear the consequences of this repression of S_1 from the structure about which I spoke earlier. In a structure, the consequences are automatic. It does not matter whether you bear a grudge against it, think about it, or believe it. It's like machines, you push a button and this has a certain number of consequences. So, if you wish this evening, I will bring two to your attention.

Firstly, the fact is that there is in this register of the Autre a signifier which is in this way repressed S_1, in a pseudo-original, pseudo-foundational position. This repression will provoke a closing procedure, the introduction of a limit into this system which would otherwise stay open – in other words, it would not know where to go, nor what it would want. In this system, the signifiers will organise a gap maintaining a dissatisfaction. And we know this will be lived as foundational, as foundational of this order itself, that is to say that it will be protected at any price. We will see, moreover, in the mechanism of hysteria something which is a defence against dissatisfaction.

On the other hand, a second consequence, by the fact of having letters of phallic nobility, this S_1 pseudo-founder gives authority to signifiers which are an expression of it. These signifiers will draw from that a certain power, but organised for ends other than sexual jouissance. Because of the fact itself of the foundational sacrifice of this pseudo-original signifier, demand will be substituted for desire. Because the total gift, in this order, is ready to respond to need and love and offers itself as a remedy of this dissatisfaction which is maintained, this dissatisfaction subsists and supports an exasperation of the demand always more pressing, to which usually an exacerbation of the gift responds.

These formulae put us on the road to a kind of nourishing which concludes always, by an anorexia. In effect, in a system of this kind, functioning on a demand always more exasperating and to which a more sacrificial gift always responds, we see how a subject produces for himself the only way to keep a minimum compatible with biological life: anorexia. By the same token, we see how what we call hysterical orality comes to be founded. It is something which presents, if you will allow me this image, as a kind of erection of the mouth going beyond what could be the erection of the breast. We can also conceive how in this system the appetite is always threatened with disgust and with vomiting. And satiation, can, in a reflex way, provoke these otherwise surprising manifestations.

This is the course, it seems to me, to be necessary to arrive at our question: Why is the body the elected place for the symptoms of hysteria? I have not yet responded, as I thought we would get further this evening. It is better that I leave a pause and stop. We can now advance the hypothesis which is probably founded on this question of the choice of body as elective field of hysterical symptomatology: I will continue this the next time, that is to say the 9th of November. Do any questions arise?

QUESTION: The expression "repression of the symbolic" is a problem for me and I wonder how you understand it?

CHARLES MELMAN: I don't think I used this term. I spoke about the repression of S_1 which is already a lot! It cannot be said that this entails a repression of the symbolic, but in fact this repression of S_1 finds itself the originator of a new symbolic order. Why? A symbolic order, it's this system constituted of material elements, proper to the game of substitution, a game of permutations, metaphor, metonymy, according to two different axes, made possible by a foundational loss. I am resuming it like that, abruptly. The history of *Fort/Da*[13] is the entry of the child into the world of the symbol. It is not a question at all in hysteria of repressing the symbolic order. What is in question, is the repression of one of these elements the S_1 supported from original repression, puts into place another type of symbolic arrangement. Why another kind of symbolic arrangement? Symbolic because it is constructed also under something which is undeniably lost and constituted by the same material elements. But it is ready for prescriptions, whether they are superego, different to the first, and to a mode of a different kind of jouissance. This is what I tried to individualise, to distinguish. In other words, we can say that to a symbolic system of the One, the hysteric brings an opposing symbolic system, his or hers in fact. "It could and should be totally different. It has functioned according to other principles, other trajectories, other finalities than those of yours. And I know that mine, it's in reality that one that the Autre wants. In other words, my system is the good one". To tell the truth, from the viewpoint of structure there is nothing to favour, there is nothing in the match, which would allow us say that one is more just than the other. We have just to appreciate the fact that they have different consequences and that is surely one of the reasons, why, the two sexual partners do not usually go in the same direction. Usually and then with the best will in the world, the best will in the world for both of them. Have I replied to your question?

QUESTION: A little – but it was principally the term of "foreclusion" in which I am interested.

CHARLES MELMAN: Listen, the term of foreclusion in hysteria: it will be necessary to devote a night to what is called hysterical psychoses. There is not the least bit of hysterical psychosis! But, when we get started of course, we can see produced things which could have the appearance of being totally psychotic. Those of my generation knew, when they went into psychiatric hospitals, totally authentic hysterics were hospitalised for schizophrenia for decades. We now have some small supplementary instruments to locate them. It's one of the first surprises of what could be our formation. Certainly, there is a certain disposition where nothing more will be asked than to tend towards that side. But it remains that the structure is totally different and we will have to give reasons why this is so. For example, the effects of repression. If hysteria is linked, as I'm saying to a kind of repression, we can see how, at the same time, it is resistant to psychosis. But it's so nice, isn't it and it gives so much pleasure when a hysteric really goes to the supposed term. This is not a term fabricated by us, doctors, it is not at all the natural term. We will have to discern why there is so willingly, a sort of complicity of the entourage so that really it will get excessive. And we will find out where this excess is capable of finding its source.

QUESTION: You began with a certain predilection of the hysterical symptom for the body. Firstly, I did not grasp why that is so. And, then I said to myself that perhaps there is a certain predilection of the body for hysterics. Rather, there is something in the sexed body of hysterics and in their sexual life, their relationship to sexuality, I don't know what, certainly something more significant, something more present. And, and at the same time you began with, this renunciation of jouissance and this gift and loyalty to the Autre.

CHARLES MELMAN: Listen, I'm thrilled by what you are saying. It's following on from what I did not deal with this evening. But indeed, it's like that. That is to say how to link this question of the choice of body to this putting into place of what I'm trying to do and which is still an introduction.

QUESTION: That is to say, that I think we cannot separate hysteria from the body, that we can say that the hysteric chooses the body. It seems to me that it's a little of the contrary, in so far as this body is sexed. That's what you said in June. You said that they have a body after all, it's not terribly upsetting, but this body is sexed.

CHARLES MELMAN: We have to see in what way it is sexed. Of course it is, but it is a little bit different. And, to immediately give the nuance for the hysteric, for example, demand takes on a character, a sexual coloration. That is not to say that it's a sexual object. What is sexed or sexual in the demand of the hysteric? We will have to be more precise about that and perhaps in doing so, show how sexuation is exercised on the body of the hysteric.

QUESTION: This sexed aspect of the demand is this not with regard to the desire of the Autre? There would be an aspect of quid pro quo.

CHARLES MELMAN: Yes. Surely with regard to the demand of the Autre, which by the way, there is the sacrifice which she imposes as a response to what she hears, as a demand of the Autre. She almost makes herself the interpreter: the *porte-parole*, the carrier, she articulates what she herself hears in the Autre.

QUESTION: What happens when, instead of repressing S_1 she is content to renounce it?

CHARLES MELMAN: Firstly, that would make perhaps conjugal relationships of another type. This does not mean this would allow anybody to realise sexual rapport, absolutely not. So, would that make something of the order of feminine abdication? I don't know. In any case, it is not a question for us of prescribing what would be most favourable coupling. It has to do above all, with ascertaining some consequences and then remark how much we are the puppets. Indeed, if something presents itself of the order of an exit, a solution, it would not be at all of the side of a renunciation which would have to be demanded of one or the other. Psychoanalytic discourse invites us also to an ethic. If we reflect a little on this, it would be worth our while to take up again the seminar on *The Ethics*.[14] The ethic to which analytic discourse invites us is surely not of the order of renunciation, but proposes, on the contrary to go as far as contradiction. In any case, the ethics of analysis is not of the order of a recipe, of a remedy. We will have a chance to speak again about the question of remedy. It's not our orientation.

QUESTION: So, what can we situate in this hypothesis, which is not totally up in the air? If we cannot situate there the natural inclination of the discourse of the hysteric, nor indeed the inclination of analytic discourse, what can be said about this situation, which would consist in not repressing S_1 but in renouncing it?

CHARLES MELMAN: In the game of discourse and its places, who will carry the weight of castration? Who will take responsibility for it? The game of S_1 is to make itself carry in the place Autre. S_1 presents itself as being full of good intention and, is disposed towards going to the end. Unfortunately, it encounters a partner, who is firstly in a strange way, ruined anatomically, and secondly does not seem to have decided to play the game. So, obviously there are problems. This is in some kind of way the song of S_1. Analytic discourse is subversive (and it the only one to do it, which is its unappreciated virtue) because it shows us that S_1 is never there except in a position of semblant. It's a semblant of S_1. No matter how vigorous, courageous, determined, ferocious, cruel, extremist, imperialist, no matter how totalitarian, it will never be but in a position of semblant. This also goes for the conclusions we can draw from those who are expressions of S_1 like he or she who is in this position of Autre.

In other words, castration is this kind of wrong way thanks to which a man and woman are able to meet and eventually do things. Good! It's this disposition between them – which joins them while at the same time unjoining them – which analytic discourse makes clear by breaking with traditional speculation. Traditional speculation is, if I may express myself like this, a kind of perpetual quarrel of management which maintains the activity of philosophy. Unless one becomes a celibate, as Lacan remarked and to give value to the morals of a celibate, that is to say a sadistic morality, who has not faced this problem posed by this kind of civility or civilisation which introduces not only the sexual, but the failure of sexual rapport?

QUESTION: You came back to your first question as to where destiny leads. And we see in the end, that a woman, in not having the penis, puts herself in the place of jouissance or in the place of the Autre. Is there no other possibility, according to your demonstration, except to repress S_1, and be a hysteric?

CHARLES MELMAN: That's really what we can assume. And yet, it is found that it's not necessarily the case and we would be totally wrong to assimilate the feminine position and the hysterical position in a facile way, even if we meet it more often than the other case. Hysteria does not belong to feminine destiny. On the other hand, what I'm advancing for the necessities of my argument, need to be corrected. For example, Lacan defines hysteria as the woman who makes the man.[15] That goes against what I'm advancing and in fact, there is a hysterical position which does not operate by this kind of repression, which consists in not worrying about anatomy and stays in a masculine position at the same level as the partner and eventually better than him, in a phallicism much more blaming, more talkative, more expressive, and much more imaged than that of the partner. This is an indication for us to introduce a certain temperance in what I'm saying to advance, that other solutions, less hysterical ones are possible. For the next evening, I will deal with what I call the economy of hysteria and on that occasion we will be able to appreciate why there is a feminine position which is not confused with this one!

Good! So, until the 9th of November!
19 October 1982

Notes

1 Plato, *The Symposium* (trans. C. Gill). London: Penguin Classics, 2003.
2 J. Lacan, *The Seminar of Jacques Lacan, Book XVII: The Other Side of Psychoanalysis, 1969–1970* (trans. by C. Gallagher, unedited).
3 S. Freud, *The Complete Letters of Sigmund Freud to Wilhelm Fliess* (ed. and trans. J.M. Masson). Cambridge, MA and London: Harvard University Press, 1985.
4 S. Freud, "Project for a Scientific Psychology" in *Pre-Psycho-Analytic Publications and Unpublished Drafts*, Vol. I, S.E. (1886–1899). London: Hogarth Press, 1966.
5 S. Freud, *Studies on Hysteria*, Vol. II, S.E. (1893–1895). London: Hogarth Press, 1955.
6 J. Lacan, *The Seminar of Jacques Lacan, Book III: The Psychoses, 1955–1956* (ed. J-A. Miller, trans. R. Grigg). London: Routledge, 1993.
7 Saint Augustine, *The Confessions* (trans. H. Chadwick). Oxford: Oxford University Press, 2008.
8 Lacan, *Book XVII: The Other Side of Psychoanalysis*.
9 G.W.F. Hegel, *Phenomenology of Spirit* (trans. A.V. Miller). New York: Oxford University Press, 1979.
10 J. Lacan, *The Seminar of Jacques Lacan, Book XXI, Part 1: Les non-dupes errent, 1973–1974* (trans. C. Gallagher, unedited).
11 S. Freud, "'Civilised' Sexual Morality and Nervous Illness" in *Jensen's* Gravida *and Other Works*, Vol. IX, S.E. (1906–1908). London: The Hogarth Press, 1959.
12 Thomas à Kempis, *The Imitation of Christ* (trans. R. Challoner). Gastonia, NC: TAN Classics, 1991.

13 S. Freud, "Beyond the Pleasure Principle" in *Beyond the Pleasure Principle, Group Psychology and Other Works*, Vol. XVIII, S.E. (1920–1922). London: The Hogarth Press.

14 J. Lacan, *The Seminar of Jacques Lacan, Book VII: The Ethics of Psychoanalysis, 1959–1960* (ed. J-A. Miller, trans. D. Porter). London: Routledge, 1992.

15 J. Lacan, *The Seminar of Jacques Lacan, Book XVI: From an Other to the Other* (trans. by C. Gallagher, unedited).

Chapter 9

Opposition S_1/S_2

Charles Melman

The Father's failure is that he is not able to make a universe. This means that his creatures are never united towards what founds desire. No matter his power, his goodness, his creatures will always distinguish each other, to occupy the positions of One or of the Autre. And even though the Father has affirmed strongly that he loves his creatures with an equal love, those who find themselves in the position Autre regularly believe that they have been hurt. The Bible, this great, realistic narrative begins exactly with such a prejudice, that is to say, this sharing which could not fail to take place between the two brothers and which ended with the murder committed by Cain.[1]

Of course, Lacan remarks that, meanwhile, on the side of the Autre, on the side of the creature who occupies the position Autre, jouissance does not fail. And there is even a supplement because beside phallic jouissance, he or she who would occupy this position Autre would therefore benefit from an access to that jouissance Autre. So, why this prejudice in occupying this position, this position Autre, if this does not show us, as might be expected, that narcissistic jouissance has primacy over so-called object jouissance? To emphasise this category Autre, is to expose oneself to the duty to please, to have to seduce in order to be accepted. This leaves us thinking about the creature who finds himself in this case, that this would not have been definitively agreed in the eyes of the father himself. When this position Autre, which is usually the case, is occupied by a woman, we find a taste for situations such as maternity which is worth a phallic stamp with the feeling that the agreement of the father is definitively acquired. It is without doubt the fact of this stamp which introduces this famous equivalence of penis – child.[2] With the feeling so frequent between a father and a daughter of a reciprocal betrayal because this stamp, this child, this recognition will find itself given to someone, other than the father. We will have occasion to come back to the problem of the relationship with the father.

Because I will continue this evening by talking about the opposition of place and value between S_1 and S_2 we see that S_1, the master signifier, only holds its power by the recognition, whether S_2 wishes or not to give a price to phallic insignias.

DOI: 10.4324/9781003167839-9

I will simplify this by speaking about S_1 and S_2 as subjects, to evoke the subject which in every case holds its topics from S_1 or S_2. In effect, S_1 and S_2 are signifiers, they are not in themselves subjective entities, but they have a representative function for the subject. We will consider how this subject can give value to his word, in relying on S_1 or even S_2. Therefore, I will remark that for a subject who claims to be the representative of S_1, this S_1 will only work if S_2 works, if S_2 consents, in other words, gives a price for what S_1, evokes in its name, even what it can eventually distribute, that is to say, phallic insignias.

To make this understandable, right away we know there are women who challenge these so-called insignias, who believe that they have no great interest for them, and who organise themselves in movements which are called feminist – very honourable, but in fact, it's they who are surprised to see this challenge to these phallic insignias not stopping in any way the resurgence in their own breast – meanwhile, if I may say so, whitened, cleansed, purified – with a division not operating any less for them, between the Ones and the Autres. We are dealing here with an effect of structure. S_1 holds its power only from the place of the Autre, functions only in seeing itself swallowed up by the consent of the proper signifier at this Autre place, that is to say S_2. If S_2 refuses the deal, refuses the suggestion, S_1 risks having a more or less ridiculous aspect.

The formula we are advancing this evening, is that if the signifier is what represents the subject for another signifier,[3] in hysteria, a reversal is attempted: the weight of the representation would bear on S_2 – from then on it is S_2 which represents the subject for S_1. The hysteric is led to this reversal by the structure which incites her/him to repress S_1. From where an effect of caesura which will recover the heterotopy between S_1 and S_2.

S_1 and S_2 are not held in the same place. To give an illustration, Achilles and Zenon do not meet because they are not in the same place. If the walk of one is sustained by natural numbers, and the other by real numbers, they could not but miss each other. But the natural heterotopy between S_1 and S_2 – with the *objet a*, means that something happens which makes the meeting impossible between these two signifiers, there cannot be any sexual rapport there – the heterotopy which makes a gap between S_1 and S_2 is interpreted in hysteria as a heterogeneity of places. It is not the same thing. Heterotopy does not in any way stop us from supposing that these two places are generated by the same punch. To give a more explicit example, if the complementarity of a closed space is an open one, we can well see how these two heterotopical spaces one and the other, are generated by the one punch, by the same trait. So, that the interpretation of these two spaces by heterogeneity aims to see them as being pertinent to two different causes. And in our habitual mill of comprehension, we are led to consider them, in some way as not being produced by the same father, as arising from different fathers.

We note that in hysteria, I will illustrate this for you a little further on, that an interpretation of this gap between S_1 and S_2 will have consequences. We will see this as a radical heterogeneity of people capable of being an expression of one or the other signifier. In this way S_1 could represent something of the order of the ego, a strong ego and he who is on the side of S_2 could represent an unknown, an X which would have to accommodate, to identify with this S_1. In this procedure, to which I draw your attention, the division produced between S_1 and S_2 is no longer an intra-subjective division. After all, this will account for the fact that the subject is divided, that he is able to speak from different places, a different locus. But, in the hysterical interpretation, it's a division, which becomes extra-subjective. As if, he who expresses himself from S_1 was no longer a divided subject.

The heterogeneity which recovers or substitutes itself for heterotopy can also justify itself in the following way. If S_1, authorises itself from the Name-of-the-Father to in some way intimate to the real, to the signifiers present in the real, to have to lend itself to jouissance, the subject who authorises himself from S_2 stays in the hesitation on the name with which he can authorise himself to call S_1.

The hysteric tries to change the course of the weight of the representation for a subject on S_2 who would represent him/her for S_1. But, what interests us is that the hysteric does not try to invest the master place on top and on the left, the place of the agent, but tries to turn it around, to subvert it, by making it from then on, from the place Autre, on top and on the right, from the place of jouissance, the place of the new mastery. And she invites he who commends himself from S_1 to submit himself there, that is to say, renounce his privileges.

To the extent that the series of S_2 (because there is no S_3, S_4 there is S_1, there is S_2 and the other signifiers are totally equivalent to S_2), is primordially the support of the body – this is it, the series of S_2, it is that, the series of S_2 – it's what supports the body – the body will take up, this place of producing signs, of producing elements with a demanding call in the dialogue.

We began with the question of the body as the privileged place of hysterical symptomatology. I try to account for this privilege from the establishing of what refers above all to structure. It has to do with justifying why, in a given situation, it is the elements of bodily signs which enter into the dialogue, in the address to S_1 – but not just in any old way.

We will try and verify this assertion and see if it lends itself to remarks which will in some way illustrate the foundation.

First point, the hysterical somatic symptom presents itself as the expression of a subject who cannot speak. This is the "beautiful indifference" of hysterics: the subject does not really know what is happening. In fact, we are unable to ask him who is there, operating this game of the unconscious which will thereby find expression. But, we have to remind ourselves that the subject cannot speak: he is in some way gagged by his symptoms, when he mimes, when he plays this scenario which he ignores and which animates him. He is so mute, so that when he arrives at the consultation, often he asks that it should be a third, a friend, a parent who will describe what happens to him. The woman asks her husband to talk about her symptoms, as if she herself is not disposed to have what she needs to do it. There is, therefore, a first question. Why does the subject finds himself in this way so mute? Why symptoms? Why, by claiming to be an expression of S_2, in this situation does it not lead him to articulate it?

We can suppose that if the subject is mute, and expresses himself therefore by this mime, by this scenario, his original problem is that he cannot satisfy the places which manage the discourse and they are the only places from which a voice can be made to be heard. If you wish to speak, you have to assert from one place or the other, you do not have a choice. To the extent that all this procedure flows from the allocation of places to which discourse is constrained – let us say, to simplify, the place of the master and slave, the place of the agent and of the Autre or of jouissance – we can conceive that the subject could value himself without a voice in the discourse, because he challenges all participation in the inevitable function as the distribution between the Ones and the Autres.

It is true that the hysterical symptom presents itself as the manifestation of a language, supposed to be unable to be translated into existing discourses. Henceforth, mutism becomes like a prototype of objects which are sacrificed, it belongs to these objects which the subject renounces, which he abandons to the Autre.

The subject invokes the name of S_2 – of an S_2 now enigmatic because, always situated in the real, as it should, it all the same refuses the place which is assigned to it by S_1 – that is to say, to have to respond at the level of jouissance. S_2 has received a call which would permit S_1 to reassure itself on the familiarity of the real. Yes, there are signifiers in the real which are fully ready to respond at the level of jouissance and at the same time of the power of the Name-of-the-Father – because that is the civilising power of the Name-of-the-Father. But, if S_2 refuses to respond to this call and at the same time becomes enigmatic, what is it? Well, because of its enigmatic character, it's he who calls S_1, it's he who invites S_1 – during the consultation for example – to speak for him, to use the majesty of his concepts, at the same time with this engagement, bearing witness to the best of good intentions.

You know how much Charcot's hysterics were well disposed towards him and were at pains to show that truly, his concepts were wonderful, magnificent and that it was a walk in the park for them to immediately get better. Sadly, this began again the following morning or shortly afterwards because this good will towards S_1 (which is a trait which interests us) turns very quickly to the conclusion that the majesty of these concepts is a little bit short. It is the hysterics who made Charcot, who gave him this remarkable lustre and at the same time were completely devoted to him. You can clearly see here in the game between S_1 and S_2, the question is to know who holds the knowledge.

In this way, the power of Charcot was dependent on the good will of his patients, who could just as well elevate him to the pinnacle as let him fall, depending on their humour.

I believe that this reminder can enlighten us on the distribution between S_1 and S_2 and remember that it's from the place of S_2, the place Autre, that S_1 derives its power. Therefore, what we see is that the subject who invokes the name of S_2 can work to the grandeur of S_1 and work for him – that is a situation which exists – but he could also work to invite S_1 to renounce its privileges, that is to say its phallic insignias. These are two apparently contradictory procedures (and it is willingly said of hysterics that they are not logical) which regroup in a totally coherent way with a single aim to try and resolve the difference, the irreducibility between S_1 and S_2. But, if S_1 agrees to this renunciation, there is a deception of the subject represented by S_2. This is regularly verified in the clinic and we will immediately see why. I think that in what I'm proposing you will refind the illustration of Lacan's formula: "the hysteric is looking for a master on whom she or he is able to reign".[4]

The problem is what comes from S_2 and here the somatic symptom, what comes from S_2, presents itself as heterogeneous with regard to S_1, that is to say, as coming from another father. Last time, we tried to evoke the ethical differences which are maintained very easily from this different reference. But if they come from another father, real and symbolic will find themselves disjointed. It is an extremely frequent interpretation according to which the real and the symbolic come from different origins.

The subject of science is he who thinks that insofar as he is a subject he has nothing to do with science. There is science on the one side, which flows along and there is he as a subject: they float, each on his own side. Science does not interest him really until he has to make a career not at the level of a subject, but as an employee, that is to say, in a situation of alienation and there is somewhere else he, as subject, which comes up from obscurity, from the unknowable. It is on this that Lacan draws our attention in an essential way from the time of his seminar on *La Lettre Volée*[5] by showing what arrives in the real, that the real is a product of the symbolic chain itself. The subject of the unconscious, it's the subject of science, it's the same. It's what we have to deal with, it's not an aberrant or erring subject with regard to the symbolic chain but a subject constituted by this chain. And as Lacan explicitly says, it's not a subject that is able to be shown but is calculable.

Why does this particularly interest us here? Because this disjunction between symbolic and real permits us to see what could be the hysterical Borromean knot, permits us to put into place what eventually can be (we will see clearly) exploited. In the hysterical Borromean knot, everything happens as if the real and the imaginary find themselves knotted but disjointed from the symbolic. And the hysterical symptom in making a fourth round is the one which knots all three, by making an appeal to the symbolic. Perhaps, in this way, we can account for the singular hysterical investment with regard to the master, to he who holds the power of the symbol, whether to celebrate this power, or to scorn him, as I said, but in any case demanding his presence. What is least tolerated in hysteria is that he who is supposed to ensure this power, abdicates it.

This Borromean knot which we can call hysterical, with this disjunction between the real and the imaginary with regard to the symbolic and this round of the symptom insofar as it attaches in some way to the symbolic, this knot could account for the fact that hysteria is never an illness, how shall I say it, a solitary one, on its own, but always brought about in a display, in a modality of a call, a call to precisely S_1 – to the power of the symbol. There is here, a totally radical difference between hysteria and obsessional neurosis.

Why this display character of hysteria? It is not for nothing, nor is it to make it look pretty and it obviously corresponds to a kind of pressure. There is a look necessary and not just any one, which is questioned by the symptom.

The subject who supports himself here from S_2 looks to be an expression of value in this Autre, in a master position, and seeks in some way to shift the power of S_1 while all the time trying to maintain it. This is the difficulty of what is at stake. But, if S_2 tries all the same to shift the power to S_2, to what father will she refer to invoke her heterogeneity? Who is the genitor, cause of this heterogeneity? It is, I believe, easy to recognise, because we saw it in relation to the pseudo-original repression of S_1 in hysteria. This S_1, in this way repressed, will be seen as being the real father, that is to say the dead father.

What does that mean, that the real father should be the dead father?[6] It's a formulation we find in Lacan. The dead father is he who engages the signifiers which invoke his name in a work of mourning. The Name-of-the-Father is obviously he who authorises you to enjoy. But, if you are dealing with a dead father, the signifiers which use his name, call subjects to this very precise exercise which is called a work of mourning. It is curious how analysts on this topic are somewhat reserved or discreet. The work of mourning is a renunciation, in general limited in time – in days gone by it was perfectly standardised – a renunciation of all jouissance, in particular, of a sexual nature. It's the time of a sacrifice until in some way, access to jouissance is authorised again. A jouissance authorised by the same father, but this time, as if by his death he had paid for the temporary sacrifice of this access to jouissance. The dead father is someone who sustains the gift made to him. It is only he who can give this possible time to jouissance.

If the father of whom S_2 invokes his name, in his position of heterogeneity, is really the one I've underlined, he who will have to be sacrificed before he can authorise jouissance, particularly sexual jouissance, well, we are in a dialectic which is no longer maintained by the imperative of desire because desire is linked to an imperative. We are in a dialectic from then on maintained by demand, the demand brought alive by this dead father. The particularity of the dead father is not to order, we give in to him because we owe him or because he loves you. And we are here in a dialectic of no longer obeying because of the imperative, but because of love.

And gladly, this dialectic is presented as progress with regard to she who supports herself with the imperative. You know nowadays that the imperative has a very bad press. S_1 is very badly recorded. He who invokes its name, it is thought, really he is being dramatic! And this is an interesting situation, this time in which we are living, with this kind of quasi-persecutory relation to S_1. Why? For very simple reasons and it's probably that psychoanalysis has had effects on this movement which is not for us to judge – I do not know why we should be the defenders of this or that – but to pinpoint things. Analysis has played its part in illustrating what Lacan dates from Sade[7] after Kant, what he called the ascent of the good into the bad. In other words, if S_1 does not keep its promises, this would be big news.

Where does S_1 lead us? Not to the end, in any case, because it fails, the so-called sexual rapport and we're up to our neck in castration. So how, these days, do we get back to S_1?

This does not obviously stop us from functioning perfectly, including all those who take exception, because every functioning no matter what, implies the label, the passage by S_1. But, up to this day, we continue, all of us, to function more or less, certainly less better than before, all the symptoms means that it screeches, it's hailing right and left – but it turns about, we function all the same.

From what does S_1 invoke its name, to function today? No longer sure of its good intentions, nor the love it has for us, there is still this movement which consists, this love, in helping to make it resurge and to see it in religion, what might be of relevance again. But today, S_1 invokes the name of science. And faced with this S_1 we gently fall into line, we obey nicely. Well, we can do that! You will tell me that there is ecology, the return to this or that, but the principal movement is this all the same. For example, if someone has not received his salary at the end of the month and protests furiously he will be told it's the computer. If the computer isn't willing, well, you will wait. Modern politicians have very refined techniques with these kinds of problems – how to lead people today – and all will gladly make reference to science with graphics on the board, percentages, curves, rates of exchange etc.

What is more enlightening, is to notice that analysts themselves participate willingly in this paranoiacal response to S_1. Those of you who knew the delights of the Freudian School (L'École Freudienne) know how much of a whirlwind originated from this: there was S_1, there was a swarm of S_1, it was the Lacanian swarm and my God – it was intimidating. Meanwhile analysts could have had a more precise judgement and avoided being carried away by this current, this passion, and understand what operated and continues to do so, to have a less persecutory attitude with regard to the master signifier. In any case, they could have been more alert to the consequences for the psychoanalytic discourse which they were supposed to promote. Because it is very clear that the revolt in some way against the master signifier, does not take us very far, it only makes us do things in another way.

I have made this detour, to make us aware of the difference between on the one hand, a dialectic supervised by the imperative, what commands desire because the master signifier is what commands desire (of course, we can consider desire as persecutory, we are not too far away!) and on the other hand, a dialectic supervised by demand, an order organised by the dead father.

These signifiers which operate there as S_2, are in the register of demand, what do they demand? Well, they are contradictory, they demand many things.

They can, for example, as I have told you, demand that S_1 lay down arms, arrange itself under the banner of this father, of this dead father, and he will no longer be made to be recognised as a son but as a member of a population of which all are finally identical. Because the trait henceforth which unites them, is the demand which ignores the sex of the beggar, or the gift, who ignores no less the sex of the donor. We are entering here into an economy of generosity and charity.

But what is also demanded by S_2 in an imperative way, because it has to do with being an expression of the power of the place Autre, is that S_1 will not give in and that it will accomplish, if it has the means, what is finally the intrinsic wish of the hysteric.

What is it? This intrinsic wish is clear, it is castration: that S_1 will finally consent to bring about castration on S_2 which will found, finally, on the side of the Autre, the at-least-One, The Woman who would found the existence of "all the women". This is the big thing, this is the final demand made to S_1, which unfortunately never supports in this way what we could hope from it. And, for a reason! That is why there is always in this disposition the imaginary of "The Woman". You know it – you will know it in particular in relationships of jealousy – this kind of certainty, isn't it, that the woman is there, she is somewhere and one would really like to see her, if one would really like to perceive her, she has just happened to pass by. One can have a glimpse here, that it would be this at-least-One who would found the order of women. It is obvious that if this castration were possible, well, it would finally appease this activity of sacrifices and gifts, repeated in total loss because they are never able to be an expression of the authenticity of symbolic recognition – except in maternity.

It's this kind of disposition which can explain to us, why the hysteric has finally the wish, that her desire should always be unsatisfied. She is always upset when she is satisfied. It's exactly what she does not want. She wants an unsatisfied desire, that is to say, founded one good time on castration, that it will not be submitted like this to totally surprising hazards which could only arrive with a bang! It would suddenly be satiation. And to say it quickly, it is clear that to hold oneself as a subject in this dissatisfaction, which constitutes one of the major resistances in analysis, is to continue complaining about it but to hold on to it.

Finally, if you wish, to conclude this evening, there is another point to verify the foundations for what I'm proposing. We know since Freud these somatic symptoms are constructed, by what? By the elements of a repressed discourse. There are sequences which speak, are repressed and consecrated to mutism, will find themselves in play, imagined, even treated as a puzzle. And it is known that for centuries these elements have demanded an interpreter who could decipher them; these symptoms forever bear witness of a call to the power of the symbolic, so that someone would come and read these hieroglyphics.

There is an example given by Freud of an astasia-abasia[8] in a young girl, after the death of her father. Interpretation: she has no more support. Meanwhile, a question remains open, why is repression so extensive as to exercise such type of thought? Why does she have to repress "Now that my father is dead I have no more support". What will find itself repressed from this pseudo-original repression of S_1 is very large. In any case, an interpretation, a reading of this symptom operated in Freud's time. Why? And why does it not work like that nowadays? Without a doubt because in Freud's time – S_1, there was then the power of interpretation – the S_1 was there in its native, growing power. It is clear that today, it's gone into ordinary discourse. Something more is expected.

Now, do we have to be content with this miraculous aspect of the affair? If it works, is it not by introducing into this discourse, this hysterical symptom, the power of the metaphor? After all, these symptoms prove to be active metaphors in a discourse, until then repressed. That's how they work as symptoms. So, what does it mean to make the power of the metaphor intervene? The power of the metaphor is important. Freud remarked to this patient, who could no longer stand upright, on the metaphoric character of her symptom and this is how this entered into the rank of things. It's not nothing. Because, precisely the metaphor, as you know, functions from the phallus. And to make it work, to expose what is there of metaphor, it is of course to put into play phallic power.

It is necessary we keep in mind that in fact, if these symptoms are cured, it is clear from all the observations we have from Freud himself that he did not cure hysteria. There is not a single observation of Freud, where he talks about a case, not only about cured symptoms, but indeed hysterias as such, as cured. We absolutely don't have one. And he himself did not embarrass himself by claiming so. Indeed, the choice of *Dora*, it should all the same, make us think, us analysts, that even though he chose Dora, the case actually did not succeed. We are confronted by a really pertinent question, to know if analysis is capable not only of removing more or less embarrassing symptoms, but if it is capable of supporting the hysterical phantasy, if analysis can have a resolution, for this.

You see that to deal with this subject is not to take up old issues, but to restore ourselves in some way, in the actuality of our practice.

A final word. Because hysteria finds itself confused with illness – what is it, illness? Does not the hysteric precisely do us the great service of informing us what illness is? Illness, it's precisely when the subject is not up to – more or less I will use this formula – accomplishing his phallic duty.

What does this mean? Take the *Essays on Psychoanalysis,*[9] the second topology. This is how Freud locates the duty of the subject, with the automatism of repetition. The subject's duty is to carry out his phallic duty, according to the order which is prescribed for him by the structure and then to disappear into the forgotten. He will have made his trajectory, believing he was free. He believed he was master of his appendage, when in fact he is, insofar as he is a subject, only the appendage, that he is in some way the servant of what leads his existence. Illness, it's what happens when you cannot keep your place in this accomplishment. Hippocrates perfectly understood that: he said that above all, what is important is not to go too near. It is necessary to let the power of nature take its course, which will re-establish the course of things. Nature has enough power to put you back on track, to put you back on the road, to put you back on your backside, if I may be so bold. What is called today, what functions as illness is nothing else but this. And there are places where really, those who find themselves out of action are accepted or loved, despite this. These places, you know them, we are here in one of them, are hospitals. These are places where one is held, where the care of those who are out of service is assured, this happens because of the creation of hospitals by the religious orders and they were assured that they were not any less loved and perhaps even more.

This teaches us that if there is such an easy, so current, so spontaneous a recovery between hysteria and illness that the "cabinet" of the doctor or the medical scene is so frequently the place where this demand comes to be exercised, it's for this: because he or she who is caught in a hysterical position, thinks, believes that he or she is not up to the measure of this so-called phallic service, reasons which belong, of course, to the interpretation of castration.

The next time I will try to deal with what I will call the general economy of hysteria. To believe that one is not up to the measure of assuming the service – to stay with this metaphor – the subject caught in this hysterical position, will find herself as the player in an interpretation of her state as an illness. Henceforth, her thoughts will be addressed to figures, to diverse representative figures, whose advice may be sought. But, it will be essentially the doctor who will be addressed with regard to this trouble and we know how much the doctor's response could be judged to be wrong, a response like: "But Madam (or Sir), There is absolutely nothing wrong with you"! It's a response demanded not to be heard but founded on contempt.

This was a bit long, so I will leave it there.

QUESTION: I would like you to explain what authorises you to put the dead father on the side of S_2 and to say that he is a-sexual.

CHARLES MELMAN: You will read Freud in the *Studies on Hysteria* and also the *Dora* case, the frequency of the father as being sick, dying or dead. It's something which deserves to be remembered, if only from the point of view of statistics. The father in question, the father of *Totem and Taboo,*[10] is of course, the dead father. The sons authorise themselves in his name and in his place from then on, to have access to women. What I'm drawing your attention to is that there was probably a time which we call a time of mourning and indeed a "work of mourning": this is a subjective stage which does not seem at all exceptional. And among these sons of *Totem and Taboo*, it is probable that some decided to give their lives to celebrating this dead father, that is to say in renouncing jouissance, in particular sexual jouissance, and to make themselves priests.

The dead father is not reserved for one of these categories. The reference as such to the dead father, the gift, what I call sacrifice, a relationship with him founded on what would be a demand by him and not in any way an imperative, but in the name of his love. This for a while, even if this time could be perpetuated by some, for whom it's a social duty. And, it seems to me, that sexual jouissance will constantly and regularly function, in this kind of oscillation for those who find themselves authorised by this father, from mourning sacrifices, from work that has been carried out and equally, by this eventual demand exercised by him, authorised as jouissance. Our culture is founded on this: the dead father is relegated by us, to times past. We are therefore outside the time of mourning and this is no longer recalled for us, except by those who have as a social task to continue, to devote themselves, to sacrifice themselves, so that we can rest at peace with him and that we, the others, in any case those who are not in such a position of sacrifice, that we can peacefully, tranquilly enjoy, because there are those precisely who continue to sacrifice to him.

There was an Italian film which was remarkable on this subject. The title escapes me, but indeed we can understand how very sensitive the Italians are to this kind of question.

It was the story of a young priest who wanted to emancipate himself and take liberties with his soutane. It is really obvious that all the parishioners make him immediately understand that really he was going too far, that it was important that he did the work. And he was put back to work, they tried then to get him back on track and it finished on the fact that all these joyous feasts held in the intimacy of different families in the village, the fact that everything got back in order and that all the different families found the tranquillity of their conjugal beds. It is quite well done.

It's this I've mentioned in my comments, in place of heterotopy this heterogeneity: this disjunction between the real and the symbolic, the fact that it is in the real, the signifiers which are present in the real, come from another cause. What I simply remarked, is that the ethic, which henceforth will animate the signifiers proper to this place, which I continue to call S_2, this ethic seems to be founded on a dead father. Not dead with this distance and with this myth but as if it had to do with the foundation of the myth itself, as if we have to work from then on, to satisfy, respond to the demand of this father.

This is what I've tried to work out and I don't think you can disentangle it from anything which is outside the consequences of Freud's work. It's perhaps not as explicitly obvious as other things in Freud, but I do not believe, in any case, that it is removed from the references Freud himself made.

9 November 1982

Notes

1 *The Holy Bible*, Catholic Edition. New York: Harper Collins Publishers, 1989.
2 S. Freud, "Dissolution of the Oedipus Complex" in *The Ego and the Id and Other Works*, Vol. XIX, S.E. (1923–1925). London: The Hogarth Press, 1961.
3 J. Lacan, "The Subversion of the Subject and the Dialectic of Desire" in *Écrits* (trans. B. Fink). New York: W.W. Norton & Co., 2006.
4 J. Lacan, *The Seminar of Jacques Lacan, Book XVII: The Other Side of Psychoanalysis, 1969–1970* (trans. C. Gallagher, unedited).
5 Lacan, "Seminar on 'The Purloined Letter'" in *Écrits* (personal translation).
6 J. Lacan, *The Seminar of Jacques Lacan, Book V: The Formations of the Unconscious, 1957–1958*. (trans. C. Gallagher, unedited).
7 Lacan, "Kant with Sade" in *Écrits*.
8 S. Freud, *Studies on Hysteria*, Vol. II, S.E. (1893–1895). London: The Hogarth Press, 1955.
9 S. Freud, *Beyond the Pleasure Principle, Group Psychology and Other Works*, Vol. XVIII, S.E. (1920–1922). London: The Hogarth Press, 1955.
10 S. Freud, *Totem and Taboo and Other Works*, Vol. XIII, S.E. (1913–1914). London: The Hogarth Press, 1955.

Chapter 10

What do we understand by body?

Charles Melman

Perhaps I was too quick and abrupt the last time and this evening I will once again, take up the problem from another point of view. When we say body, what do we mean by this?

This question gives rise to an embarrassment insofar as the "body", the signifier body, is precisely what, by its very nature will give an answer to every question. One is tempted to say that it's the last response furnished by the real, a response of which the more appeasing character will at one and the same time put an end to all questioning and give the guarantee that it has to do with the right response. Because, as we know, all questions come from the real and exist only because the response is already there.

Why is it that this body, this signifier body, will respond to every question about the real? Of course, because in the real, thanks to this body which we can grasp, there is an "enjoyment". When this kind of response is produced, we can only be quiet, it's not the right time to discuss things because the last response is there, no matter what the question.

The proselytising of jouissance was advocated, for example, by Wilhelm Reich,[1] a person not without merits even if he went a little off track at the end! Why did he so completely fail in his intention which he wanted to be revolutionary? Because this kind of response – in the real, there is of "enjoyment" because of the body – that's exactly the religious response. This is what says that the real has been managed for us, has been "cultivated" for our jouissance. As we know, Eve was created to distract the first man from his boredom. What this means, it has to be said, is that jouissance is not in any way an insurrection against the father. It is, on the contrary, the celebration.

If "body", the signifier body, illustrates the category of the real by its resistance (it resists by its thinness, its density, its compacity, which it opposes in the taking) the jouissance of drug addicts seems to organise itself differently: by investing on the contrary on what is smoke, pulverising, liquid. It is as if this kind of jouissance treated the real as an imaginary, beyond which it would have to catch the *pneuma*, the pure breath, the impalpable, always fleeing, which would support him. This puts us on the road which, after all, specifies the category of surplus jouissance. Perhaps it is not a bad way to get

DOI: 10.4324/9781003167839-10

our bearings in the clinic of addictions, to pinpoint that this mode of jouissance denounces mediocrity, insufficiency, the limitation on jouissance promoted by the father and aspires to an infinite jouissance. We know that the only term capable of bearing witness to this is death. It's a way of accomplishing the cycle of one's existence, in avoiding what Freud pointed to us to with regard to the second topology, that is to say, being the appendage at the service of the father.[2]

If the body is what, from the real, is opened up to jouissance, the hysteric, to come back to our theme, is a witness, from her side, for this service that the body should give, that something is not right, there is something wrong. And in the final sense, what this body represents as a response of the real, she substitutes nonsense, that is to say what gives her this appearance, this simple appearance, that she is a little bit mad.

In fact, what *makes* a body? How does a body hold together? We will not be content with metaphors of compactness, of thinness, of density, of that which resists being taken.

Because we always refer to structure, I will advance immediately a kind of response: what makes a body, its nothing other than the chain of signifiers S_2.

But, there is here immediately a totally necessary restriction. Let us imagine, that at the beginning this chain did not exist. It is a concatenation of signifiers whose order is determined randomly, signifiers which follow each other, without anything linking them, without anything fixing the possible space of metaphors and metonymies, a space without which they could not produce themselves. Let us say, a chain produced by a machine in a naïve state (and I will explain this term later) spontaneous, innate, without consistency. The elements which compose it, lend themselves precisely to falling apart, to pulverisation. This can be observed in the clinic, for example, in certain cases of schizophasia brought to term: in the mouths of these persons, signifiers succeed each other, broken, nothing links them anymore and this is not without strange effects on their physical body: tonus, vasomotricity, skin quality, physiognomy, mimicry, even vegetative functions. If we suppose that originally the chain of signifiers present themselves in this succession because of chance, what is it that gives consistency to the chain? What gives it precisely a body? What is it that holds all the elements together which ensures that there will be a possible game, a certain freedom which makes metaphor and metonymy possible, without meanwhile prohibiting all these elements to stay fundamentally linked to the others?

We have to admit that what gives body to the chain of S_2, it's precisely S_1 and more exactly what falls between S_1 and S_2, in other words, *objet a*. It is castration, which in some way orders this chain of S_2. Castration puts a limit into place, which the chain cannot reach and towards which, henceforth, it tends towards. It has a direction which is that of a quest for jouissance. With castration, this opening is managed, this place which makes possible the game of metaphors and metonymies and which specify, for each speak-being, what is called his style, is nothing other than his mode of access to jouissance, his way of arriving at it. What fascinates us in a literary style, is what we hear there, we perceive that it has to do with certain modes of access to jouissance. You have no doubt heard Lacan's remarks on the realist school, even the naturalist one,[3] where the principle of metonymy dominates. And as we know, it's a huge mode of access to jouissance.

What we mean by body is nothing else, but this concentration of signifiers which, without our realising it, leads us towards jouissance, and which is gifted with this wisdom which we ignore, and in which meanwhile we place our trust.

Here, two problems arise. The first, is that if the chain of S_2 finds itself thereby oriented by castration at one of its extremities, it will mean that it will be an infinite chain of signifiers. It would be great to have a certain number in the dictionary, in the treasure house of language, the chain will increase itself, modify itself, it is open to all enrichments, to all creations. That's how it is, it is not closed. And if it is infinite, even though it is organised by castration (that's what makes a chain) still, it is not all phallic. Signifiers respond to us from the real, detach themselves on a basis which despite everything, always stay a little enigmatic and menacing, even if we are protected by this certainty in which we live, that the real has been equipped to serve our jouissance, that it is the garden that we would like to equip for our frolics. We function like that but it's enough to read any investigation or inquiry or an ethnographical report to see that in cultures which do not have such a relationship with the father, the real is not at all of this kind. It is not a universal procedure about which we can generalise. Indeed, for these populations the real does not offer itself in any way on the basis of a familiarity, of reassurance, while we always identify it as good and made for us.

There is something enigmatic in the functioning of the body. This chain is not all phallic, because it is infinite you can never catch it in its entirety. And this is indeed the kind of relationship we have with the body, we cannot enjoy it entirely. As Lacan used to remark we can only ever have a little bit.[4] And this bit of the body is obviously conceived from the categories of the imaginary. That's what the phantasy comes along to support. You know that, in the theory there was this distinction of the partial object, introduced by Abraham,[5] which assumed that a total object existed. To speak about the whole object, it's obvious to believe in an all-phallic power. There is no total object, we always have to do only with objects which remain partial, if one wants to say that, they only represent a part of the body.

What interests us with regard to hysteria, is what makes the good standing of the body, its density, its good functioning, its wellbeing, a body which works well, which on its own, which one does not have to worry about, it's what I said a while ago, it's the consistency which assures a limit. From then on, this limit will orient it, the signifying chain will regulate this body in an assured way, things which are perceptible at the level of the tonus, of vasomotricity, exonerations and at the same time, the right measure of its exits as well as its entries. It will regulate the spontaneous automatism of its exchanges, things work. As I've just said, this consistency of the S_2 is in agreement with their relation to S_1 and what falls between them, between S_1 and S_2 is what links them; not only the S_2 between them, but what from then on links an S_1 this one and not another, to S_2.

Moreover, what is articulated by the subject as truth, is precisely the origin of this place managed by the fall of the object. That is to say, that the word articulated from this place will reproduce the original agreement, the first agreement which knotted S_1 and S_2. There is no truth except this one. There is no universal truth, no generalisable truth, no truth for everybody. There is, for the subject, only this truth which counts. That is to say the word articulated in a place and articulated in such a way that it will resuscitate, bring alive this original gap which was creative of the link between S_1 and S_2, it's foundational gap.

If S_1 and S_2 shatter like fragments of glass from a broken vase, if they coincide perfectly, are we going to say, that's it, that's the truth? Well, indeed, psychoanalysis recounts totally stupefying things, absolutely not! That's indeed the problem. Certainly, this perfect shattering, we can encounter it in the clinic: when the subject finds himself at this place of S_2, at this place Autre, at this place of jouissance – I always recall the four discourses – when the subject finds there an idealised image of himself. At this exact moment he is certain that that's it, that this clings, that it's exactly it! It's her, or it's him. It carries a name, it is called erotomania. And you can always try and deny it!

But the logical difficulty to which analysis introduces us, is that S_1 and S_2 when they are here produced, resurging in the name of what would be the original gap allowing the truth be articulated, their truth which is there (it would indeed be them), it is not in stumbling that they are in agreement. It is because, precisely, there is this gap between them. But, it is not just any old gap, not just any old fault – it is not enough to be in the wrong fault to be in the true one, that would be too easy! It is the fault specific to this gap, the genitor of a given subject. This one and not another. That is why Lacan repeated it so many times that in analysis there is no typical case.[6] Even if there are large clinical forms of the kind we are talking about, there are always only subjects with their singularities.

With regard to the place about which I speak, where we could finally speak in truth, it escapes us, because it's really that of the unconscious. We cannot speak about it in our own way and decide: now, today I'm going to speak to you in truth, this is my day of truth. Not at all! It's the moment you least expect, a little something will be produced, the lapsus, the witticism, whatever you want and that will be its emergence. This place where it speaks in truth indeed, it speaks in its fantasy, it speaks as it pleases. And, that is why the Freudian formula: *Wo Es War soll Ich werden* "there where it was I have to arrive",[7] is really problematic. It means to say that you can come along and live in your house. I don't have to tell you that it is a big dream and one can spend one's life managing the house where one will be well. Insofar as one has an unconscious, that is to say insofar as one is a speak-being, what is your home will escape you. You live there? Well, you will hardly have time to return there, and it's gone! You have stayed there and then you have left it, and that's it. But, meantime, it is there.

But, let us return to the relationship of S_1 with the body, that is to say this chain of S_2. From this S_1 are we not the master of this chain of S_2? But, of course, this body, we do not make it say whatever we want, this body will only accompany us, only if we obey it. That's what's really annoying. To take the first metaphor which comes to mind, it will be more the horse rider you will have to manage and learn to follow the horse. This brings us to the dialectic of the relationships between S_1 and S_2 of which I've tried to make you aware by asking you from where it is commanded and who orders. But this commandment exercised on the body, not only does it not go on its own, but it cannot work on its own. It needs the consent of S_2. In other words, from S_1 you cannot say just any old thing, otherwise you will obviously be denied, denied by the body.

For example, when as an adolescent Gide[8] discovered to his great surprise, that the sight of little boys caused manifestations in his own body, what did he do? Well, he begins, obviously, to put S_1 into play, he acts like everybody else. He was well brought up, he engages in the battle, in mortification, in prayer (in any case for him, I do not generalise about Gide). Up to the moment where he understood that in this battle, he lost, what? He loses his soul, that is to say his truth. Even if his truth reveals itself as strange, as we say, against nature. Is it his fault if the very honourable and, always a little sad, Madame Gide, whose husband seemed to be more occupied elsewhere and with other things, had so invested in a child, that he, André when she lost him, when he grew up, grew hair, when their intimacy was shattered, she had to mourn for this? It is this lack in the mother for the young Gide which constituted for him his own gap.

This is an example to remind you that our body, for us it is the Autre. There is no need to go looking I don't know where, it is there primordially. We will not do a bad arrangement with it on the condition that S_1 of which our word is an expression will stray congruent with this Autre. Congruence, this means, two things will meet as necessary. Lacan made *falloir* and the *faille* equivocal (it is necessary and it is a fault)[9]. If S_1, which you claim the name of which you invoke – of which your word is an expression, which you invoke as an expression of you as a subject, is not congruent with S_2 which constitutes you as Autre, there are produced effects, which in the first place are those of repression and then symptoms, neurotic symptoms.

What we encounter here in the game between S_1 and S_2, it is what we can call the opposition between two kinds of knowledge. Let us take the four discourses which are so essential for us – I'm developing them by giving meaning to writings – it is possible to give others, but, I will give this one – there is in this play between S_1 and S_2 an opposition between two kinds of knowledge. It's a theme I mentioned during the study day on the psycho-analysis of children. S_2, the chain of S_2, it's obviously knowledge. Let us not say that its primordial (you see, its immediately this kind of slippage) it is the kind of knowledge in which we all have confidence, each one of us. Obviously, there is a category of people who do not have confidence in it, these are hypochondriacs, and it's an interesting point to note with regard to this rather obscure category. But in general, we all have a kind of transference more or less spontaneous on this knowledge which is in us and which works for us.

This chain of S_2, when it is consistent, is supported by a spontaneous knowledge. It is not necessary to go to school to be a possessor of it, but to be possessed by it. It's a knowledge organised on the principle of diachrony, of historicisation. It's an anti-conceptual knowledge, it objects to all that is general, it opposes itself to the savant, to the doctor, to he who is supposed to be the depository of a knowledge. You thereby have currents, I don't know how to qualify them, let us say metaphysical, ecologists. ... And there are analysts who will tell you that the end of the end of analysis it is to entrust yourself to this knowledge, it is to do what you would dare say in the name of this knowledge. There is no need for this to have read many books, nor to be too bright. A very precious knowledge was put into you because it's this knowledge which invites you to jouissance and what you will say will have authority in itself. What more could you ask for?

This knowledge opposes itself to another kind of knowledge which is on the side of S_1, male knowledge, conceptual knowledge, which proceeds by generalisations. This is a misleading knowledge because it will lead you to nothing at all: the chain of S_1, it can be written in all its purity, in a mathe-matical writing and then afterwards?

The opposition is clinically totally perceptible. People who function in this S_2, and for different reasons think that they cannot invoke the name of S_1 may have the impression of being an obstacle to scientific learning, of there being a totally irreducible barrier.

Locke[10] has this idea, I could not find the reference for this evening, of a language precise enough not to have to refer to any general term, any con-cept. This language, singular enough to get around the kind of difficulty I mention here, would perhaps be made only of S_2. If this kind of language is obviously thinkable, sad to say, it would be the tower of Babel, everyone would use his own particular language. We can also put a parallel between S_1 and S_2 in terms of conflict: which side will dominate? We find the same kind of speculation.

But if the good functioning of the body is regulated by this limit, what is it about the body of the woman if it founds itself essentially that in the struc-ture, this concatenation of S_2 which we've just said, is not all-phallic? It does not function in its general equilibrium like that of its partner. I do not want to go into the details which would risk being odious but there is an indisputable biological witness: the body of the woman has a much bigger longevity than that of her partner. It is as if the man who claims to be all-phallic, as if he were pressed to go to the end of the procedure, as if he were pressed to go to – the bottom of the hole. I will use here a metaphor, it's not obligatory because of that. You know that in the Borromean knot, there is a link which appears strange: the jouissance of life, opposed to phallic jouissance. There we can see that phallic jouissance, stretched in some way because it is under pressure, in the quest for the exit. The woman, a jouissance which is not all phallic, she believes in it – but a lot less, it poses for her, all the same, other questions.

Are we going to say for the hysteric that this is what happens? Exactly not, something else altogether happens. The feminine position distinguishes itself from the hysterical position. Why? If, as I'm saying, what operates for her (or for him) it's the repression of S_1, not that she decides this, but, because in the structure which is offered to her, is that she will not have the right, in some kind of way to invoke S_1. And the father to whom she refers, this dead father with this work of mourning not completed, demands in some way this kind of repression. If there is repression of S_1 and therefore a suspension of castration which operates between S_1 and S_2, we can well see from then on, the chain, the famous chain presents a relaxing of the tension which vectorised it. And the hysteric finds herself hesitating between what would be for her a term, an aim, a limit, hesitating between a possible exit, an exit other than castration because it is from this she suffers.

That's how a certain number of consequences properly called somatic, register themselves. The fundamental feeling is one of dis-ease, of illness in the body, of a body which does not work. But, also in the huge registers that I mentioned earlier, for example, that of exonerations and of entries which will find themselves hit by a kind of uncertainty, of excess or of a failure of renunciation. It's indeed one of the big signs of hysteria. One is entering into a totally bizarre economy, as if there was no longer any spontaneous economy, as if there was no longer this unconscious knowledge, to regulate all that, to decide for it as if it were necessary to decide for it.

I finished last time by saying that the state of illness is extremely simple to define: this specifies someone who is in a state of suspension with regard to phallic duty. That's exactly what can be said here about the body. Not being any longer orientated, attracted, called by castration, the body goes through a period of floating and of dis-ease, an incapacity to accomplish what I call phallic duty.

In hysteria, it's generally not a phase which lasts too long, it alternates with periods dominated by sublimation. That is to say, absolute radical castration, and from then on the chain of S_2 finds itself effectively vectorised. Vectorised by what? Precisely, by the body itself, in that the hysteric would have had to renounce it, have to make a gift of it, this offered body, prepared as a support of jouissance for her partner, to make a gift to the Autre, to this dead father. These times are, on the contrary, marked by a hyperactivity. As if by this exoneration the body would find itself guaranteeing the well-meaning look of the Autre, of this dead father. The problem is that this kind of activism, where one feels well, even very well (in these movements, things work perfectly) this kind of activism fails in the long run. Because the Autre does not always respond, it has the air of not being ever completely satisfied, content enough, the sign of recognition on its part late in arriving. Except, that the illness itself is interpreted as a sign of recognition, the illness a testament that this body was given as a gift to the Autre. There is a little paradox in these cases which I call activism, what is at work, is S_2 and not S_1. S_2 functions as a master signifier, in its address to other signifiers. But it is an S_2 which succeeds with what it reproaches S_1 of never having been able to accomplish, an S_2 which in this case would be a successful absolute castration. Because what is reproached to S_1, is that it is always too feeble, never able to assure the castration of its partner.

Another remark, during a session, on a previous evening, I had spoken about the real of the body as being marked by a topology – for example, this sagittal division between one dominant side and the other. In general, we are not ambidextrous, the laterality of the dextro dominates. We are fundamentally asymmetrical. If painters and artists wish to testify to as how human a body is, it's enough that they make it asymmetric.

It happened that the next week there was on the medical page of *Le Monde* a really astounding article by our dear colleague Madame Escoffier-Lambiotte.[11] It's to her we owe the fact that the article written by Lacan on the events of May 1968 was put in the rubbish bin and, as he himself did not attach great importance to his productions, also consigned it to the bin, this means we will never have it. The recent article in *Le Monde* is entitled "the sex of the brain". What interests us here? It recalls recent works, American of course, which remind us that the two cerebral hemispheres have different tasks. One could establish a chart of cerebral hemispheres by the injection of radio-active substances, and the study of local variations on blood circulation and on the absorption of glucose, that is to say on oxygen consumption. The reading of all that by ultra-violet rays permits the establishment of a functional chart of the brain with zones of a square millimetre. You could provoke a kind of activity for a subject (activity of language, orientation, emotion) and see the zone of the cortex which functions at this exact time. These procedures have allowed us to establish that the chart is not the same for man and woman. For the man, there is a dominance of the left hemisphere, what commands the right side and where the centres of language are found. On the side of the right hemisphere, we find the centre of spatial orientation, emotional responses and then what are called global. non-verbal tasks – in other words what you would do and which would not be a thought, not be articulated by an explicit discourse. And the moment, this totally fascinating procedure shows us is that for the woman, lateralization, dominance on one side is far less clear. Instead of working with one hemisphere she has a tendency to work with the two. All this is very well explained, it's because the body – the calloused body, by which the influx passes from one side to the other – is more developed in the woman and therefore the woman is liable to a greater plasticity. The philosophy which Madame Escoffier-Lambiotte takes from history, is that man has one, and that the woman, has two. This means a lot of letters from readers of *Le Monde* today!

This would explain also, and this is interesting why dyslexia is much more rare in girls than in boys (statistically, there are five boys for every girl), as well as other difficulties with language. Because the girl uses both sides, it is necessary for bilateral localisations for a woman to be hit by an aphasia, for example, while, for the boy, it's enough for the localisation of the left hemisphere.

Why tell you all this? When I talk about this real of the body, this sagittal division, this may appear difficult for some of you. Well, it's biologically functionally verified. If we follow our thoughts on this, for the woman, the side from where it should dominate, causes a problem. It happens that it can dominate from one side, then from another, from the side of S_1, then from the side of S_2. She would have, in this way, a happy egalitarian tendency! We are all the same touched to know how much the experience of biologists are in accordance with Lacanian categories. We won't believe ourselves that we have found the good fragment, but all the same, it amazes us!

To conclude, I would like to take something up which I have already spoken about, long ago at the École Freudienne. For the hysteric, the trait is not sagittal, but horizontal, cervical. As if the body as a possible support of the partner's desire had to be repressed, at the same time as the S_1. As if the activity which, from then on is proposed and which vectorises in a rigorous way, the chain of signifiers represents an attempt at exoneration of this body, always running, until fatigue is reached, which marks a limit. Fatigue, here functioning at the level of jouissance, of an always imperfect jouissance: always failing, because it does not allow in a definitive fashion to know what this wish addressed to the father would entail, that is to say, a radical castration, as radical as that of her partner – and which would allow from then on this partner to meet, The Woman. It would of course be the only possible way for there to be The Woman, in the same way, on the other side there is The Man.

In other words, all this enterprise in which the hysteric finds herself, is not detachable from this kind of worry, properly speaking, sacrificial and altruistic founded on the attempt to respond correctly to the partner, that is to say to allow him to meet *the real woman*. That's where I will finish this evening.

QUESTION: Earlier, you spoke about the signifying chain which would be supported by knowledge. Do you not think that the signifying chain itself constitutes this knowledge?

CHARLES MELMAN: Of course! It's the signifying chain which organises knowledge, which means that there is an organised knowledge. It is not representative of knowledge, any more than there is thought on one side and our word on the other. In the same way the chain of S_2, is knowledge. I cannot see how a body, could be something other than that. And if we take all the metaphors in which the body is utilised, it is every time a call to what is held together and to a certain wisdom that it holds. If the word "body" comes under your pen it will always be that, which opposes itself to what I will call lack of limit, pulverance, dissolution.

JEAN BERGÈS: Lacan speaks about the hysterical "cutting" of the body.[12] But, because you speak about limits, where is the frontier of "cutting"?

CHARLES MELMAN: I would like to say that for the hysteric this cutting resumes once again the cutting of the phantasy, which founds a part of the body as an object of desire. This part, presented as homogenous with those constitutive of the image, to be the image, cause of desire, is presented as an ill area. There is a kind of reversal here. The hysteric presents what is linked to the procedure which founds a part of the feminine body, as ready to support the desire of the partner. This desire, proper to jouissance, is a failed, missed jouissance. And indeed that's what's presented as an ill area. There could only be illness there, in functioning in such a stupid manner. And, I have to say, that without discussing the way in which Lacan puts the problematic of hallucination into place, in his text on psychosis (the kind of utterance "I've just come from the butcher")[13] I would like to bring it nearer to what is the fundamental question, what operates by cutting, by a dissection. Far from this body functioning in a unity of movement, of its vectorisation, of what is being asked of it, there are bits and pieces. What is proper to hysteria, contrary to hypochondria it's always a little bit which varies, which displaces itself – it's not melancholia, for example.

QUESTION: But are there not cases of hysteria where the whole body is proposed as being ill, in anorexia or in bulimia, for example?

CHARLES MELMAN: We have to see if we can say that is the whole body. What happens more in hypochondria is the general functioning of the body is presented as failing. In any case, we can understand well, why it's at the level of an economy of exchanges that it is found broken, because what is found there questioned, she does not know too much what she should do, nor to what she has a right, we can present things like this. And, as we know, this will go into the problematic of excess, always of excess in one sense or another.

QUESTION: With regard to the real body you made reference to the tribes who do not function in the same way as us. Could you develop this?

CHARLES MELMAN: I would say that we have a peaceful, easy relationship with the real, which is easy. What comes to us from the real, what we can look at was made for us, so that we can take jouissance from it. And the first pages of Genesis tell us this. The myths in which we function are essential for us. It is good, it was seen that it was good, and therefore it was made for us. You dislocate yourself therefore in your world and a little extra thing could emerge for you. In populations which don't have this kind of – aberration – the relationship with the real is much more persecutory and one could say of a paranoiacal style. But our categories are not the same for all these cases. In the relationship to the real, there is always a fear, there is a necessity for identification.

But, you, you will say: Oh, it's just something small, it's a thing – and you won't need to say anything else. You don't need to give it a name. You will see little flowers, we are all nearly illiterate in botany, but we have no worries at all. We know that the little flowers are there so that things will be pretty and there will be a nice scent. Look at what happens with these populations, these people in their rapport with vegetation for example, it's a different relation. There is a necessary procedure of identification, which, by the way is infinitely more knowledgeable, wiser than the other kind. Finally, I won't go into these ethnographical things which are very wise, very complicated, very difficult: there is a separation of what is good, what is not good, what has to be avoided, there are areas of the real which are forbidden, where one should not go. The real is inhabited by beings we do not know, which can be made known, but which will often gladly represent maleficent, hostile wills. It is therefore a mode of apprehension of another style. It is constructed differently.

QUESTION: You have spoken about the problem of disgust as if it were yes or no, but is it not a mixture of the two, which means that it cannot be tolerated?

CHARLES MELMAN: It's still a little ambiguous. It's true that there is a big dividing: this is good, that is not good. This is edible, that is not. This is poisonous, that is not. But I'm thinking of certain texts where this kind of division is not so radical and where in the interior of what may be good could appear subdivisions, or even mutations. I'm thinking in particular of Pierre Clastre's book[14] where this kind of situation is fairly well developed. But no matter what, I always use if this as an illustration to help us understand that our rapport with the real has no natural support. It is an artificial relationship. That what we call nature is a construction. It is a construction we owe because of our reference to the father.

QUESTION: In fact, this brings up a differentiation, between animism, paganism and monotheism?

CHARLES MELMAN: When we authorise ourselves from a father creator of the world, etc. this has effects. We are within it, it goes without saying. What I'm saying is that our rapport with the real is of a certain kind, a certain mode and that the real for us is constructed for our jouissance, for our agreement. It was made so that we can enjoy it there. That's great, it's cute. But, when psychoanalysis intervenes with its history of castration by saying that it is broken, that it doesn't work, it is clear that this is not without creating problems.

16 November 1982

Notes

1 W. Reich, *The Function of the Orgasm*. New York: Touchstone Books, 1974.
2 S. Freud, *Beyond the Pleasure Principle and Other Works*, Vol. XVIII, S.E. (1920–1922). London: The Hogarth Press, 1955.
3 J. Lacan, *Dialogue avec les Philosophes Français*. Société Française de Philosophie, 23 February 1957.
4 J. Lacan, *The Seminar of Jacques Lacan, Book XX: Encore, 1972–1973* (trans. C. Gallagher, unedited).
5 K. Abraham, "A Short Study of the Development of the Libido", in *Selected Papers on Psychoanalysis*. London: Routledge, 1988.
6 J. Lacan, "Variations on the Standard Treatment" in *Écrits* (trans. B. Fink). New York: W.W. Norton & Co., 2006.
7 S. Freud, *New Introductory Lectures on Psychoanalysis and Other Works*, Vol. XXII, S.E. (1932–1936). London. The Hogarth Press, 1964.
8 A. Gide, *The Immoralist* (trans. D. Watson). London: Penguin Classics, 2008.
9 J. Lacan, *La Troisième*. VII Congress of the Freudian School of Paris, Rome, November 1974.
10 J. Locke, *An Essay Concerning Human Understanding* ed. P.H. Nidditch). Oxford: Clarendon Press, 1979.
11 Dr. Escoffier Lambiotte, 1923–1996, medical doctor and journalist who was the Medical Correspondent for *Le Monde*, 1956–1988.
12 J. Lacan, *The Seminar of Jacques Lacan, Book XVI: From an Other to the Other, 1969–1970* (trans. C. Gallagher, unedited).
13 J. Lacan, *The Seminar of Jacques Lacan, Book III: The Psychoses, 1955–1956* (ed. J-A. Miller, trans. R. Grigg). London: Routledge, 1993.
14 P. Clastres, *Society Against the State: Essays in Political Anthropology* (trans. R. Hurley). New York: Zone Books, 1990.

Chapter 11

A Christmas seminar

Charles Melman

I'm going to give a Christmas seminar. I will try to give everyone what he desires. The only problem is what everyone desires, as you know, is precisely what he does not want. So, I will try to distribute from now on, what everyone wants. But, you know also that what he wants is exactly what he does not desire. To introduce things like this, is to speak about the difficulty there is in distributive justice, because this division is that of the subject, founded on, dissatisfaction. The subject supports himself only by dissatisfaction. That is why he holds on to it so much. That is why this dissatisfaction is the strongest resistance at the end of analysis. The subject holds on to his symptom because it is from this and from this dissatisfaction that he ex-sists as a subject. And it is from this that he is able to enjoy it, as if he were another. He enjoys obeying the law and this dissatisfaction heightens for him what he imagines at the same time to be a filiation.

If we begin with what supports the subject – the subject of dissatisfaction, that is to say, the hysterical subject, there is no other, that is why to speak about hysteria is really to speak about everybody because in speaking about the subject – what makes a commandment for the speak-being, the king of domestic animals as we know? Nothing other than a place. This place is managed by the failure of the signifier, in its attempt to take hold of the lost object. And, we have to underline the paradox that this lost object does not obviously pre-exist the signifier because it is the signifier, in its very attempt, which constitutes it.

What makes a commandment for the speak-being is a place or rather: a definite hole, not to stay in a rather vague image, as the symbolic is unable to reduce what covers the imaginary of the phantasy.[1] The imaginary of the phantasy is necessary, to give a meaning to what the Autre demands, would demand of us. It's this object demanded by the Autre, which founds the desire of the subject. The condition of the speak-being is without doubt to imagine what the Autre demands of us, faeces for example, so that henceforth we find ourselves filled by a phantasy, supported by such an object.

To write about the human condition, it is not necessary to engage in a study or in a phenomenology of cowardice, it is more essential to interest

DOI: 10.4324/9781003167839-11

ourselves in the way the phantasy constructs us. Therefore, what makes a commandment for us is a place, a place which we imagine is occupied by a real object, the *objet a*. In advancing this, I believe I'm being faithful to the intelligence of language. If we look in Ernout and Meillet's dictionary, the etymology of the verb *facere* which gives us our "faire" (to make) we find, in a first meaning, an original one, "to put, to place, to pose", to put into place. From where the second meaning, which does not go without saying either: "to place oneself – to pose oneself" (or "to put oneself"). From where the third meaning and in this way is derived the meaning of "faire", *facere sacrum*, "to make a sacrifice", in other words, beginning with what is placed on the altar, *facere* has passed to the sense of "to make", of which the original sense is to make a sacrifice. And then, without any difficulty *facere* comes to mean the act *par excellence*, and brings a whole series of derived meanings of which the most frequent are to "talk", to "excite", to "work". As we can see, there is an intelligence in the usage of a language which can reassure or comfort us on our way.

From this place, possibly occupied by the *objet a* (because the phantasy is not an obligatory condition, one can be in a certain rapport with language, without being caught by the phantasy, but let us leave that) the signifier One takes its authority. Why? Although it's not as an authority that it operates, or a kind of magical accomplishment, it is because this place will vectorise the signifying chain, will lead it. Therefore, it will be from this place that the signifier One, which is written S_1, will take meaning and from then on an imperative value – of the task always to be accomplished, since the speak-being will never reach his term because he misses the object. In what I'm describing for you, with the establishing of the signifier One, you will recognise the super ego. The super ego reminds you every morning that your task has not been accomplished, that you should do it.

The problem is that the meaning which S_1 takes, in being animated by this place, finds itself strangely doubled and contradictory. As you know, logic constructs itself in eliminating contradiction, (the propositions A and not A cannot hold together, it's one or the other) as all reasoning is done in a general manner. If you wish, Socrates thinks about the incompatibility of contraries. And yet, what the superego illustrates for us, is that a perfectly contradictory consistence functions at the heart of the speak-being. In fact, what are the two meanings which S_1 brings with it?

The first is well known. S_1 commands castration for the subject, for the speak-being, beginning with a renunciation, a transfer of the object. But we see in the clinic (I will give examples), that because a pact was not made with the Autre, this demand of a renunciation is able for example to go as far as emasculation, or even demanding the gift of life. It's here it will find the articulation of the famous archaic superego, which Lacan takes up by the way as the desire of the mother to reintegrate her product.[2]

What happens for Schreber?[3] He is prey to these signifiers, to this signifying chain, without any pacification by transferring something of himself. He fights for months until he has this illumination and understands that he is inscribed in the order of the universe, what the Autre demands of him is emasculation. He makes this pact with this Autre on the condition of feminisation, a shaky pact which in not finding any symbolic sanction, is maintained only by an imaginary location. He is obliged to rig himself out and always be in front of the mirror. You can see how close this disposition is to Lacan's Schema L.[4] Seeing himself in the mirror Schreber is able to imagine the benevolent look of the Autre, and this procedure allows him, to find a subjective position for a while. He writes in the preface to his book that this is also an attempt to be recognised by an other, in the legitimacy of his get-up, in comforting him on the absurd constraint of the mirror, and thereby benefiting from a recognition by an other of this new feminine nature as conforming to the divine order. Lacan says that the Abbot of Choisy[5] could not think without putting into place the same kind of procedure. This is the first meaning exercised by S_1, the invitation to an unlimited castration, resumed in what is called the archaic superego.

The second meaning is apparently in contradiction to the first. This S_1, on condition of an intervention linked to the paternal signifier, commands the speak-being to enjoy. That is to say, this transformation means that the second S_1 can be named S_2 to describe the fact that not only is it second, but it occupies a different place to S_1, that its topology is therefore different. Henceforth, this S_2 finds itself offered to jouissance. I'm saying that this procedure is linked to the intervention of this paternal signifier, that is to say what links castration to a duty of a jouissance, nevertheless invited to go to its term. Castration, is, to be more precise, the fact of having to renounce the impossible capture of the body of the maternal Autre. This is impossible, as the Autre constitutionally infinite, will not be captured. When this happens in practice, incest, which is the fact that the Autre loses this characteristic of infinity, has subjective consequence which can be somewhat disturbing. This is the totally absurd and eminently contradictory character of the superego. As we learned from Lacan the superego says "Enjoy the fact that you are a being who changes, who takes over who is submitted to the order of hearing, you have to enjoy, and you have to enjoy to the very end, even though it is prohibited by me."[6] No matter what, a woman, will occupy this Autre place whether she wants to or not. The speak-being does not choose in this affair, this has nothing to do with her feeling or her arbitrary freedom, she will find herself in some way caught in representation: she is led to represent this power in a two-sided way. Her eventual consent to present herself as an object of jouissance, that is to say as a response to the provocative imperative of the superego, ensures that she registers herself in paternal law. But this eventual consent (it is not obligatory) willingly doubles itself with another side: a reminder to the partner to castrate himself more, because despite her efforts and her risks to hold this place of an offered object, presented, agreeing to sexual jouissance, indeed, her union with her partner stumbles over the failure of sexual rapport. There is always in some way a virtual game here, which is always possible. For example, I will take very nice examples obviously, the invitation to the partner to work harder. I will remind you of this little thing in Lacan, which seems to have been enigmatic during a soirée the evening before: the proletarian, returning home, called his wife the bourgeoise because, whether one of them wanted to or not, she took her place where the very process of exploitation is articulated. Whether or not she consents to offer herself as an object of jouissance and/or at the same time invite castration, a woman inevitably occupies this mistress position, she is the representative and the S_1 seeming to hold her power only through delegation. Is it necessary to show the number of times, where the husband presents himself only as the representative, the instrument, the megaphone, the delegate of the spouse?[7]

You will refind here if you wish, this other formulation which is the hysterical wish (that is to say the wish of the subject) as it happens, a feminine one: "to have a master on whom she could reign".[8] You see the game: S_1 the master she arouses, creates, maintains, to whom she delegates a power, but on whom she can rule from this place, from this space. And, we also know if the master in some way shies away from this reign, he becomes like a tyrant.

It's therefore from the Autre that the power is exercised, all power, even when a subject engages with a transfer of the *objet a,* which in some way makes the case worse. Why? The Autre on its own, is of the order of indetermination, unpredictable, unlimited. The transfer of the object, by the speak-being, even if this transfer is purely symbolic and even if this object is purely imaginary, introduces an order into the Autre, which from then on knots the subject to his jouissance. But, spontaneously, a confusion is made obviously between the Autre and the small *a.*

In other words, when we treat the Autre as a small *a*, we are persuaded that there is in the Autre someone who guides us, who leads us. It is not too much to say that if it is true that for the speak-being, this is how all power moves along, makes a commandment, the art of governing is always done from this place. It is precisely this confusion between the Autre and the little *a* the speak-beings that we are, will enjoy this very exploitation. You will refind a formulation of Lacan in *L'Etourdit* where he says, "The slave is a serf",[9] not of the master – it's I who adds this but the "serf of jouissance" and it is really this which supports him in his servitude. There is obviously here a condition, which the men of the art of governing know very well. In order to govern, it is necessary for the slave, so that things can work, to be persuaded that the other enjoys his sacrifice. In other words, that the other is a free man. A free man, someone who is not submitted to castration, who escapes and therefore the jouissance of he who occupies this place will profit from all that the slave sacrifices, to find himself in this way satisfied.

This is a perfectly verifiable supposition. What is peculiar to the master, to this free man is to be in the shade of the phantasy, that is to say to bore himself (I'm following here indications which you will find in Lacan's texts) not to know what he wants, not to know what he desires. This free man is in a very particular rapport with regard to the symbolic – a rapport of a game – and not of an I. (There is an equivocation *Jeu* and *Je* in French) because it is not the phantasy. I would go so far as to say that the game, it is this, to use the symbolic, but in showing how one can never be taken in by it, never smitten by it. In other words, to ensure that this rapport with the symbolic never goes beyond the dimension of caprice. Of course, there are obviously subjects who get themselves into the game, that is to say, they seek just how far that can go. We find here the face of this archaic superego: this can go as far as the gift of life. It is not really any more in our mores, but you know for example that in the 19th century the great distraction for the masters, was to finish by a duel, the measure of which they were not able to assume. What does this mean? This means that one gives to the Autre the last thing which remains.

A little digression which is perhaps not futile. It is quite amazing that someone of the quality of Winnicott[10] could theorise the analytic relation itself as a game, that is to say as a kind of manipulation of the symbolic but without engaging seriously with it: it was only at the end of the day a way of playing! You see how that clashes with what I'm saying. We have to see here the attempt by Winnicott to resolve, to put an end to the difficult question of the transference and its resolution. Like as if one said to the patient "You see it is like a cricket field, the 'cabinet' of the analyst or the couch, we are here only to play, isn't that right?" Lacan does not veer in this sense at all, he, on the contrary thinks that the transferential relationship is the most authentic and the most decisive, the most definitive in the relationship of the subject to the symbolic order. Lacan did not at all think that the analytic procedure was for laughs.

But, to stay with any kind of problems of government, it is really clear that a regime could fall down at any time: when the masters become jealous of the jouissance of the slaves. At the risk of being bored, they would really like a taste, a little bit of sandwich – Louis XVI had his establishment and Marie Antoinette her nursery, that's how it went. Inversely, a regime – it does not matter its forms or its aberrations, it's of absolutely no importance – only holds when the discourse of the master is applied there without any regard for the good of the serf, but in the affirmation of jouissance which the serf can assure for the master. That the serf can take his own good there sometimes, this is not the business of the master. In these cases, it holds well, it holds really well. Those among you who nowadays associate with true masters, know that their personnel adore them, no matter what their political colour happens to be.

Is this inevitable? With these unhappy problems with which analysts themselves are confronted, do we have to follow Freud who constituted the I.P.A. as a society of patrons?

Is it necessary to say that if we wish among ourselves, as analysts, that things will work, we will have to take adequate measures? In this affair, utopia has nothing to do with it. It is important to be realistic, which has only one meaning for an analyst, that is to say the conformity which the structure will or will not make possible. Do we have to make the great social bond last forever?

We could be tempted, but there is a small problem, which is that this famous division between S_1 and S_2 is intra-subjective. And what is amazing, is what functions as a social bond is ordered from the inter-subjective distribution of this division. But if this intra-subjective division will found the model of the intersubjective relation, then the social bond will be knotted as if it were the relation with the Autre which gave the model of the relation with a fellow. One will take the value of being all, all One, all master, and the slave will guarantee by his work the jouissance of this master, which could not be then anything other than purely narcissistic. In other words, the exploitation of this slave will assure a service he will take on himself which will henceforth be the fault of castration.

Why castration as a fault?

The slave cannot respond to the master in a mirror position where he will be like a master himself. That would be, after all the proper response, it would give satisfaction to the master who may feel this in a disobliging way that the other, the small other, his fellow, is always deficient, is never really up to it. But the slave cannot do this because if he himself were in a position of mastery, that would abolish his relation to his master – from the mirror stage, a symmetry is impossible. He cannot guarantee the illusion of mastery from he who takes up this position, except in working to satisfy him. Why the "illusion" of mastery? We know that the word of the subject works itself from a place which escapes all mastery, that this mastery is constitutionally flawed. It is the place of truth in the four discourses that speaks about castration which the discourses try to resolve. In the discourse of the Master, it's the $, that is to say the subject, the hysteric.

But we benefit from a discourse which helps us to go a step further and affirm the illusory nature of this mastery, that is to say, points to this place as being that of the semblant.

And yet, what interests us in all this, is that the social bond which we know no matter what, is thereby founded on a denial of castration. The work of one is charged with assuring the totalitarity, even the totalitarianism of an other. And we can understand how the denial of this castration, insofar as it is foundational of the social bond, supports, between what Lacan calls in *L'Etourdit*,[11] not only two classes but two races, an exacerbation grounded on a mutual dissatisfaction, the mother of conflicts without any end because equality, always imagined, always dreamed about, is a utopia. Why? Because it is not authorised by the structure, which only authorises two places which are fundamentally asymmetrical and unequal.

Then, what did Lacan wish to say when he spoke about a new social bond which would be in some way, consistent with analytic discourse?[12] Some people understand this from a text where Lacan says that it has to do essentially with the relationship between analyst and analysand which is a place of two people.[13] Others say that it has to do with a text in *L'Etourdit*, where Lacan seems to say that it has to do with a general social bond.[14] What, indeed, could that be?

Firstly, it is clear that psychoanalytic discourse does not in any way put the two places in peril, that of the agent on top and to the left and then that of the other or the object.

These places belong to every discourse. But to say that the place of mastery, the place of S_1, the original, is also that of the semblant invites us, if we agree, to occupy these places only with a certain lightness and not to participate in denial of castration with an obstinate perseverance, unsociable or too engaged in the bond with the other. Because it has to do with restoring the division between S_1 and S_2, as intra-subjective, and to live it first of all as intra-subjective. It is necessary to extract a kind of ambiance on what would be the best place. That people who are from one side aspire to go to the other and do everything to achieve this, even succeeding, is really the sign that on each side things are not going too well. Therefore, the problem is not to engage in value judgements, nor even "therapeutic" points of view – jouissance is found on the side of the slave. It has to do with knowing if analytic discourse is capable of making a guess as to what a social bond could be – which is not nothing, obviously. From then on, that which founds "the line" destined to occupy one or other side is interrupted, because this discourse does away with the idea that there is a nomination which would in some kind of way qualify you once and for all. In the past, this nomination could be hereditary, transmitted from father to son. Or it could be arbitrary and you were named by such and such an authority to take up a position there. Today, this nomination has taken a scientific side, those are named as masters who give witness to a knowledge, of an acquisition of knowledge, of capacities, of a talent which makes them apt to occupy this position. As we know, this functions in an optic "of progress".

It is inevitable that analytic discourse will come up against this kind of procedure. To conclude, let us examine what it suggests. You know how it is conceived – in the place of the agent, on the left we put the *objet a*. These are the diverse objects of our phantasies, which will command us and reveal themselves as such. This is what you obey.

But another reading is possible. Let us take the voice, the totally pure voice as it can be heard in certain circumstances, for example, in the glossolalia which we are soon going to study. This voice will take its place here among the objects, only if it will respond to what in the Autre is a fundamental silence, a first silence. Proust wrote[15] a note to his mother scolding her because she had spent an evening with a man. And his mother made him say "there is no response". That was an extraordinary trauma for Marcel. Yes, what commands, it is this, it's that there is no response.

Then, if the message received is what is found in the position of the other at the top and on the right, the $, if there is a distinction made between The Autre and *a* because there is no response, the question becomes: what does it want itself insofar as the $ would want it?

- And, there is at the bottom and on the right, the S_1, at the place of what is produced if one holds the analytic discourse, that is to say by an address to the Autre. No longer objects assumed for jouissance, but nothing other than S_1.
- The same ones as those which constitute, which found it and are constituted only by unary traits.
- And then what is in a position of truth, at the bottom and to the left, that is to say S_2. That is to say that once the turn has been completed what remains for the subject, well, it is to accomplish his jouissance S_2. That is without doubt the meaning of Freud's *Wo Es war soll Ich werden*,[16] it is also the meaning on what the first Rome discourse concludes:[17] to bring the subject to the term where he can realise on what he depends. This will not have been a useless detour – there were schools of philosophy which came to that conclusion without having to do all this legwork – if we consider the context henceforth, a new one, of this kind of relationship with the partner, or with a fellow, no matter who, that such a way allows us to introduce.

The next time, that is to say the 11th of January, I will begin from here, to take on board a general economy of hysteria.

14 December 1982

Notes

1 J. Lacan, *The Seminar of Jacques Lacan, Book XIV: The Logic of Phantasy, 1966–1977* (trans. C. Gallagher, unedited).
2 J. Lacan, "Family Complexes in the Formation of the Individual" in *Encyclopédie Française*, Vol. 8. (ed. A. de Monzie). Paris, 1938 (trans. C. Gallagher, unedited).
3 S. Freud, *The Case of Schreber, Papers on Technique and Other Works*, Vol. XII, S.E. (1911–1913). London: The Hogarth Press, 1958.
4 J. Lacan, "On a Question Preliminary to any Possible Treatment of Psychosis" in *Écrits* (trans. B. Fink). New York: W.W. Norton & Co., 2006.
5 Abbé de Choisy, *The Transvestite Memoirs* (trans. R.H.F. Scott). London: Peter Owen Publishers, 1973.
6 J. Lacan, *The Seminar of Jacques Lacan, Book XX: Encore, 1972–1973* (trans. C. Gallagher, unedited).
7 Lacan, *Book XX: Encore*, "Even though it is prohibited by me" (Charles Melman).
8 J. Lacan, *The Seminar of Jacques Lacan, Book XVII: The Other Side of Psychoanalysis, 1969–1970* (trans. C. Gallagher, unedited).
9 J. Lacan, *L'Étourdit*, Lacan 1972 (trans. C. Gallagher unedited), unpublished.
10 D. Winnicott, *Playing and Reality*. Foreword by F.R. Rodham. New York: Routledge, 2005.

11   J. Lacan, *L'Étourdit*, Lacan 1972 (trans. C. Gallagher, unedited), unpublished.

12   Lacan, *Book XVII: The Other Side of Psychoanalysis.*

13   J. Lacan, *The Seminar of Jacques Lacan, Book VIII: Transference, 1960–1961* (trans. C. Gallagher, unedited).

14   Lacan, *L'Étourdit.*

15   M. Proust, *In Search of Lost Time* (trans. A. Mayor, revised by G.J. Enright). New York: Random House Inc., 2014.

16   S. Freud, *New Introductory Lectures on Psychoanalysis and Other Works*, Vol. XXII, S.E. (1932–1936). London: The Hogarth Press, 1964.

17   J. Lacan, "The Function and Field of Speech and Language in Psychoanalysis" in *Écrits* (trans. B. Fink). New York: W.W. Norton & Co., 2006.

Chapter 12

The economy of hysteria

Charles Melman

Our weakness is that we always have a tendency to think in terms of object relations while the foundational relationship is constructed not with the object, but with the lack of an object.[1] Henceforth, we have to do not with behaviour, but symptoms – to speak about object relations represses the existence of the symptom. Also, there cannot be an analytic anthropology, just a clinic. And, if the philosophers have presented our relation to the world as being founded on the dominance of the shadow projected on to the bottom of the cavern, psycho-analytic practice is without precedent, when it shows that it is the lack of the object which constitutes subjectivity. Also, we will not be surprised that it is subjectivity which takes this lack of the object into account and that it defines itself as being always guilty, guilty of being here, guilty for existing.

We can understand hysteria as the demonstration of efforts made to try and regulate this account. And, from the determination of the subject by the lack of the object – beginning with the phantasy,[2] I will suggest a formula which may permit us to articulate a large part of the economy of hysteria $ \Diamond a$. It is $ one side, the a on the other, knotted, joined one with the other, by the inferior part of the lozenge, which we can read as $ vel a. The vel which is noted V is exclusive, of course. In so far as one is a hysteric, one is a subject, one is asked to put oneself on one side or the other: either $ or else a. This alternative is the big way in which the hysteric will try to resolve the impasse of her fundamental guilt and I will immediately give a first expression of this.

Either, $, that is to say a pure subjectivity, in other words locatable and expressible uniquely by the affirmation of its exteriority, of its ex-sistence. By the same token, the affirmation of a radically strange rapport, with the darkness of a world to which nothing attaches this $ and, as an effect, a kind of affective anaesthesia (it can go as far as being bodily) which contrasts with the manifestations of invasion, of an affective submersion capable of provok-ing an identification – it does not matter what, an image of someone etc. It is as if this identification is a mode of entry, a way of transitory participation in this world, the only method to assure a presence there. This subjective posi-tion, pure, exterior, detached from the link to the object a, as you can find it, if I believe what somebody told me, in a recent film, *E.T.*, which seems to be

DOI: 10.4324/9781003167839-12

constructed entirely around this game which causes a lot of tears – there is good cause for it indeed.

Or a. On the other side of this *vel*, there is the position of the *objet a*, that is to say an engagement with the world from the relationship to the Autre, a taken position, concerned by the desire of the Autre, which also addresses itself to one's fellow. But this engagement has the particularity of being total, that is to say to exclude, at the moment it is produced, all division, all subjective detachment.

As if the alternative were either a separation: a division without engagement, or else a total engagement excluding from then on all subjective division, all detachment, all distance. Besides, it is not unusual, this alternative – of which one could say everything or nothing – is produced alternatively in the same person, without some paradoxes in his behaviour. In any case, it seems to me that we consider it as the matrix of attempts made by the hysteric to cure herself of castration. Let us try and enlarge a little on the consequences and manifestations.

To live her subjectivity as perfectly estranged from the world is one of the faces of the beautiful soul.[3] It has to do with a refusal to see herself in the image of her fellow and in the economy her fellow holds, whether it has to do with a libidinal economy or very simply a market one. But, by this very refusal a privileged filiation is affirmed, a particular election in so far as it is an exception, with a father who finds himself complicit in this refusal. (I will develop this point a little later on). This subject affirms, constructs his exceptional character on denial or on the repression of every desire, that is to say on the gift that he will make of his desire to the Autre. We have already seen that. What will allow us to advance a little, is that this mode of imaginary rapport with one's fellow finds itself preformed by the mirror phase. It is one of the paradoxes we encounter, the mirror phase is constructed on a fundamental dissymmetry, because the image of the other, the small other, only takes its brilliance, and at the same time its formative power, from being supported by the *objet a.* You will find this in the example, always quoted by Lacan, the birth of *l'invidia*, of envy, pointed out by St Augustine as a child looking at his brother at the breast, that is to say in this exact position where he will be supported, organised by this object *a.*[4] This dissymmetry is the same for each of the partners, because for both of them the image of the other is held up by this brilliance but these relations do not hold in the time of specular reality, but in relation to this time with the structure. And yet, in this relation which organises itself in this dissymmetrical mode, the particularity of the hysteric is to take part. She (or he) takes part in what could be a conflict of separation, of war, a battle for mastery, for recognition. The hysteric leaves it straightaway to the other, to her fellow, who from then on is imagined as perfection and as master of the image, and represents herself (or himself) as animating a deficient form, indeed somewhat enigmatic; fragile, threatened with break-up. And this, because of a failure to make oneself recognised as another, as a small other, by this fellow henceforth invested.

What is commonly called the coquettishness or the seduction by the hysteric (him or her) can find its first origins in this disposition. This attempt to make herself recognised is impervious, it does not depend on the good or ill will of this fellow. But this presents a double risk. To sin by default, in failing to capture, to keep this fellow will confirm the inadequacy of the imago in question (her own). But it is one of the paradoxes, to triumph would reverse the roles and risk tipping the mastery to the side of the hysteric. We will see later that this is a risk, for precise reasons, which is not avoided. Discord borders, therefore, on both sides of the relationship to the other and the margin is thin. That can give a particular style to a behaviour constituting back and forth, apparently contradictory, the hysteric "does not know what she (he) wants". Because it is fundamentally about a demand for love, and when it is eventually satisfied, it is not unusual that it proves difficult to tolerate.

This latter is marked by the stamp of a fundamental misunderstanding, because what is demanded is nothing other than a recognition and this demand appears strange to someone, for whom it is not a question. This demand for recognition cannot of course be heard except by someone who finds himself in the same position.

What is outlined here is a very original economy. The interesting point is that in this dual dissymmetrical relationship, the hysteric renounces the conflict from the outset, to engage in a movement which resembles, a gift made to the other, to her fellow. What is given, as *objet a*, the hysteric renounces (in so far as *objet a* holds her image) it is obviously what she has not got. It is therefore a gift of love which is proposed instead of war, with a call to reciprocity, to equality in the renunciation. But from then on, it is the slave – to take up the famous couple – who holds the recognition, with the possibility or not, of according this gift of his love to be who will dub himself master.

Cinema and literature have exploited the question, to a large extent, as to which side mastery is really situated in this ambiguity of relations between master and slave. This economy of the gift validates itself from a support taken in the Autre, from a reference to a father who is no longer the God of the armies, but is the God of true love. He does not order, but consents to make masters of His creatures, at the price of His own humility, at the price of His own weakness, at the price of the gift of His love. This arrangement may call to reciprocity, incite the creature to sacrifice his mastery for Him. And the circularity of the system allows us to catch the representation of this God constructed on pure love, which commands us from His gift. This representation can gladly take the traits of the child, his weakness. And in familial organisations constructed on the lore of gods, no matter what their explicit references – we know how the child can be the pivotal organiser of the familial economy, under the mode of being a token of this god.

A new sliding operates: the subject supports himself from a position of exteriority, of strangeness to the world, that is to say from a solitude which leads him to enjoy the feeling of his own uniqueness, especially if he always has the complicity of a father, imagined as homogenous because this dead father himself is supported from a position of exteriority. It is in his place, in place of his father, that the subject, organised in this exteriority is supported. And one of the difficulties in taking up the question of hysteria, is the hope of keeping a mystery around the existence of the father. To deal with the subject, in dealing with hysteria, is, by the same token to deal with the father and it is to here raise a cover which should not be done without reticence. This father can be that of a revealed religion, or a private religion, or an intimate religion.

It is by the reference to a father, in this organisation, from this uniqueness, the subject finds himself exposed to a collective identification. The unique but decisive sign is that the members of this collective recognise each other not by the fact of having it, but I will simply say, by the fact of not having it. It is precisely a mode of the hysterical dialectic. I do not wish to immediately introduce our categories but the problem is the following: the hysteric can recognise herself only in a collective identification with participants in some way marked by this trait, marked by some lack. If we refer to Freud's paper on "Identification",[5] it is, for the friend of the boarder, that this lack amounts to not having received a letter from her boyfriend. It can be all we imagine, but that is the condition of belonging to a collective. From this all, collective epidemics are organised when this fault takes on the aspect of a coarsened collective demand.

We here encounter this fundamental arrangement which, for the hysteric will therefore divide speak-beings between those who come from the category of having and those from the category of not having. This kind of inter-pretation will construct the division between the sexes – and not the contrary. This is a totally new situation, because henceforth, we have to deal with a unique category, those who have and those who do not have.

This kind of inequality is resolved by an economy of a reciprocal gift, but also by therapy. I mean that the privileged relation the hysteric has to the doctor can be understood as marking the passage from frustration to priva-tion. The interpretation of frustration, as it were privation, – the real lack of a symbolic object – introduces us directly to the terrain of medicine, with the expectation that this will connect what, from then on, is nothing other than an accident, even a malformation.

This affirmed extra-territoriality of the subject, that is to say the renuncia-tion of what could sustain his desire, is worth an existence, the same time deprived of a project, of an intention, an orientation. Here is an existence destined to find itself tossed back and forth, in a wandering which is not only subjective but also geographically realised.

In the same way, the mode of rapport with a fellow, with the other, finds itself taken in this failure of determination, of orientation, of vectorisation, marked by an unpredictability, a risky character of affects, such as humour – to the surprise of the messenger as well as to the one for whom it is destined. Because, as I have said, the dynamism of the project is restrained, between the repetition of an effort to be recognised by one's fellow and the risk of a flight from then on, which this effort could finally end.

The feeling of solitude and uniqueness can be interrupted by a collective identification, an identification with others who find themselves marked by the same failure. The meeting permits a birth to the world, with the attachment to one's fellow, representative of this ex-sistence. The subject finds himself comforted with the idea that he who is the truly loved one of the father, the truly chosen one, is really the one who has renounced this object and has made of it the gift of love.

But I mentioned in relation to the mirror stage, the frustration reverses itself into a voluntary sacrifice, which henceforth becomes the sign of a real mastery, because the collective identification is the witness of what is indeed finally demanded by the Autre, and on that condition one is his loved and chosen one. Mastery is the more true because it exercises not only from S_1 who authorises the fellow but from the object itself, on whom S_1 confers its authority, this object a of which the hysteric invokes the property in the Autre in its name because its sacrifice is instituted there. There is then the possibility of laying down its authority and in asking for the organ itself, even the instrument of the Autre, of his voice, for example – all these instruments, all these organs have obviously a phallic connotation. By this reversal, one passes to the other side of the small V, from the side of the object a, and installs itself there as a totalitarian project, that is to say the demand for a realisation of totality. What's more, this identification, exercises itself with regard to S_1 or he whom it represents, by demanding that S_1, is up to it.

This movement of oscillation, which in a disarticulation of the phantasy, means that the subject takes hold as much as from the side of $ and poses himself in a pure exteriority, as from the side of object a, permits us to regroup the large forms of clinical hysteria, according to two modes which are apparently paradoxical. One form which I would say is depressive, is ravaged by a lived frustration as an infirmity, affirmed as irreducible. And, another form, hypersthenic is ravaged by the fact of authorising itself from the organ, even imagined from the other and assuring jouissance by responding to it as it likes. I've already said that these two big forms, depressive and hypersthenic can, in a way that is not exceptional, succeed each other in the same subject.

In any case, what holds together the dynamism of the hysteric is the guilt of castration. This taking hold of oneself, as $, of castration is mainly made from an altruistic preoccupation. It has to do with protecting one's fellow, who is thereby put in the shade because the weight of failure is taken on oneself, but also protects the father by conserving children for him, who would be up to the mark. It is the same worry to protect the others who will make the hysteric run away, whether or not he is successful in his quest for recognition, because his image risks contaminating them by looking. From where this putting aside, this voluntary retreat judged to be salutary.

In this way, hysteria participates in private or social dialogue with his friend, her friend, or in the collectivity, in a paradoxical situation. He/she feels it is an imperative to have to face even though he/she lives life as pure imposture in a specular reciprocity, putting to her account the category of the semblant and lending to her fellow human being the category of the true image.

This kind of habilitation holds what is felt as the role of the substitute, of a replacement – a role destined to take the diverse forms of supposed objects of desire of one's fellow, to keep oneself in this specularity – shows the finesse and the subtleness of the hysterical position (and her predisposition to the activity of an analyst). This apperception of the form called in such and such a circumstance tends to be an expression of – in the category, in some way, of making function – as what compensates for castration. This could go very far, because the hysteric could propose herself as a substitute for those who seem to be failures. And, in the demand for the totality which I evoked earlier, she can be led, when she is a woman, to take the place of the male partner, because the poor chap finds himself irreducibly castrated, that is to say timorous. Or else, and this is not a slight paradox, that of the dear professor whose knowledge is certainly very elaborated, very beautiful, but who remains impotent in the face of hysteria, for example. That is not to say that this necessarily pleases him, this role of function-making, this replacing those who bear witness to the mark of castration.

I think we can see there the trajectory of diverse possible moments of an elaboration, or of a dialectic which, since the recognition of oneself as marked by a failure, brings to this position, where there has to be, on the contrary, a substitution for those who find themselves marked with this kind of insufficiency, with this kind of failure. But, what makes the failure of the enterprise (in general, because there are exceptions) is the fact that the hysteric only accedes to this position on the condition that her replacement is not "titled". This stays at the level of function-making for an extremely simple reason. As the hysteric does not have the ultimate testimonial of this recognition by the father, there is this fear that to find herself with a title will jeopardise this phallic organisation on which she depends, this is a totally banal thing.

When Lacan says "the hysteric it's the woman who makes the man",[6] this can be heard in different ways: because of her position, it's she who supports the man and who "makes" him, or else, or it is she who puts herself in his place, and she has to do this because he does not hold on, as he is supposed. There is the worry of looking after those who are only taken as an interim, in the majority of cases this does not veer towards feminine homosexuality for example, even though here are cases where it does, where finally the titularisation is passed.

I will conclude this evening with this. The formula $ \$ \diamond a $, presents an interest in collecting the kind of dialectic I've mentioned. It appears to be capable of taking into account the diversity of the clinic and of the to-ing and fro-ing of the hysteric, of a primordially altruistic worry, which animates her economy, but also the two great forms which are apparently paradoxical, because contradictory, which are: an exteriority branded as radically hetero-geneous to the world, and a total participation without a recoil, without division. As if the oscillation were played between the refusal of all affirmation, the refusal of all *Bejahung*,[7] and on the other hand what presents itself as being the absolute affirmation.

I propose, next week, a re-reading of *Dora* to try and clarify what we dealt with today. We will also take up again the privileged rapport with the father and that of the rapport with the woman. So, that's what I wanted to say to you this evening.

QUESTION: You have separated two major clinical forms. In the depressive form, I can see clearly how the goal is to protect ones fellow or to protect the father. But in the second one, the hypersthenic? I understood better when you talked of a way of putting into place a substitute which would try and supplement castration.

CHARLES MELMAN: It's not in any way contradictory. In the second case, it has to do with ensuring that the jouissance of the father is complete, to ensure that it would be an adequate jouissance. I will immediately give you an image with regard to the oedipal situation which will make the thing, perhaps – too clear. What is not tolerable is that the father, the real father in fact, is castrated. It is interpreted as a failure in the economy. And the demand that the jouissance of the father is total, without limits, is totally homogenous with the structure itself – the at least One etc. This is a supplementary reason, so that the castration of the real father can be heard as unsuitable, as a local accident. If the jouissance of the father were without a limit, the failure introduced in this economy would be lifted.

QUESTION: But, a jouissance without a limit, is it not to wish the father dead?

CHARLES MELMAN: You are right, but this is about the he who is already dead. The reference by which the real father is failing, it is the dead father, in any case, already dead. And then, the unconscious does not embarrass itself with this kind of, it is not even a contradiction, this kind of risk. This does not stop it making it coexist, to hold together the ensemble of impossibilities.

We can see how the ambition of the hysterical position is to cure not only herself but her fellow. And that is why there is this fundamental affinity of hysteria with the caring world. It is a therapeutic attempt, totally apt at repairing and interpreting the diversity of failures, and envisaging what measures of sacrifice and devotion to take. Of course, this also happens in the hypersthenic form, this is the position taken by Bertha Pappenheim after her psychotherapy with Breuer. It has to do every time with making a diagnosis, repairing what does not work and henceforth on devoting oneself to remedying the issue at the price of desire. There is also willingly in hysteria, this aspect of vocation – obviously to be heard as the articulation of what would be the voice of the Autre.

QUESTION: I'm aware of this kind of "aggrandisement", the dimension which you show to be universal of the structure which the hysteric has with the world and that this at the price of her desire. Is there also a universal position other than this mode of distribution in a hysterical style, in religion as well as in politics, etc?

CHARLES MELMAN: This is the essential question. Analytic discourse reverses this position because it proposes another articulation where desire will command the game. Therefore, totally other than renunciation.

QUESTION: In the trial at Moscow, how did the military revolutionaries get through, no matter their structure (obsessional, perverse, I don't know what else) from activism to militarism to self-accusation?

CHARLES MELMAN: The subject does not have to have committed any crime to be fundamentally guilty. Subjectivity is constructed on guilt, and it is with guilt that its ex-sistence is maintained. And therefore, it is experimentally the easiest thing to make him adjust to anything, all it takes is a little time. You are speaking about what I'm speaking about, it is the subjective position: what happens from the minute that subjectivity orders discourse. The manifestations, the expressions which follow, we put all these into the category of symptoms. This allows us to tackle them in totally different ways, not only an accident, coming from the bad or good will of the subject, but as a consequence of structure – and thereby making of the symptom that which speaks the truth of the structure and what it imposes on the speak-being.

11 January 1983

Notes

1   J. Lacan, *The Seminar of Jacques Lacan, Book IV: The Object Relation* (ed. J-A. Miller, trans. A.R. Price). Cambridge: Polity Press, 2020.

2   J. Lacan, *The Seminar of Jacques Lacan, Book XIV: The Logic of Phantasy, 1966–1967* (trans. C. Gallagher, unedited).

3   J. Lacan, "The Function and Field of Speech and Language in Psychoanalysis" in *Écrits* (trans. B. Fink). New York: W.W. Norton & Co., 2006.

4   Saint Augustine, *Confessions* (trans. H. Chadwick). Oxford: Oxford University Press, 2008.

5   S. Freud, "Identification" in *Beyond the Pleasure Principle, Group Psychology and Other Works*. Vol. XVIII, S.E. (1920–1922). London: The Hogarth Press, 1955.

6   J. Lacan, *The Seminar of Jacques Lacan, Book XVIII: On a Discourse that might not be a Semblance*, 1970–1971 (trans. C. Gallagher, unedited).

7   S. Freud, "Negation" in *The Ego and the Id and Other Works*, Vol. XIV, S.E. (1923–1925). London: The Hogarth Press, 1961.

Chapter 13

The ex-sistence of the subject

Charles Melman

What can be said of the subject is that he ex-sists and it is this ex-sistence which makes the consistency of the symbolic chain. We cannot say that this chain is articulated by the speak-being but only that the subject is an add-on, caught there, clinging insofar as he renders it consistent. That is to say that the subject testifies to at least one of a repressed signifier, *Uverdrängt*, he testifies to this signifier, which in the chain makes a break and at the same time gives it its consistency. In other words, this signifier *Urverdrängt*, if it is the cause of the cut, is the subject himself. No matter what, we know because of our work, that this ex-sistence finds itself filled with, holding on to the world by, the *obscenity* which is its cause and which is, as you know the *objet a*.

If there is produced in hysteria a repression of desire, maintained by this *objet a*, because this desire was renounced, or because it was denied or refused, this abandonment of desire which fills ex-sistence in the world will mean that this ex-sistence can no longer support itself except by its own heterotopy. Henceforth, from this place of ex-sistence, the subject, reduced to a glance, perceives the world as strange and cannot any more recognise himself in creatures who appear to him as being "cursorily improvised men" and animated by a complete farce (which Schreber called *Menschenspielerei*)[1] the scenarios of which appeared to him as vain and vile. But, such a glance works itself from this subjective position, everyone after all will, recognise his own. This glance of the eye becomes properly hysterical when it is put forward in a master position, in an organising position of this world itself. It is therefore inevitable that everyone, no matter what their position or their neurosis, will be able to recognise in the clinic of hysteria traits which are to do with him, because these are the inevitable complements of every subjective position. And, if one has a psychoanalytic clinic, we know that the couch forces the analysand to speak from a subjective position, in other words, the analytic operation is in itself hystericising. What's more, it is enough to remember that from the minute the analysand begins to speak as a master or a teacher, analysis cannot take place: it is one of the forms of resistance.

I became aware of this in writing about this putting into place, of a question which is not without interest and which we are accustomed to avoiding

DOI: 10.4324/9781003167839-13

and turning around. It is still a really serious question and which was in the past, discussed by very serious people. They met at a Concilium[2] to question whether or not women had a soul. It is a question which today we can reformulate in the following way: Does feminine castration exist? We are able therefore to isolate what is a subjectivity specific to the feminine, a word and a desire which is proper to her and permit us to immediately identify her: here, a woman is speaking. You know, there were for example, recent speculations on what could be a feminine writing. To be even more precise, *die Urvedrängung*, primary repression, is it different for her than for a man? Or is it only through an identification with him that a woman participates in the *Urverdrängung* of her man? In some way, she would make her own of the castration of her fellow, by participation, by sympathy (in the etymological sense of this term) but in always keeping the possibility of feeling this eminently alienating character – at the same level as her ego – of this castration induced in some way, by the game suggested by her fellow.

What does Freud say about whether there is a specifically feminine *Urverdrängung*, or an empathetic participation with the castration of her fellow? Freud engages with the question by saying that libido is the same for both sexes, which means that it is from this libido the same organ, finds itself the imaginary representative, but this very same organ, finally this unique *Urverdrängung*, identical for both sexes, will be the cause of dissymmetrical effects. This will organise his subjectivity for the man which will be felt as a fault in having, while for the woman, the fault will be felt as a fault in being – if we resume this distinction which is always pertinent. For the woman, it manifests itself in the worry about being recognised, and if it is what vectorises feminine desire, at the same time, the desire to reach it will be forbidden. Here, we find ourselves with one of the modalities of the hysterical impasse. We can therefore conclude, with assurance, that there is no specifically feminine repression, but a difference with regard to its subjective consequences, not with regard to the modality of the object, but of the desire which vectorises it. And this, without counting the specificity, properly feminine of an Autre desire, that is to say, other than phallic, but which presents, contrary to the precedent, the difficulty of being unfounded. Because of this desire Autre, there is no *Urvedrängung* here, which will organise and make a cut.

This all comes back to consider the paternal blessing, that is to say, castration – because it is nothing else – as being equally standard for both sexes. But it is not rare that a woman is unable to have the advantage of a narcissistic guarantee in this distribution, in some way different to the tasks brought about by this paternal blessing. A woman may willingly think of herself frustrated in this distribution, even left feeling orphaned.

The question debated at this Concilium persists with the same virulence, not only in the private life of women, but also among their spouses with demands, calls, wishes. If we can conclude that a woman has indeed a soul, the problem is that this soul will find its accomplishment only in renunciation, which allows her to consent to make of herself an object, totally absurd, totally private, totally particular conditions which organise the phantasy of a partner. And this, always according to the apparent wish of a father, her own, who does not allow her be recognised in her being, except by another man – I mean by this that the father himself cannot assure this favour. One of the difficulties we see illustrated in Dora's case, it is that this soul was given to her in some way only to be removed from her. And this procedure does not seem to be without consequences.

So, let us talk a little about Dora. Because these questions, these kinds of questions, Dora after all, most certainly put on the map.

Dora's history, I hope you have all re-read it, appears like a *murder party* [in English in the text]. Everyone tries to resolve the enigma, not only to know who is the guilty one, but also the victim. We have to say that Dora herself tries to resolve the enigma, before going to see Freud. I will allow myself to say that all in all, the history of Dora seems to be that of a *mal-entendu* between Freud and Dora herself. Freud seems to believe in the possible natural harmony between a couple (for example, he who would unite the young and beautiful M.K. and the adorable Dora, all the while encouraging this couple) while Dora herself is a witness to the failure of sexual rapport. It is she who says this in some way to Freud and she does this in the context, of the family history, where the woman is most particularly regarded and denounced as a vector of death.

In the *Dora Affair*[3] (we can call it this, it is a superb piece), Freud begins with his conceptualisation of hysteria in 1899–1900. He waited a bit, the case was published in 1905. You know, for Freud, hysteria is linked to a repression of sexual desire, as it happens in the woman, repression itself due to a precocious sexual excitation that is to say in childhood, at a time when the child did not have the adequate organic means to satisfy the flow of this drive, this heightened excitation. This means that the quantity of excitation finds itself converted into the somatic (because of this it is called "somatic provenance") at the time of puberty, that is to say when new quantities of excitation come to the fore. Although the subject has at his disposition the means to satisfy his desires, the old ways are taken up by new phenomena of somatic conversion.

The aim of the treatment, therefore, is to lift the repression which has accidently happened in childhood and allow the hysterical woman to have a satisfying sexuality. This is Freud's theoretical position, at the time he was dealing with Dora, and he will enforce this illustration at the time of this observation, that is to say to show the good foundations of his thesis.

But what do we see in the scenario of this affair? We see certain pivotal personages.

We have first the central personage who is the father. He was in Freud's "good books". He is a very interesting man, a captain of industry, a man who has succeeded socially, even though he had been ill, mainly with TB. On the other hand, this man is grateful to Freud to have known, when he came to consult him after visiting numerous doctors about paresis of his lower members, to ask him the necessary question about his sexuality. This allowed Freud to identify the cause of his paresis as linked to tabes [dorsalis] and he gave him anti-syphilitic treatment which had a totally miraculous, marvellous effect, as this man could use his limbs again and is, therefore of course, very grateful.

The mother equally, a really interesting figure, distinguishes herself on the scene by having nothing, if it is not as Freud tells us, of the housekeeping syndrome, that is to say being the good wife of a syphilitic husband, who spends her time cleaning her interior.

The older brother is incidental, but he has illnesses which he has passed on to Dora, who of course always had them in a more serious form and Freud recognises immediately what this means: this means that sexually it was he who initiated Dora, and about which she thought that this had embarrassing consequences for her.

Another interesting figure is the paternal aunt, the sister of the father. There is obviously a privileged link between him and his sister, a mistress, it seems, who is very unhappy in her marriage. She constitutes, in a certain way a feminine model for Dora who identifies herself and her troubles with this aunt. This aunt will die in the course of events, leaving cousins.

And, then our Dora who is obviously intelligent and extremely pretty. Octave Mannoni thought that Freud's choice of first name for Dora as being linked to Pandora, she who had all the gifts. Why not? Because it is certain this is a young girl who merits such a*dora*tion – you know that Freud willingly used the French language, which he knew well in his own associations, even in his own dreams. And, of course what is really important, is that she was sent to Freud, by her father. She herself demands nothing, but at a certain time she's had enough, she becomes a pain in the neck for him. And, because Freud knew how to ask him this question about sexuality and he knows full well that it's all about this for his daughter, her father sends her to Freud. Dora, for her part thinks the symptom is not hers but that this symptom is somewhere in the situation. It is really because of that it's a *party*, where one looks for the victim and the guilty one. But, in the end, she consents, to go see Freud.

Dora is characterised in her symptomatology by the fact that since childhood she has had respiratory symptoms, the same as her father. I mean by this that she considers herself since childhood as being worthy – I do not know if we can say the daughter, but in any case, as worthy of being the dignified child of her father. It is likely that she has a certain knowledge that her troubles are linked to the sexual excesses of her father in his youth, before his marriage.

And, what interests us is that Dora, before she was brought to Freud, had found her equilibrium between the father, Mme K. and M.K. (I will not go into detail about all these personages in the text). How does she organise herself? You know that she became the friend of Mme K. and at the same time something like the eldest girl, the eldest imaginary daughter of the couple formed by her father, and Madame K. – a platonic couple, because she knows that her father is impotent, whereas Mme K. suffers from lethargy. This couple is a union of two ill people who support each other. And Dora, in this scenario? She looks after everybody a little bit. In particular, she makes herself the tutor of the K. children, because their mother has a habit of abandoning them, as she did not seem so attached to the children she has with her husband. This is, for Dora, an ideal family because it is founded on love, a pure love, a disinterested one, sacrifice, the gift, chivalry. In some way, the sublime character of this organisation will wash away the excess crimes of the father's youth.

And, in this stable situation which seems to suit everyone, and then bang! The edifice falls down. What was it that causes the fall of the house of the K's? It is not new that Monsieur K. passes to the act. He makes tender gestures to Dora, but he also has come on strong, there have been caresses, which are not in any way equivocal. But what is not right, is that this time Dora feels the need to tell her father something, which she had never done, like the big girl she is. And now, something happens which is intolerable for her; her father does not believe her. Or rather, he does not want to believe her and Dora knows exactly why: if he were to believe her, he would have to respond as a father, that is to say destabilise a situation where he finds his comfort. And, here suddenly, Dora finds herself, sold, betrayed, treated like a servant, like the governess who took her holidays two weeks earlier from the house of Madame K., that is to say, treats her like a nobody.

And yet, the peculiarity of this situation is that Dora only finds her satisfaction and her equilibrium in this position of an imaginary child, the ideal child of this couple. Why? In this place, she could think that it is she, alone above and beyond Mme K. who is the loved one of her father. And, at the same time, that it is she who being the imaginary child of this couple, is loved above the love that Mme K. had for her father. She occupies a perfectly unique position in her phantasy, through identification with Mme K. and the waiting for a transmission which operates for her because of Mme K. and assures her femininity. I will come back later to the problem the hysteric has in relation to the woman. This waiting on a possible access to femininity, through the intermediary of Mme K. because she has nothing to get from her mother's side, this expectation was, course essential.

But, two things happened before Dora decided to speak to her father and therefore broke all this organisation. Firstly, she finds out that the governess has received the advances of M.K. (who must be a little frustrated, all the same, in the scenario of this story) and has decided to leave, because she realises that she has been subordinated, as we say, in other words, that this will not take her very far. And, on the other hand, when Dora, in objection to his advances, says to him that he is married to the charming Mme K., M.K. responds "I have nothing for my wife" (This has been translated, it is only a detail, it is not essential) in French as "My wife is nothing to me". In the German text we find, "I have nothing with regard to my wife". You will notice that the father would have already used the formula with regard to his own wife when he came to see Freud. "I have nothing with regard to my wife". This situation reveals to Dora, firstly, that she is not a unique object, a privileged one, then if M.K. has nothing for his own wife, all the effort, all the expectation she has to obtain from Mme K., what would permit her an access to femininity, would find itself obviously disavowed or would make it redundant. But, indeed, what does he want? Here M.K. tears the game apart.

Freud himself is not against this type of exchange – which it has to be said, is not banal. The laws of marriage are not to give your daughter in exchange for a mistress, this kind of thing does not happen anywhere. The laws of marriage always have to do with successive generations. It has to do with assuring fecundity for the generation which comes along afterwards. And it is very interesting to notice that Freud himself in the end, disapproves of Dora. He thinks that in his affair Dora resists M.K. in a typically hysterical fashion. After all, it would be preferable that she would give in to this beautiful young man rather than being a hysteric.

Dora is looking for an exit from the situation, she herself is looking for the method of moving forward, which will allow her to get out of this knot. We see her trying a whole series of identifications. It is surprising when we read this story to observe that Dora identifies herself with practically everybody. She is looking for her place, she is looking for what would be for her, a stable ego, in all this affair. We see her identity with her mother, with her father, with her aunt, with cousins, with M.K. And, of course, with Mme K. In this story, Mme K. is her feminine ideal, because she has met someone who is loved by her father as a woman, and with a love which was until then, a platonic one (even if she could have some vague doubts about what in fact had really gone on) a chaste love, that is to say a complete love, which is not compromised by anything.

We have seen Freud's position. He totally holds to his representation of the mechanisms of hysteria: it is always a repressed desire. His diagnostic, is that Dora loves M.K. but that she represses her love. He won't let go of it. He says "In my attempt to lift this repression, I thought that the loved object was M.K. There was in this hysteria and perhaps in all hysteria, a dominant homosexual fixation and I did not recognise this in time, in other words, I made a mistake".

In this way, Freud understood what the countertransference as it is called is about. We know the way in which Dora treated him: by giving him his fortnight, like a servant who would not merit it, but to Freud, who only wished that Dora, would, put herself in the position in some way of having to serve M.K.

This evolution is marked by two beautiful, interesting dreams, which are brought to the observation. The first has to do with the passage from inside to an outside, and, the second from the outside to the inside. That is why I began with the problem of ex-sistence for the subject.

I will recall very succinctly the first dream. The father jumps up at the foot of the bed, in the night, with the worry of defending his children against a fire. You have to read these dreams in German because it is much more precise. For example, at the beginning, in *einem Haus brennt es*, is translated as *"there is a fire in a house"* – this is right, but the word after word (in German) is more alive.

> *A house was on fire. My father was beside my bed and woke me up. I dressed quickly. Mother wanted to stop and save her jewel case, but father said: "I refuse to let myself and my two children be burnt for the sake of your jewel case. We hurried downstairs and as soon as I was outside I woke up"* "Jewel-case" in German is *Schmuckkasten,* which is quite near *Schmutzkasken* which means "rubbish box".

Let us interpret this first dream, with our own risks, with a key to dreams, that is to say, as Freud says, in a chapter on *The Interpretation of Dreams*, with the authorisation in certain cases to interpret dreams by using the symbolic. Therefore, the male organ would never be represented in a dream by a hollow container for example, but by whatever you like, a tower, a bell, etc. – as if there was in the language of the dream a coaptation between the forms and the symbolic, as if the imaginary seems to lend itself to a certain coercion by the symbolic.

"Something might happen in the night so that it might be necessary to leave the room". I will permit myself to push things here so as to stay in the outline of this dream: as if the father would have wanted to defend his children against the risks of the family foyer – there is the fire at home, there is a danger for the children and it would be better to stay outside. "Something might happen in the night so that it might be necessary to leave the room". And, this is taken up a little later but it's not translated into French. During the night, some unhappy thing may occur, so that we might have a reason to leave, to get out. And the father would like to protect his children while the mother, she only thinks about her jewel case, as if she could only think about how to satisfy her lubricity. It's actually very explicit in the associations. This dream is built on a certain denial because it seems as if it is the father who carries the unhappy outcomes of a lubricity during his youth, while the mother does not seem too concerned by that. Here the father watches so that the children could be out of the loop.

We know how Freud proceeded at the time: He gave explanations to Dora about the Oedipus complex and told her also, that in her symptom, she revived her love for her father so that she could defend herself against her inclination for M.K. And it is here that is produced the second dream, which is not unconnected to the explanations which Freud gave her.

Dora is outside, in a strange foreign village, where she recognises neither its streets nor its places. And, here, she has a house where she lives – outside – it's her place – she finds a letter from her mother, saying to her; "Daddy is dead, you can return". And, even when she reached her house after certain difficulties – she had difficulty in finding the train station, to get there etc – the concierge said to her "Mummy and the others are at the cemetery". (It's fairly ambiguous). In other words, the house is empty.

Freud also explained to her that dreams were always the realisation of a desire. Here, in any case, Dora can return to her own place, be inside this time, leave her position of exteriority, of ex-sistence. She can be intra but on condition that they will all have disappeared: they are all at the cemetery. The father is certainly there as he is dead, but the concierge told her: "The others are also at the cemetery". Therefore, she is quiet and goes in search of a book. What we have in this second dream is an evocation of the Sistine Madonna at the Dresden Museum, in front of which she stayed for nearly two hours and this picture reminded her that some days before hand, or the evening before, she had gone to see an exposition of the *Sezessionsaustellung*.

In other words, if we make use of our key of dreams, with what that nearly brings about, we can attach ourselves to these properly topological aspects concerning the vacillation of inside and outside, that is to say, the place from where a word may come out, for her. The dream concludes on a model of participation: to be inside, introduction, but obviously at the price of a certain mourning, for that of her father – Freud indeed found that it was her own fulfilment which appears here – but at the price of a position of the Madonna, already the place she occupied in the K. couple and to which she holds on this time, to which she is determined to hold on, to which she promised herself to hold on, but at the price I repeat, of all these renunciations, all these mournings.

All this means that, in terms of this story, we are really obliged to question ourselves as to what Freud's desire is in this story, including this conceptualisation itself. It is clear that Freud's desire was to match a couple, as if the lifting of the hysterical symptom is the mode of a possible access to the matching of a couple. It is, as if, at the price of the lifting of the hysterical symptom, a happy rapport is possible, in any case for him, in the imaginary, between this beautiful young man and this beautiful young girl. While for this beautiful young girl the history of her family, including that of the Ks, was evidence of a totally major discord between men and women.

The history of these two families, including her aunt, was registered under the sign of the fact, that between man and woman, things do not work. And it really seems that what engaged Freud's desire, was, on the condition of curing hysteria, that could be rapport between a man and a woman.

This brings us to two important crucial problems for the hysteric. We see them drawn out in Dora's story. These are the relationship with the father and the relationship with the woman. Can we therefore, in Dora's history, say that they are typical?

If the hysterical position maintains itself from ex-sistence, with regard to the father, from then on this position is displayed with a possibility of reversal, faithful to the formula which I mentioned the last time $ \$ \diamond a. $

- Or else, beginning with this ex-sistence, the affirmation of not belonging to the line of the father, not only of the real father but the symbolic father; To be a perfect stranger to the world, in not having anything to do with it. From whence, why not say it, a certain taste for betraying him because, if he conducts himself in this way, in not being able to look after his creatures, it is well for him, he only has to learn this and that will teach him! Even the wish to castrate him, which is a current symptomatic mode of expression, really banal, but it has to stop, this kind of production and of descent, has to stop once and for all!
- And then, always from this place of ex-sistence, a reversal founded on the consideration that this place of ex-sistence is after all, a position which finds commonality with the real father, who is held less from ex-sistence – with an interpretation of the disorder of the world linked to the fact that this real father could be under the "whack" of privation, in short, that he is ill himself. I will move on. I will not take up again the place of ill fathers in the observations of hysterics. In order to cure this ill father, this father in a state of privation one has to give him what one does not have – love. But, to give him what one does not have, it is the organ which is at fault in this case. And I will pass over the frequency of impotent fathers in all the observations with which we deal. There is therefore, a kind of reversal by which instead of looking to castrate him in some way the hysteric will make, as I said the last time, of him her organ, in so far as this is put to his disposition, put to his service. In other words, if M.K. had received a little bit of psychology, he would have not been taken in like that. It would have been necessary that he would have some small little somatic symptom. It would have been necessary that instead of being a young man full of health – he would have made a mistake and all would have been well for him!

And, finally the question of the relationship to The Woman. I will say it again, *La femme*, The Woman, because surely, there in this belief in the existence of – at least – One, she who is able to put into place a specifically feminine castration. As a result, the girl would have an oedipal situation totally symmetrical with that of the boy. That would permit him to accede to a purely feminine genealogy, generated by The Woman, guaranteed by a feminine castration. It is on this that we habitually conclude on the so-called homosexuality of Dora, which does not seem to be anything other than an attachment to Mme K., as if she were the one who would eventually be able to play this role for her. Dora was expecting something totally different from her, when she told her father about the goings on of M.K. instead of being simply treated like a vulgar fool so as not to risk disturbing the activity between Mme K. and her father.

Dora's story concludes in a way that does not include any removal of hysteria. It was recognised in the United States, by an American doctor listening to her many years later, that she had somatic symptoms, hysterical symptoms. She was not feeling too well, obviously and Freud does not tell us anything else: he absolutely does not tell us that he cured her. Therefore, the question remains active, pertinent for us. In this kind of scenario, what can we envisage as a cure for Dora and what means would we take for that? If Dora had found her equilibrium in a sublimation, even if she relied on the Madonna, what will we suggest as a method of cure? Analytic discourse suggests another kind of arrangement, which is a question for us. In what way is the introduction of analytic discourse, capable of suggesting to Dora something other than a cure by this method of sublimation? This is a question I will not avoid, but, which for the moment I will leave unresolved.

The next time, the third Tuesday in February, I will deal with what is called hysterical psychoses. And in March, I will deal with masculine hysteria.

QUESTION: Is what makes the difference between the father and the analyst the difference between the discourse of hysteria and the discourse of the analyst?

CHARLES MELMAN: Yes, you can indeed say it like this. But that is not the position taken by Freud. There's the interesting point.

QUESTION: Everyone tried to pass her on to someone else. Her father tried to give her to M.K. but it didn't work. He tried to get rid of her in passing her on to Freud, who in turn, tried to pass her on to M.K.

CHARLES MELMAN: Exactly! This story disturbs us because it is precisely the hysterical question. She stops things from turning. (She) stops things going round because precisely she is never satisfied. Do not be too dramatic! She satisfies herself, with it in a certain way. We do not see why it did not last in this position where she made herself the eldest girl of the couple of father and Mme K. Perhaps, who knows, she would not have evolved too badly in the end, if perhaps – all the same, it is a kind of economy which is not exactly the classical familial economy. It was not, all the same, nothing, from her sublime position, she had a perverse response from her father, from Mme K. and from Mr. K. "Listen, don't go on and on about this, get on with this yourself, and you too will receive your just desserts". You are indeed very right to notice that in any case, the analytic response is not in any way, to take things from the side of a paternal benevolence. Have you not all felt that the expression by an analyst of a paternal goodness has activating and accelerating effects manifested on the symptomatology?

QUESTION: Equally, a severity?

CHARLES MELMAN: Of course. There is an appeal to the father from a hysterical position, but if this is manifested a little much, it will face serious criticism.

There is therefore a position which can only be an oscillation on the part of the analyst because he cannot imprison himself in either one or the other of these representations.

QUESTION: Why did he not think of getting her married, the father?

CHARLES MELMAN: You are right, but he was a liberal man, and in that, Freud was happy with him. He said to his daughter: "You see, I'm not afraid and I was not afraid, you, don't be going on too much".

QUESTION: He did not take too much of a risk, this fellow!

CHARLES MELMAN: He did take risks. Syphilis – in Vienna at the beginning of the 19th century – where he had a social position. He led, it seems, a quite liberal existence. There was, all the same there, a kind of exchange between two women with very friendly relations with M.K. to whom he sent his daughter to have some peace, and it was done I would say, without hiding himself too much.

QUESTION: Does not the miraculous cure of tabes diagnosed by Freud, pose in reality, the problem of masculine hysteria?

CHARLES MELMAN: Listen, I totally agree with that. But, if I remember rightly my questions as an intern, I think the treatments prescribed by Freud, were not without effects, and it appears that the syphilis was serologically verified – All the same, I believe if the father was not a hysteric, the position offered to Dora was. In such a context, from where can she be an expression of a possible access to femininity? Not from the side of her mother. She could find a response in a certain way in the woman loved by her father and she tried that. And, then it did not go beyond a certain limit, beyond this sublimation. In any case, Dora's hysteria had every reason to function.

18 January 1983

Notes

1 S. Freud, *The Case of Schreber, Papers on Technique and Other Works*, Vol. XII, S. E. (1911–1913). London: The Hogarth Press, 1958.

2 Herbermann, C. (ed) *Ancient Diocese of Mâcon, Catholic Encyclopedia New York*. Robert Appleton Company. 1913.

3 This chapter mostly deals with the Dora case, see Freud, S. "The Dora Case" in *A Case of Hysteria, Three Essays on Sexuality and Other Works*, Vol. VII (1901–1905), S.E. London: The Hogarth Press, 1953.

Chapter 14

The polymorphism of hysteria

Charles Melman

As Lacan remarked, it is clear that what could make us work is the, "I don't want to know anything about it".[1] The difficulty is that normally we regulate our "I don't want to know anything about it" in a communal way. We are, by the same token, sure to partake in this, to taste it in our community. And, if a member of this community pushes the button a little bit further, this will of course, produce waves. This, by way of telling you that I am not without questions with regard to the sense of what I can do here and the eventual waves I can provoke. But even if sometimes these are not too pleasant for me, I receive assurances that I touch a certain real, because, the proof of it is that it turns out to be disturbing.

This preamble, because the minute I have to deal with certain questions, I'm asking myself as to what it means to take things with which we are dealing by way of the clinic. In front of an auditorium of philosophers in a conference, taken up again in the *Écrits*, Lacan renounced the "forced card of the clinic".[2] Why should the clinic be that of a "forced card"? I'm asking myself that question to try and figure out what might have annoyed him in this. The clinic has the aspect of a forced card to the extent that it leaves the subject to whom it addresses itself, without recourse, up to the question of the *passage à l'acte*. And I have found, also, that I have provoked certain passages *à l'acte*, indeliberately (or indeed, even deliberately, who knows?).

As far as psychoanalysis is concerned, is there a place for us to take on board what we have to deal with under the angle of the clinic? What will justify this work, is that its destination is clear. For those of you who would like to get interested in this, it has to do with dispelling what is maintained, as the instability of the subject. The subject would constitute a kind of sombre zone, a dark continent which would derail and always go against rational attempts to account for himself. Meanwhile the clinic of hysteria is witness to the fact that the subject can never of course be shown, but as Lacan says, offers himself up to a calculation. Despite the mysterious and irrational power with which we would like to charge him, the subject does not escape reason. The subject is demonstrable, he is accountable. And you know what Lacan says: he can always count himself as *plus one*.[3] Whether in the cartels he was

DOI: 10.4324/9781003167839-14

counted thanks to *one* who functioned as a *plus one*, he was taken as the leader, as the spirit, as the inspiration for the cartel, something, which was obviously not Lacan's aim.

In exposing the subject to rationality, it is shown that he does not absolutely act in an unpredictable, surprising, mysterious or opaque way, but according to a certain number of known, locatable ways, which can be spoken. But, at the same time, the projector is pointed at what permits the subject to sustain himself, to ex-sist himself as a subject, that is to say on the paternal function. This is a huge question which, remains, for psychoanalysis, unresolved.

You can take this whichever way you like, this prudence, these explanations, these precautions before I engage today on the clinic of hysteria. We shall see how the polymorphism comes down to a structural matrix – held by the constitution of the subject, a structural matrix, totally elementary, totally rudimentary, totally simple, capable of engendering this apparently different range in the clinic of hysteria.

I will immediately put my master card on the table. This polymorphism of the clinic, of the hysteric, explains itself easily by the care which hysterical passion holds – that is to say that from which the hysteric suffers and which animates her – the care of resolving the clinic of the hysteric insofar as the subject regularly attributes the blame to this.

The malaise of the subject finds its origin from the moment we situate the mirror stage, that is to say from the time of the image of the other, of the small other, appears to the subject interested with a quality, with a brilliance, of an assurance not symmetrical with his own. And, that is always how the other image will appear to him, even if it is his own in the mirror. This constitutive dissymmetry of the meeting with the image in the mirror will drive the hysteric to renounce these qualities for herself.[4]

Why is the hysteric led to such a renunciation and, at the same time, I think it has to be said to an identification? Because I will go so far as situating the time of this initial renunciation to the fact that the hysteric will find herself exposed, offered to ulterior precipitory identifications, to indentificatory fluculations, which could be not really expected, could be quite surprising, so why this renunciation to invest oneself as a support of this image? Why, in fact does she give it to the other, to her fellow by renouncing it herself?

As we know, the mirror stage, which Lacan accounts for, perfectly explains the constant division of the subject with his own image and the always ambivalent and aggressive relationship which he holds with it, in so far as this image constitutes the subject, in what is properly speaking an essential alienation. By this I mean that this alienation is constituted in the image of the other – it's really in fact the primordial form of alienation – and, at the same time constitutes this subject, in the fact of having to renounce what could have been, because of this alienation, to reveal to the subject what his being is. There is always a nostalgia for isolation, for solitude, for the desert island or the retreat from the world which would permit a revelation of what would be the specificity of being because he would not have to lose himself anymore, would not have to submit himself to publicly imposed figures.

The mirror stage marks this division of the subject with regard to his own image. But, it leaves in suspense the fact that in a dual meeting, one of the subjects is led to renounce making himself the support of this master image. He resituates from then on this master image in a realised alterity, effectively realised: it will be the image of another (male or female) in regard to which he will find himself in a rapport, no longer of division but of separation, which is not at all the same thing. Therefore, in this original dual meeting (I call it this to testify in a mythical way to this so-called inaugural time), the subject renounces for himself this master image for the good of his partner and finds himself given over to, abandoned to a bodily malaise, which is really noticeable in the clinic, which translates itself in its tonus, just as a much as in its attitudes, even its gestures. This is a rudimentary clinic, even if it is not perfectly demonstrated.

With regard to this alterity, to this image from which he is thereby separated, what is this subject looking for? Of course, it is to make himself recognised, that is to say to admit himself to the same level as his fellow, as a fellow. And for that, there is only one unique way: he searches to put value on the *objet*, the concealed, secret object which could also support his appearance.

That's how the qualification of seductress, or more pejoratively, the one who gives you "the come-on", said to be the hysteric, has an essentially lay origin, if we could say it like this, essentially a non-sexual one. It has to do above all with the wish to make herself recognised as a fellow by the other, the small other, from whence the facility of interpretation in the register of seduction. And this attempt is generally suspended on an attempt at sublimation, in establishing with this small other a fraternal and egalitarian rapport, that is to say mutually narcissistic. All in all, the hysteric tries to repair inequality, the arbitrary sharing which finds itself inscribed since the mirror stage.

The difficulty with this operation, is to realise an equilibrium which would be fair. It does not matter if her parade is not taken in a competitive way or in an aggressive rivalry, a pretension at possessing more brilliance, more qualities than one's fellow taken as an effort at participation in the community: an attempt to realise the impossible of symmetry and reciprocity in the mirror. Her exhibition will always be in some way tempered, because it has to do also with preserving the image of this other, of not bringing prejudice to it. In return, the hysteric has the feeling that it's her temperance which permits the image of the other to be maintained. With, at the same time, this care to protect one's fellow, to maintain him, not to mortally wound him, not to break him, because of what this brilliance could show from the other side.

But, this care makes the image of the other responsible because of the very limitation which the hysteric imposes. Altruistic care leads to hysterical speculation, the accusation of limitation of the other as a cause of what would be ultimately his own constraint, his own limit, because the aim of the procedure stays as an impossible reciprocity.

In the usual case, it's only in the position of a pure mirror that the hysteric could accept this master position, that is to say the whole position attributed to the other. She will not occupy this master position except in a transitory and delegated way – I will come back to different moments of its evolution – that is to say, "this time, it's you, this time it's me".

Why? Because she fears that her facticity could be put in danger if it's she who has to represent it, the phallic order on which her subsistence depends. Let us remark that facticity is not the same thing as semblance: the latter is always swallowed by the other, whereas facticity is in some way delivered up to the capriciousness of the subject.

We know that the worry of making oneself recognised goes inevitably – should it not be in the need to recognise oneself, because one can only recognise from the recognition that one has obtained – by the devolution of a sign of phallic belonging. If one can recognise a fellow it is solely because he will be up to value certain traits, even if it is only one, which would demonstrate that it arises from a phallic order.

What is of the order of the semblance is only recognised as such, because it has gone through castration, recognised by the symbolic father. The hysteric (I will speak about this in the feminine) knows very well that the men she is dealing with are semblances of men. She knows this perfectly well and this raises many questions for her. Why semblances? And why are they recognised by the symbolic father? She sees very well that they go through castration, that is, from castration that they hold this value, this trait. But, if the semblance is on the side of the male partner, we can see how the hysteric, no matter whether she is anatomically male or female can only try to be an expression of the phallic order, on the condition of giving value to a position which could never be taken up, except from feminine facticity.

A huge question arises. The economy, the dynamism of the hysteric, are entirely taken up with the constraint of resolving castration and this beginning from an inaugural event (which I call inaugural in a mythical way) the incapacity to respond in the mirror to a call from the partner. The impossibility is linked to the failure of non-sexual rapport. I mean that what symbolically orders this imaginary phase is that there is no sexual rapport and as a consequence, the prevailing wish of the male partner is homosexual.

It is from this being torn between things, that we can grasp why the dynamism of the hysteric will be taken in a kind of contradictory movement. This dynamism aspires to castration in order to get recognition from the partner, a recognition at the level of one's fellow, a recognition of the title of fellow and also by the imaginary father, let us call it like that. But it has not got to do with castration in the competition, to know who will own the best goods. On the contrary to say this in a more brutal form, it has to do with who is the better, or more castrated: he who has sacrificed the most to the other and therefore is supposed all the more, to be recognised by the other and loved by the other. In sacrifice, as a mode of competition with this partner, the hysteric is successful in general in turning to the sublime, that is to say, that this castration will no longer be symbolic, but real. For example, if it has to do with a feminine subject, it makes sure that the anatomical difference is explained here by a castration, which would go as far as being verified in the real.

It's here that the paradox is produced which gives this contradictory aspect to the dynamism of the hysteric: In order to achieve this sublimation, to become so perfectly ideal for the other, the hysteric sees herself, imagines herself as a pure object of a wish supposed to the Autre. Or again, at the price of this castration, brought in this way to its term, to its absolute, she accedes to a field which ends up as a totality, this field which in an imaginary way, realises the *objet a*. Because, the object *a*, of course, does not lack anything: it is obliged to function itself in a register which would not be at fault anywhere.

The hysteric is capable of juxtaposing castration as an ideal on the one hand, and the demand for a total realisation on the other hand. Of what? Of the rapport with jouissance as much objectal as narcissistic.

Let us remark, to take a little bit of breathing space *en passant*, that this identification with the *objet a* – I will later give the structural support – finds itself detached from all worry about representation. I began earlier, with this suffering of the rapport with one's fellow, of this passion to remedy it. But, this identification with the *objet a* detaches totally from the worry of representation because no-one will ever be able to perfectly agree. Also, it can be accompanied by an absence of the worry of appearance, of the worry of appearing in the world, or at least to have to be recognised. And, there is obviously, a certain pride in this method of detachment.

Because there was "A Philosophy of Furniture", we should outline "A Philosophy of Clothes". This has already been done, but for analysts to take it up again, in a different way, it would be quite interesting. Lacan, himself had a philosophy of clothes and we were amazed by the care he took to stand out from our humility with regard to clothes. I will call it like that. It was not always like that and those today who would wear fabrics of the 18th century, would appear totally gaudy.

Since then, we have acquired a kind of discretion, which has to be taken as a great sign of pride, contrary to appearances. A sign of pride; if we did not have to worry anymore to make ourselves seen, of making ourselves recognised, it's because we are never certain of the very fact of our sacrifice, of the benevolent look of the Autre for us. And we would not be any more at the level of the problems of ribbons, trimming and lace.

With this dynamism, the hysteric finds herself oriented by a double pole, a kind of needle which oscillates rapidly from one to the other, up to the point of almost juxtaposing the demand for an absolute castration and the worry about the establishment of an order, not knowing limits.

Obviously, the child exposed to this contradiction has some difficulty in locating himself and in grasping what is asked of him. There are recent American works explaining why schizophrenia happens to people who would have received, in their childhood, contradictory orders from their parents. I would really like to know if that spared them much and all the same we are not all schizophrenics.

In any case, it's through castration as such, that this will be accomplished and by an identification with the *objet a*, that the hysteric finds herself in a position to make, to live as the instrument of the Autre. And, henceforth, she devotes herself, as the organ of the Autre to occupy the different positions where it seems possible to compensate for the fault in titles, because these positions are, in general, occupied by the holders. Because there is castration and therefore suffering, one of the hysterical interpretations is that the holder is not up to his job, and she therefore has to substitute herself for him. I said earlier that the hysteric is careful not to occupy the master position, because of a fear of putting the phallic order in danger. If she becomes its representative, it's because she is sensitive to the register of facticity which maintains her. But, after she has identified herself with the very instrument of the Autre, diverse potentialities are possible.

One of them consists, of course, in substituting herself for the failure of her partner. The hysteric knows very well that Man does not exist, to the extent that there is no true man, because those whom she meets regularly are always at fault. As far as the imaginary father is concerned, there is at-least-One who escapes castration.[5] One of her questions is to ascertain why the ideal father has male representatives who are just as careless with regard to what he has to a right to expect from them. It's here that the hysteric realises what Lacan calls "to make the man", the place in which it seems this same man wants to keep her.

It has to do, for her, not to realise herself as all man but as a whole man. And she distinguishes herself from her male counterpart by the fact that when she occupies that position (this could also be for the male hysteric) – of castration – she has nothing to do with it! Because, henceforth, she proposes herself to the very image of this imaginary father, that is to say she realises a filiation which would not be degenerate.

And this is a mode of formation usually and solidly found in heterosexual couples, in these couples, where a woman occupies this place. To tell the truth, I do not see why this has to be repeated, it's one of the things which the structure demands, calls, regulates. Castration, inherent to every instrument of the couple will find itself lifted by this substitution to a man – who otherwise is the vector, but who only maintains his virility himself, by identifying himself with castration.

As we know also, it is not infrequent that to "faire l'homme" (make the man) infers a homosexual position, an attempt henceforth, to realise oneself with another woman, the possibility that in the end she will be a real woman.

There again, it will be a mode of union which will exclude, which will not be tolerated by castration. And now, to remember that the longed-for woman, because after all there is nothing good to be hoped for from a man – this is what in the past the child hysteric would have no doubt wanted to hear from her own mother. In the observation of Freud's young homosexual woman,[6] it is really patent that it has to do with the young girl, showing her father that she, with regard to a woman, has a desire and that she will go the whole way. In other words, it's not castration that can stop all that, she doesn't even need her instrument, she can do without it, and perhaps even that is much better that she can do without it. And she testifies, before her father's eyes, that in the register of chivalry, she is ready for supreme sacrifices, for the greatest. And, indeed, when the object shies away for more or less good reasons, she does not hesitate to sacrifice herself and to offer the good that is most precious, her life.

There is another possible interpretation of castration for the hysteric. It's this: if castration is thereby active, if she suffers as a result of it, it's not so much the male partner who is responsible for it, but the knowledge which is exercised there, in a master position and which would be a knowledge – in any case this is how it is interpreted as – lacking. Castration is attributed to this, to the knowledge which exercises a master position is not the good one and the hysteric is totally disposed to substitute her own . For that, there is no need for a diploma or a certificate because it has to do with demonstrating that every one of us is animated by a practical knowledge, an unconscious knowledge, this knowledge put in us by the Autre, even the knowledge of the Autre. On the condition of giving value to this knowledge as true, it should be possible to resolve castration. This gives rise to the denunciation of the knowledge of doctors, of pretend sages. Instead there is glorification of the knowledge of humble people which was indeed put into us by a benevolent providence, and which the glossary could only spoil – it's because of this glossary there is failure. The point has been the focus of long controversies for philosophers and in the early days of religious thought. Wisdom was denounced as madness against the benefit of natural wisdom, native, spontaneous, deposited in each one of us. The question has known a totally different future, with what seems to have been established, very early on.

You see how I'm trying to show how the hysteric may, beginning with a certain identification with the imagined object, with the organ of the Autre, come to occupy the places of discourse of the master, the places of discourse which here I will not call the university, but of knowledge – with a problem for the subject S_2, to which we will have to return.

And, then there is another discourse which the hysteric is perfectly called to occupy, because we can say that in hysteria, what represents S_1 for S_2 alternatively, or else $ for a! We can ask the question why did Lacan not say that S_1 represents a for S_2, while in fact he said that S_1 represents $ the subject, for S_2. In any case, in what I'm trying to illustrate as the possible identification of the clinical polymorphism of the hysteric, with what I will call this antagonistic couple, which regulates its dynamism, I hold to the following: for the hysteric, S_1 can represent alternatively, in a very close fashion just as much a and it's from a the identifications, which I mention here, find themselves upheld.

So, it is really obvious that there is going to be a discourse which will lend itself perfectly to this identification, and it is analytic discourse. To the point, moreover, that this could lead one to think that the hysterical position and the analytic position find themselves confused, that they are the same. But I think that we can distinguish them by remarking that these cases are identifiable in situations, where the analyst identifies himself in his function with this object, takes himself in reality for this object. There are different objects but let us take the voice, for example. An hysterical tonality properly called, could be recognised to the extent that this voice will propose itself as vector of a message, of a wisdom, of a pedagogy why not, proposing itself as a resolution for all. We will recognise in hysterical tonality traits of type, which will respond to what I called earlier hysterical passion, that is to say, the concern to resolve castration.

A question may be legitimately asked here. What is it that permits us to distinguish this discourse held, for example, from a hysterical identification of those which would be real discourses – I don't know how to call them in opposition to those which would be a borrowed discourse? There are some traits altogether sufficient to help us recognise the essential dimension of the pseudo.

Firstly, the hysterical position in the affirmation of this discourse, distinguishes itself in being of value for all of us, that is to say, in posing the postulate of a totality which deletes the dimension of the Autre, to put forward the idea of universality. Henceforth, the Autre in how it is questioned by these discourses, is not any more that of jouissance, but what is called conformity.

Then, these discourses will willingly, take a character which we will call pseudo-paranoiac. Paranoiac in appearance because every putting into question of what holds it, is lived as an attempt at identify. And, pseudo-paranoiac because it has nothing to do, in any way, with a true paranoia.

There is also a trait which is essential, it's a complete identification with the enunciation, as if these enunciations offer themselves without the division of the subject. The saying would come directly from the Autre because there is this possible identification as an organ of the Autre, but he who is the vector, the subject, presents himself as not being in any way divided, with regard to what he enunciates, as he is entirely identified with the I of the enunciated. There is this disposition particular to language which does not miss having a certain number of effects properly speaking somatic: dermographism, stigmata, a certain number of otherwise surprising manifestations, which could explain themselves as testimony that the subject is not divided.

But, if there is no division of the subject, there is alternance in his utterances, and will reappear in what I called earlier, separation. Speech is engaged at such a moment as if there were no subjective division, as if there was total engagement of the subject with what he enunciates. And, then there are very brusque ruptures and suddenly the word is articulated from the place of the subject. Sometimes, a word without a subject, sometimes a subject without a word, and this phenomenon of alteration could clarify what we can well call the double personality of the hysteric. In fact, two absolutely different, split, divided lives can co-exist together, one made of sacrifices, of rigour, of devotion, of honesty, of care about superior interests, an irreproachable life and then the other, separated from the first, maintained by phantasies to which the preceding situation would lead to renounce the sexual for example. People who are perfectly worthy and respectful lead double lives, with sometimes awful public or private acts, and we can sometimes see these apparent paradoxes, in a rather embarrassing way, with regard to the modesty of one or the other, in front of the judge. And if, in the first time, that of sacrifice is entirely organised in the altruistic concern to preserve the little other, and to assure the jouissance of the Autre, it seems always as if in this apparently contradictory economy of the hysteric, the second time is compensated by a private jouissance no less complete.

I'm a little bit long this evening but I would like to finish with this. I spoke about pseudo-paranoia. Why speak about pseudo? We can also describe in hysteria, phobic forms, perverse forms, forms which take the shape of obsessional pictures, but why every time pseudo? And there are even forms which are so precise that we hesitate with the diagnosis. For example, in the case of phobias, at the point where Freud spoke about hysterical phobia, which Lacan challenged: he thought that a hysterical structure had nothing to do with phobic structure.[7]

Why for example, in dealing with a perversion, will we say: that's a real perversion or this one is hysteric? There is a very simple way of accounting for it. Of course, perversion constructs itself, no less than hysteria in the concern about resolving castration. It's always, in this way that neurosis is constructed, and obsessional neurosis is also a defence against castration. But, the perversion, which we will call authentic, is itself, what constitutes the phantasy. So, that in hysteria we can call perversion "pseudo", because it's one of the modalities the subject could perceive as a way of resolving castration. It will be a borrowed phantasy and we will have the surprise of seeing, that the so-called perversion can be perfectly abandoned to the advantage of a totally new disposition, which because of such and such a circumstance, may appear better.

The inexhaustible concern to resolve castration accounts for the lability of the clinical pictures. The phantasy which upholds them is like a shell, invested for a while as one of the modalities which permits the vivacious concern to deal with castration. For the same subject, we can identify them as pseudo, because of the dimension of facticity, a chance facticity, which will eventually justify engagements all the more important for the subject, rather than this dimension always more painful and weighty.

This is where I will stop this evening.

QUESTION: When you say that the hysteric knows that the man does not exist, how can we not think about the formula "the woman does not exist". The signifier "The woman" is foreclosed. Do you think this is the same for the man?

CHARLES MELMAN: Of course not! Let us reassure ourselves. The hysteric searches for the reason why it doesn't work. One of her interpretations is that there are real men. What's more – it's true, but this does not stop man from existing, but only as castrated, by renouncing making himself equal to this original father of the myth and structure. He can identify himself, uphold himself from he who would escape castration, but at the price of being himself only of the order of the semblance. The distinction, all the same, sensible, between the semblant and facticity could also lend itself to confusion. There is here an open door to organise the constellation, to organise the way in which things could turn around. She reverses the proposition from which she suffers by saying "The good men, the real ones, we'll await their arrival!"

QUESTION: The man is not all man for her but this is not what interests her in the least.

CHARLES MELMAN: Man is every man, that is to say in a certain way, one is as good as the other. But, he is not all man. And, it's really that for the hysteric, which does not work. Because there is a possibility of linking her suffering to the fact that the man is not up to it and in order to keep going, there is only this strange castration. She holds on to it, because of it she is able to hold herself up as object of a prize, but at the same time, this castration revolts her, because it is linked to her in-existence.

QUESTION: Why is this renunciation posed as a primitive time, at a moment of the mirror stage?

CHARLES MELMAN: This renunciation, which is assuredly a mythical time is essentially imaginary. I began with that but it is watched over by symbolic conditions of the structure and by the real. It's first and foremost an altruistic worry. A sharing has to be done, it's me or you. That's how the dual encounter is presented. One of the big dimensions of altruism, is the concern to give to the other what one does not have in order to protect him, to accord him this privilege. Are we going to put it uniquely in the register of altruism? It's also, it has to be said, in the concern about an Autre jouissance, that is to say, to expect from even this renunciation, a kind of supposed jouissance imagined as a superior order to that of the master. The worst, this is indeed true, because jouissance is on the side of the slave. Lacan pointed this out many times and admirably![8] The master, is destined for boredom, the culture of narcissistic jouissance which is reserved for him, has its limits. What operates in this sharing also includes a choice of jouissance. Lacan will go so far as to say, that of which the serf remains serf, it's above all the jouissance which he monopolises.

All these elements have to be taken into account, as to what makes the determination of this choice. Of course, the minute he makes it, the consequences are not thought about, I mean to say, for what has to be paid. It is obvious that suffering is also part of jouissance, it's one of its poles, one of its extremes. There are all those factors and the concern about a certain competition in the love expected from the Autre. In fact, the relationship with the Autre is always lived in a mode of exchange, that's how we are, it's our system up to this day. In exchange for agreed castration, there is a venture expected, in the form of love and therefore, at the same time, recognition, eventually more secret, more complicit. All this intervenes in the balance.

QUESTION: In a previous seminar, you exposed the effects of renunciation as a structural moment where the subject precipitates himself. You referred it most noticeably to the possession of the penile organ which would delimit either on the side of S_1, or on the other side.

CHARLES MELMAN: I indeed brought up the question, if it is anatomy which makes destiny. That's also an element which could intervene. What could intervene there again, is not to find oneself responsible for what fails (because this causes huge guilt for the subject, to live as being responsible for what fails) is to not find oneself endowed with the instrument which would bear witness to the will of the Autre, by its reality, by its erection.

If erection plays an important role, the functional role of the instrument is very well questioned by the games of feminine homosexuality. They testify that the instrument can in certain constellations, be treated as not being indispensable and indeed, the contrary. Long ago, I knew a woman who for many years worked as a brothel madam. She always specified to me how much it was not a question for her to use herself as a fake and she boasted about how she had a drawer full of love letters, that many a man would not receive. Moreover this was true.

The question as to whether anatomy is destiny has to remain open and should be more precise than what we're doing at the moment. In any case, if it intervenes in the choice I'm talking about here, it's possibly with this concern only that the image could be left to the other, because it would be more useful to resolve castration it would work better if the other endorses it.

That being said, as I have developed it, this can be evaluated differently.

QUESTION: When you spoke about total identification of the subject with the enunciation, I don't understand.

CHARLES MELMAN: Yes. It's an important question which deserves to be taken up in a more detailed way. With regard to the signifying chain, the position of division in which we are generally, puts us into a certain shade, leaves us with a certain availability, a certain freedom. We are there, but, of course, but we are not totally there.

We have to mention what happens when we are totally there, that is to say, in this division. And we have to ask ourselves about the strange somatic effects which can be described in hysterics (and would otherwise, stay enigmatic, not understanding, why it comes along in this way to inscribe itself on the body) but also, with it has to be said, emotive effects. Why, for example, the articulation of an apparently banal indifferent phrase, which, it has to be said, sometimes is simply heard, why would it provoke this kind of emotional surge? This kind of submersion, with sometimes very different somatic effects.

But, if we wish to deal with these phenomena, it seems that there is an access here: to envisage how much the hysteric finds herself in these times identified with her utterance – the hysteric will not tolerate any renunciation, any dialectic, this utterance presents itself as a kind of valuable segment in its integrity, in its totality. We could equally think if the signifiers have this power with regard to the body, it's that, by the failure of division at this moment, the real of the body finds itself there – this has to be elaborated in a more precise fashion – perfectly in submission, with a vectorisation of blows, of stoppers, traces, marks, burnings, operated by the signifier. This appears to me to be a possible access to account for these phenomena. It's a fairly important point to establish something more clearly.

QUESTION: I had the impression that you were speaking here, not of division but of duplicity.

CHARLES MELMAN: No, not of duplicity, but, of separation. We could say duplicity to mark the character of aberrance which I mentioned earlier, but the term, sadly, has a moral connotation, pejorative, and I am not sure which term would be the better one.

QUESTION: But, when you said that the hysteric is totally in what she says, I heard, that, in this moment, she is not divided, but is in duplicity.

CHARLES MELMAN: It is that she is at one and the same time, entirely in what she says, and yet not divided but radically separate. It is not at all the same thing. And, this is without doubt, one of the disagreeable aspects of the situation, to be at one and the same time in an enunciation which aims to stop this disagreeable feeling, and at the same time a complete separation (not a division) virtually put in place. This will only go to provoke a redoubling of the vigour of the enunciated.

JEAN BERGÈS: You don't believe in what you made allusion to when you speak of a mythical time, before the mirror, before there was an ego and when there was only the imaginary.

CHARLES MELMAN: Listen, I think it is difficult to make these categories function in isolation. You will find that with Lacan, they function in a chronological order. There is in the *Écrits* a whole putting into place of concerns, especially of the effects of the imaginary, before the discourse of Rome.[9] It could only be a procedure of exposition and 1 believe that it would be difficult to talk an initial time about, purely imaginary.

If there are no other questions: I think we will return here again on the 8 March.

15 February 1983

Notes

1 J. Lacan, *The Seminar of J. Lacan, Book XX: Encore, 1972–1973* (trans. C. Gallagher, unedited).
2 J. Lacan, "The Subversion of the Subject and the Dialectic of Desire" in *Écrits* (ed. J-A. Miller, trans. B. Fink). New York: W.W. Norton & Co., 2002.
3 J. Lacan, *The Founding Act*, June 1964 (trans. C. Gallagher, unedited).
4 J. Lacan, "The Mirror Stage as Formative of the *I* Function as Revealed in Psychoanalytic Experience" in *Écrits* (trans. B. Fink). New York: W.W. Norton & Co., 2006.
5 J. Lacan, *The Seminar of Jacques Lacan, Book XVII: The Other Side of Psychoanalysis, 1969–1970* (trans. C. Gallagher, unedited).
6 S. Freud, "The Psychogenesis of a Case of Homosexuality in a Woman" in *Beyond the Pleasure Principle*, Vol. XVIII, S.E. (1920–1922). London: The Hogarth Press, 1955.
7 J. Lacan, *The Seminar of Jacques Lacan, Book IV: The Object Relation* (ed. J-A. Miller, trans. A.R Price). Cambridge: Polity Press, 2020.
8 J. Lacan, *The Seminar of Jacques Lacan, Book XVII: The Other Side of Psychoanalysis, 1969–1970* (trans. C. Gallagher, unedited).
9 Lacan, "The Mirror Stage".

Chapter 15

The hysteric and her father

Charles Melman

I will take up again what I went to Brussels to discuss, under the more or less correct title, "the hysteric and her father". I will speak about this to you because in preparing the seminar, I became aware that it was a continuation and a search for what is sometimes in contradiction to what I said there.

That is why I prefer to give you the first stage this evening (with perhaps elements that you will find new and introduce some new questions) so that by next Tuesday you will be able to see in what way it can be corrected.

I did, first of all, and of course, I will do it here again, undertake psychoanalysis by way of the clinic. Lacan spoke about the "forced card of the clinic"[1] and this for a very precise reason, the clinic is always, written from the position of the observer as if he, the observer, was not in the loop. It is a way of looking at his fellow as a phenomenon and forgetting that exteriority – which does not allow oneself to be considered as a fellow – is in itself a phenomenon.

But, hysteria gives us the chance, which justifies our enterprise, to study this exteriority in a new way. Because everyone can recognise the elements of his own subjectivity which is at work in subjectivity itself. Each one of us, no matter what his preferences or his neurotic talents, finds himself concerned by the discourse of the hysteric and may be led to support it.

I would like to draw your attention to this. Michel Foucault[2] attributes the birth of the clinic to a displacement of the look. You know the definition of Bichat:[3] "Good health, it's the ensemble of forces which resist death." It is the fact of putting the look in the very same place as death, which permitted the birth of the modern medical clinic. It's essentially a radical displacement with regard to Hippocrates, for whom, on the contrary, death was the ensemble of forces which battled against life, and it had to do as a result of this, of putting the life force into operation so that the treatment could operate and not go too near it.

Now, well, it's still the same for the Freudian clinic. If you pay attention, you will see that Freud operated this second topography with exactly the same kind of displacement – without of course wanting to. The look from then on is put in the place of death to consider life, health, as the ensemble of forces which resist it, but are made to lead to one it. It is not uninteresting that a little later than Bichat, Freud operates this same return.

DOI: 10.4324/9781003167839-15

Therefore, from this exteriority where we can place the observer, the question poses itself of this exteriority, which is not in any way natural, but appears in history. Lacan calls this moment, here again very precisely, the emergence of the Cartesian I.[4] We know that the Cartesian I is supported by this extra territoriality, which authorises one to doubt everything, everything of which subjectivity will extricate itself to affirm itself as truth.

We don't, in general, have many of these texts to accompany us, and I would like to make you aware how far away we are from what founded up to now the speculative tradition following on from Aristotle, in establishing this point, this totally new approach to truth. For Aristotle, truth was to be searched for in the realisation of being. With the emergency of the Cartesian I, what is no longer anything but a pseudo-being has to rely on what would be a non-deceiving God. The question, however remains for us here, it's even the obsessional question, *par excellence*: God, after all, does He not deceive us? Because we can't exactly put our hands on the object, does God not separate Himself from us? For Lacan, truth, from Descartes onwards, is only he who says, "I think", that is to say he who says "I". Truth, from then on, comes from he who speaks. The problem is that this truth will say that the world is only a semblance, that the world is uncertain. The object and the ego, finds itself no less exposed to this systematic doubt, which means that the Cartesian I also inaugurates the pain of existing.

I will take up again Lacan's articulation, the truth of this existence, it's, therefore, suffering.[5] We qualify hysteria as this truth, henceforth it wishes to affirm itself in a master position. And, for us, it's primordially this, hysteria: the pain of existing, insofar as it shows itself, insofar as it wishes to make the law.

This introduction, which envisages an audience less prepared than yours, aims to detach hysteria from contingency, to illustrate it as a fact of structure, to detach it from its link, too much in common with the feminine sex and to remind us that it is a type of discourse, that is to say as a way of knotting the social bond.

To advance into the question of the rapport of the hysteric with her father, we can remark that this exteriority in which the subject is held is not a metaphor, because it's a repression operated by everyone, thanks to the example of original repression, which maintains subjectivity. What functions as $ maintaining itself thanks to a repressed signifier, a repression which is itself only possible because there is an original repression, an *Uverdrängt,* of which Freud said very clearly, constitutes the point of call for repressions to come. We could say it in this way that our subjectivity *is* this signifier which finds itself barred, whose literal materiality insists on making its return in the name of the repressed.

Our subjectivity has a material support in this signifier, which founds its subjectivity. What is important for us, is that if it manages this place which supports the subject, we do not need to shilly-shally, it's the one who takes up for us the divine name. Here, yet again, this is not a metaphor. There is at least a signifier which is at fault, which is lacking, and for us, this signifier of original repression takes on the value of the divine name. Let us remember, that if it were revealed, the sacred tetragram remains unpronounceable. You can play with these letters, but in an original tradition, you will not know how to pronounce them, therefore you will not be able to pronounce them (other than the fact that you will not have the right to pronounce them, but I will not enter into these kind of considerations).

But this should permit us to remark that this retreat of the subject, this non-linkage, this side of being outside the groove, that is to say this "dé-lire" (punning on "lire" and "delirium"), this exteriority is not in any way crazy, because it takes hold in the very place, put in place by what is recognised, what is celebrated, like the original father, like the foundational father. From whence this kind of support of solidarity, which the hysterical exigency of power finds, which is hardly a sliding, proposes itself as the voice itself of this imaginary father. She wins it in this place, henceforth force and passion, to offer herself as inspired, as coming from this beyond, even speaking in his name.

You know in pathology, the frequency of mystical deliriums. It's not an accident, or because they copy one from the other. Mystical deliriums have a certain rapport with this putting into place on which I'm working on. They find their inspiration from a very precise place which I try to isolate and which I try to show that it comes from the subjectivity of each.

We see very well from then on how the voice of the deep, how the voice of guts, the voice of the heart, the voice of feeling, can be presented so easily as vibrating the voice itself of this imaginary father.

This introduction tries to give value to the type of solidarity which unites the hysteric and her father, their privileged and constant relation. By the same token, the most extravagant and spectacular manifestations of hysteria could be, with difficulty, qualified as psychotic, if it is true that by its structure, hysteria implicates the Name-of-the-father. Of course, this is not without therapeutic consequences and this is a point which I will take up later. If we remain coherent with the concepts which inspire us, can we speak about psychosis with regard to hysteria, even with regard to manifestations typically "psychotic" in hysteria?

How could we say, if this is accurate – this is a demonstration which has to be made – that the hysteric, by her status alone, implies a privileged rapport with the father? I spoke here about the imaginary father, but we have to still reflect on the rapport to the Name-Of-The-father which implicates hysteria.

We can remark that all the relations of the hysteric with this imaginary father will be oriented by a unique question. I will present it to you in the following way but there could be other formulations.

This imaginary father, he is not castrated. I evoke here also the father of *Totem and Taboo*,[6] who has all the women, this father who Lacan puts in place, this at-least-One $\exists x \, \overline{\Phi} \, x$ that is to say, he who authorises in some way the totality of men, on the side of the male. It's funny anyway, it is often said that there is here a logical error, an arbitrary sleight of hand by Lacan, this – at-least-One.[7] Russell asks how a totality can only be held up by an element which of itself cannot be[8] understood in this totality, and shows the properly logical foundation of this writing. It's the history of the catalogue of catalogues which do not contain themselves. We can well see where Lacan has gone to look for support.

The question posed by the hysteric to this imaginary father would be the following: if he, not castrated, if he escapes castration, how is it that his creature is able only to resolve this on the condition that she herself should be castrated? Can we really hold that the true filiation of the father should be marked in such a way by the sign of castration, while he is perceived as having all the powers? There should be the sign of a lack here, of a degenerescence which he would need to rectify. And that is how the hysterics' protestations will be addressed to the master – it's the writing of hysterical discourse – the master insofar as he is a representative, authorises himself from this father. Because a master is, after all, never anything other than this: he who affirms – this is the big political tradition – that he holds his power only by authority. The hysteric will question him about his impotence, this so-called legal representative of the father.

The first of these masters – for her, pseudo-masters – which she will question, is the real father, by this I mean he who is at home, the incarnate father. The hysteric cannot admit that he will be so much beneath the imaginary father of which he will affirm himself meanwhile, as the representative. Because he is impotent, incapable of giving to his daughter, which would be the smallest of things, a recognition of phallic membership – a child, for example, which she has to go looking for, most commonly, to another man.

I've already mentioned the case of Freud's young homosexual. The evolution is totally transparent. It's after the "refusal" opposed by her father – because the child, it's the mother who will have her – she will take up a virile position. But not the image of this pathetic father! A real male position, because for she who would be the object of her loves, she will show herself, capable of going to the end, of sacrificing her life. And, as we know, the modalities of this sacrifice, will illustrate a certain relation with this birth, *das Niederkommen* which is produced at the home of her parents. Here, in any case, we see the genesis of feminine homosexuality.

Therefore, with the protestation provoked by the suffering which this real impotent father gives, we know the kind of solutions the hysteric will attempt. For example, as we have just seen, by substituting for this failure of the father and to make the man. It's a frequent solution, chosen less for pleasure than for duty, and accomplished in the concern to show oneself the representative of this imaginary father, an authentic representative because the real father, really is a little bit too timorous.

This will give clinical pictures where femininity finds itself marked by certain traits of virility. In fact, let us not forget, this imaginary father has traits usually of sexual ambiguity, because, to have escaped castration, he has also a feminine side, a feminine face. And, for the child of this hysterical mother, this mother without a fault, the analyst will be able to show us that this is not without consequences.

If this way of substituting oneself for a lacking father and to make the man is a solution in some way intra-social, a way of secularising oneself, we can call extra-social another mode of very frequent response. It has to do with refusing the world of this real father – in other words to refuse to participate in what we call reality – in cultivating a position of exteriority. This in the general denigration of those who people that reality, these shadows of such cursorily improvised men, these castrated people, to have instead a kind of intimate relationship with the imaginary father, a complicity which could be more or less anticipated on the occasion of certain existing elaborations, or else will stay totally secret. Contrary to the precedent, which participates firmly in the world, our second disposition is an attitude of a more paranoiac style. Every invitation to participate in reality, that is to say in this world, will be lived as corrupting, all participation will be prohibited. Why prohibited? There is surely here an essential point which has to be taken up again.

I will not develop everything but there is still, beginning with this exteriority and this denigration of the corrupting world, another frequent position which permits an interesting reintroduction to this world. It has to do with returning this hatred of the world into love, in the attempt to give to these shadows of men so curiously improvised, to give them what oneself does not have, to give witness to them of the greatest love and the greatest charity. Therefore, these curiously improvised men find themselves marked, because of this exteriority no longer by castration, but by privation. We also have to say why. From where the idea that the gift is healing, and we know that the therapeutic vocation is strongly linked to such premises.

Therefore, in this context, the real father will no longer be denigrated but loved, not for what he has – because he hasn't got it – but precisely for what he has not. Loved for example, in what is interpreted by him as an illness and we have already seen in the observations of Freud the frequency of these ill fathers, impotent, delinquent, syphilitic, dying. In this case, a worldly participation is authorised, is possible, but only insofar as one is the benefactor. This recalls the history of the famous Bertha Pappenheim, who could return this extraordinary demand in an activity of multi-directional benevolence (oblative love), not without conserving, and it's interesting, a hatred of men, I mean to say a hatred of what could be called the virile pretensions of men. And, this is never without some consequences, all these little stories. If you look up her history, for example, in a recent book by Lucy Freeman entitled *The History of Anna O.*, or in an article by Lucien Israël[9] which is a few years old, or in other more recent ones, you know that she was engaged in considerable activity, of social work in the Jewish circles to which she belonged. The biographies also noted that she was strongly opposed to Zionism, at the departure of Austrian families in Palestine, and that she maintained this attitude up to the very end, even to the time of the *Anschluss*, in a type of protestation, it seems, against the pretension of these types of people who wished to see themselves as soldiers and founders. She was someone who was quite influential in the community at the time, and with her endless bounty and her generosity, she was it seems, responsible for a certain number of inconveniences which were produced later – to tell the truth, this kind of oblative love, I will take it here under its most salient aspect, never fails to have some inconveniences, even if it stays at the private level.

I give here the large traits of the kinds of options, hysterical positions of exploration orientated by the relationship with this real father, this real father denigrated or loved, to remind ourselves that all these movements are regulated by the attempt to remedy the fact that The Woman does not exist. If this famous father had been capable of making her exist, there would have been no need to give oneself all this trouble! It's exactly her failing, this Woman, which causes all this movement. And these many diverse styles will always be upheld by a unique and contradictory economy because she will confuse the demand for castration by her partner, which would be brought full term, that is to say to the sacrifice of desire, and parallel – I wish to say, at the same time, because its contradictory only in appearance – the demand of a jouissance without limit, also sexual, by the way. We have to say why.

But the hysterical position has to do with making heard the voice of an imaginary father, escaping castration, we can see that it's enough for this voice to detach itself from the constraints imposed by the castration of the listener, of one's fellow. Let us remember, from the minute we engage in a dialogue, we put between our interlocutor and ourselves a certain number of laws. Mutual recognition, good sense shared, are linked to castration which permits a certain *malentendu* to function and two people are able together to not hear themselves in "communication". But, it has to do with making heard the voice of an imaginary father, from the minute he is renounced with the constraint of letting himself be heard which the listener imposes, this voice engages itself in madness. Madness is what it is called here, where hysterical psychoses are seen to be essentially linked to moments of evolution where a word is found, for no matter what reason, which is liberated from the incidence of castration. You can observe there delirium, mental automatism, hallucinations, subjective straying, anything you wish for!

It has to do with our knowing if the moment is reactional, it is an attempt, amongst others, to lift the castration of the partner and to make heard the voice of this imaginary father (a mad voice if not castrated) or if it has to do in the hysterical phantasy with an accident as may be produced. The problem is that it is enough that the entourage, with the best reasons in the world will identify her as psychotic, so that we will isolate her as an excursion or as an accident which can be made without a return and will begin to evolve in her own way in what we know in ecstasy: being known as the holder of the word of this imaginary father, does not go without a certain ex-tasy.

But, if the hysterical position implies the activity of the Name-of-the-Father is it possible that we could speak of hysterical "psychoses"? Are we not, first of all, startled by the fact that if the entourage consents, we will not engage too much, they will be transitory manifestations and that at more or less longer intervals, these patients will find their feet again?

The day after this conference, we saw a remarkable case of a young woman, undoubtedly hysterical, who had an episode in a paranoiacal manner – I say manner, but all the picture was typically paranoiacal, at the end of a few weeks this paranoiacal picture had fallen and things fell back into order. What was rediscovered, as an "exciting" circumstance, was an intervention of her father, benevolent but – in a very paternal style. But, in this extra-worldly position, which I spoke about earlier, she organised herself in an exteriority where she was not able to participate, to integrate herself into a social or an affective reality. The father had the concern, the goodness to give her the material conditions to permit her not to find herself anymore on the wrong path. He got her a place to live, gave her an address, a place for herself, a socially fixed insertion. It was at this time, in the days which followed, in what we can really call a transgression, that she fell into a typical paranoiacal epi-sode: she was followed on the street by men in cars who wanted to proposi-tion her, to treat her badly etc. There was no hallucination, only interpretations. The police were called and they did their investigations. There were a whole lot of serious things. But, she could, under certain conditions and to the extent that she put herself into a certain exteriority, find her place again and her life took a calmer course.

These are episodes which should question us a lot. This is the way I'm trying to follow, to lead us to know how to separate, even though they could be very alike clinically, psychotic manifestations from the hysteric and psy-chotic manifestations belonging to other structures. We also need to empha-sise that the patients who were presented to Charcot and whom Freud saw, today without a doubt, would have been identified as psychotic. That's also to be noted. At the time, they were well able to recognise these as hysterical manifestations.

All of this reminds us that hysteria is, in the final resort, the expression of the suffering that there is no father universal enough to encircle the speak-being into a "whole". That is really the problem for the hysteric. Henceforth, she can, of course, engage herself in this kind of prophesy of a father who, would be comparable, of reuniting all of us, in the end!

We would like to say that the hysteric is essentially a party pooper. Why? Everyone is not equally invited to the feast, according to the estimation of the point of view of the hysteric, because certain ones are too ornate.

It's this kind of injustice the hysterical symptom commemorates by attach-ing itself to suffering, and by refusing to renounce it. This suffering is really the only testimony that there is, for the hysteric to exist, because for her a representation is really only a masquerade.

It has also to be said, it's the only way of valuing a *plus de jouir* (a surplus jouissance) a greater jouissance. The first clinicians were of the opinion that these great hysterics had always a side a little too ambiguous and seemed to bear witness to a jouissance in the act of accomplishing itself.

There is also in hysterical attachment to suffering a way of holding on to this jouissance, brought to its term maintaining the value of an image supported by the *objet a*. The proximity with the said object takes account of the hysterical call to a certain exoneration of something which encumbers, to a certain amputation, to an intervention which would put an end to the excess which she feels as supporting her body. But it's also the source of jouissance, the proof of which is that she confines it to a suffering presented as a scandal, a prohibited suffering because it was not necessary to go that far.

The analyst is confronted with solutions which the hysteric may find in the treatment. In presenting things as I have done, it does not go without saying, which makes it necessary for us, I say clearly, to take up the questions again and to elaborate on them.

In this work which I have presented, I have stayed, I would say, too discreet. I spoke about the imaginary father, I spoke about the real father. I advanced quite rapidly, that the subjective position, the $ sustains itself necessarily from a rapport with the symbolic father. I think this point has to be taken up again so that we can assure ourselves in reality, that hysteria cannot veer towards psychosis. This mode of relating to the father has to be developed, that is what I began to write for this evening's seminar, when I began to realise that this meant you had not heard it.

There are also certain questions which you asked the last time: what is it that precipitates hysterical destiny? In other words, why is it in this inevitable sharing in the dual relationship – it has to be one or the other – what does it mean for some of us (male and female) that one swings to one side or the other? What are the constraints which push to the side of hysteria?

This is what I wanted to say this evening.

QUESTION: You do not speak of the mother of the hysteric?

CHARLES MELMAN: It's a great injustice! There is in the feminine position a difficulty which belongs to the relationship to the mother, and pushes in some way towards this exteriority, to this extra worldly position. I will speak about it next time.

QUESTION: If a subject presents a clinical picture for a sufficiently long time which does not correspond to his structure, does this not put into question the very notion of a structure?

CHARLES MELMAN: I have tried to say the opposite. What dominates is the structure. We have tried to explain why psychotic episodes can be produced in structures which are undeniably hysterical, to try and move forward a bit better. In these cases, it has a very strong status, a mode of realisation which is very captivating. The case about which I spoke to our Belgian friends – there are telepathic communications which are done without any connivance – it's really an amazing illustration of these kinds of things.

With regard to Dora[10] our principally hard-wearing case, it is really certain that something important played in such a way, so that she could enter into this extra-worldly position (this extra-territoriality which is her own when she plays the nurse in the K. household, when she looks after the children, when she plays the eldest child, etc.). When an occasion comes along to participate at the party, to enter into circulation, into exchanges, it takes the form of the dream. The dream she has afterwards, this famous dream with the memory of the prolonged stay before the Madonna, to remind us of the position of exteriority which she wishes to conserve. We have to believe that for her, this mode of participation, of invitation to enter into the round finds itself prohibited. Why can she not? We have to talk about this. And, if she ends up by realising it, if she ended up by marrying and having a child, it's under the mode of what I called earlier a party pooper, by saying all the time that it's not working, it's not working. I won't teach you anything new, if I add that this is a mode of participation which is not rare.

QUESTION: In the case of hysterical psychosis, can there be auditory hallucinations?

CHARLES MELMAN: Of course, I believe that there can be, from the moment when the moorings of the phantasy are broken. Let us say that the phantasy orients, like a compass. If this compass does not function any more, the game of metaphors and of metonymies are delivered up to a capriciousness which is not oriented any more, because what founds sense finds itself dispersed, broken up, in bits. Then, many stars begin to constitute so many points of call and points of dispersion. We see in certain clinical pictures at very precise moments, there begins to be many kinds of sunshine and the place of the subject becomes very mobile, very erratic, so he can no longer find himself. It seems to me, that we can observe there all the manifestations of psychosis, including auditory hallucinations. I don't wish to contradict myself here and leave you thinking that psychosis is available to everyone? If each one of you would like a little excursion, a little experimental verification – I'm giving you the recipe – we can try a little access this evening? Why is this not impossible in hysteria? Why does the hysterical structure lend itself to it? It is not shown that the others lend themselves to it, nor that one can in a voluntary way engage oneself in releasing oneself. In general, certain drugs are needed. There is a little adjunct needed to get there.

QUESTION: Can the voice say disagreeable things, for the hysteric?

CHARLES MELMAN: Sadly, ecstasy is not impeded. It's not ecstasy because one finds oneself invested with one's own flattering thoughts. There are voices of support, but it's not exclusive.

QUESTION: You reminded us in speaking about the position of the subject that hysteria is also in the masculine as well as the feminine. Yet, the descriptions which you have then given, seem to me to be more about hysterical woman.

CHARLES MELMAN: Absolutely! Masculine hysteria seems to be a witness to another kind of rapport with the father and I will speak about that.

QUESTION: In this kind of picture, can we find very repressive pictures of this kind of delirious melancholy?

CHARLES MELMAN: To be faithful to what I've just said now, we have difficulty in seeing how a delirious melancholy can be produced. But, this has to be verified. And, if this has to do with a hysterical structure, we have to hear this by taking up the points of reference, which we try to give about this.

QUESTION: We have the impression, that clinically a true psychosis and a "hysterical psychosis" are not that really distinguishable.

CHARLES MELMAN: You are right. The next time, I will try and give a trait which permits us to distinguish them and which is not, moreover, very constant. There is very frequently, the expression of a certain prophesising, that is to say a presentation of the imaginary father, or a realisation in the real of what would be his voice, for example. And, then there are the antecedents, the putting into place, and eventually the evolution. But, there is still this trait of which I spoke.

QUESTION: What makes this pseudo-psychosis fall again, so quickly?

CHARLES MELMAN: If it is, as I say, an excursion, we can see how, after an exploration of the voice in question, a return to the case at the beginning, is put into place. This happens after an access in many hysterical manifestations. And we can conceive the psychotic moment as an attempt, among others to resolve the question which is put to him/her.

QUESTION: Is this kind of experience good for the subject, as a kind of attempt at self-cure, or is it, once the excursions has finished, everything enters into order as before?

CHARLES MELMAN: Yes. It is a question of a labyrinth which was explored, in any case at the beginning of a case of hysteria.

8 March 1983

Notes

1 J. Lacan, "The Subversion of the Subject and the Dialectic of Desire in the Freudian Unconscious" in *Écrits* (trans. B. Fink). New York: W.W. Norton & Co., 2006.

2 M. Foucault, *The Birth of the Clinic: An Archaeology of Medical Perception* (trans. A.S. Smith). New York: Panther Books, 1973.
3 X. Bichat, *Physiological Researches Upon Life and Death* (trans. T Watkins). Philadelphia: Longman, Hurst, Rees and Browne, 1816.
4 J. Lacan, *The Four Fundamental Concepts of Psychoanalysis* (ed. J-A. Miller, trans. A. Sheridan). Paris: Éditions Seuil, 1978.
5 J. Lacan, "Science and Truth" in *Écrits* (trans. B. Fink). New York: W.W. Norton and Co., 2006.
6 S. Freud, *Totem and Taboo and Other Works*, Vol. XIII, S.E. (1913–1914). London: The Hogarth Press, 1955.
7 J. Lacan, *The Seminar of Jacques Lacan, Book XX: Encore, 1972–1973* (trans. C. Gallagher, unedited).
8 B. Russell, *Logic and Knowledge*. Nottingham, UK: Spokesman Books, 2012.
9 L. Israel, *L'Hysterique, Le Sexe, et le Medicin*. Paris: Masson, 1997.
10 S. Freud, "The Dora Case" in *A Case of Hysteria, Three Essays on Sexuality and Other Works*. Vol. VII, S.E. (1901–1905). London: The Hogarth Press, 1953.

Chapter 16

Psychotic episodes in hysteria

Charles Melman

We say that the mirror stage individualises the moment where the small speak-being alienates himself in the image. Whether that be his own or the other it is, as such, inverted and beautiful as the mirror sends this image back to him for the Autre.

This time marks the symbolic coordinates which are all the same locatable, puts these into place and gives them their decisive character. These are commanded by the introduction of the little speak-being into a language where the lack of being of the real Autre, his mother, for example, returns the message of his own failure to him. So, can we recognise even if it is retroactively, a time no less isolatable than the mirror stage, a time of the introduction of the small speak-being into this language, where he can regulate his own words on the castration of the Autre? Can we also recognise a time when the word he speaks returns his message as if coming from the Autre in what could appear to him as the most intimate, the most approved part of his subjectivity? This word is able to vibrate his own ears as the expression of an irreducible alterity, introduced into him to defend with his whole body, against which he can do nothing – except to keep quiet.

What I would like here, at the beginning, is to note really strongly that the mirror stage, designating this constitutive moment of imaginary alienation is no less isolatable than the time of an alienation which would permit us to call here symbolic and real, at the same time.

To receive one's message from an Autre, from an Autre marked by the lack which animates him, through castration, the little child will be able to hear his own word – which could appear to him to be the most approved, the most assured at the level of the I, the I of the enunciation – as being no less than the expression of an alterity. That is to say, an expression of alterity coming from this Autre which finds itself at the same time introduced into him, his body defending it, whether he likes it or not, and against which he can do nothing. Except, of course, to close off, which can be produced in certain cases.

You can find this time I'm talking about in Lacan. It's essentially around the *fort/da*[1] (repeated many times) that he wanted to locate it but he never named it as such. I think it will be, fairly easy for us to isolate it, in the same

DOI: 10.4324/9781003167839-16

way as the mirror stage, this stage, where alienation, or indeed alterity find themselves regulated by symbolic coordinates. This is a time which has to be recognised as such. Because there is always this quest for a self-identity, the assumption of a subjectivity which would be the most intimate, the proper, the most true, this location makes possible a certain pacification, a certain temperance in this quest which sometimes takes on fairly excessive demands. A number of other conclusions come from this but it's not within my remit to talk about them today.

This evening's subject is the occurrence of psychotic episodes in hysteria. We know that to hear one's own enunciation, that is to say the most intimate of one's desire, as a voice perfectly alienated, is produced readily among those speak-beings who refuse to recognise the world, because of the fact that they cannot find themselves there in a master position – this position of mastery being nothing other than symbolic recognition, nothing which would be of the order of reality for example. The question of the father is central for at least half of us speak-beings, those who do not benefit from this authority of mastery, for whom this is suspended.

To take up again this question, central to hysteria, we begin with three points:

- The first is the point of origin, constituted by what finds itself transmitted by the primordial introduction of the Autre, that is to say primary repression.

And two other points which are characterised generally by the taking up of a position:

- We have a point which the hysteric will take up within the rubric of dis-avowal[2] – I will explain what I mean by this term as we go along – which is the symbolic father.
- And what I mentioned last time, a point taken within the rubric of deception, which is the real father.

These points, which form a kind of triangle, are organised, beginning with the following question: why does the little girl, whose phantasy is put in place in a no less virile way than that of the boy, have to renounce the expression of her desire? Her desire is no less virile, because there is no other expression of desire – on the contrary, we would indeed have a witness from women's existence. The place Freud individualises as the phallic phase, notes that "everyone has it"[3] and that the phantasy of the little girl is put into place in the same way as that of the boy.

Let us remark in a little bit of a lateral way that the consequence is, there is really only true incest, with the mother. There is only this which is capable of producing some difficulties of a subjective order. The other kinds of incest –

than that of the boy with the mother – are usually without notable repercussions. This bears witness to the fact, *a contrario*, that the phantasy for the little girl is indeed the same as that of the boy.

Why do enterprises in which she will engage with regard to this father – which are no less and even more so than the boy around castration – why do they not bring along with them this symbolic recognition for her by the father? Everything happens as if a paternal nomination arbitrarily given to some speak-beings accords the privilege of following his enterprise and are able to desire by identifying himself from his name. These are the authentic ones and "ready for duty". But, for others nomination is suspended, they have to give their proofs by renouncing this desire and finally, in a problematic way, make themselves recognised by the father. There is here an ambiguity and an asymmetry. And we know these proofs; it is always only by being a mother that a woman will find herself definitely recognised, that is to say nominated.

Things up to now can seem simple in their arbitrariness. But they can be taken up in a curious way when we state that the name "woman" comes meanwhile from the paternal function, if it's true that this name is destined to bring along the real, in order to make it right for sexual jouissance. The real, henceforth is not only this unknown and disquieting land, eventually populated with strange vegetation, not named, unknown and menacing beasts (this is the landscape which so-called adventure novels exploit). But the real, by the operation of the paternal nomination is inhabited by this creature, a woman. Therefore, this real has been civilised by the father. I will come back to this.

For the boy, the paradox is that he cannot lay claim to his filiation except at the price of castration, which we know by heart. He accedes to it only on the condition he renounces it. He accedes to virility only on the condition he has renounced it properly, that is to say renounced his mother and this is the price he pays for symbolic recognition. Whereas the girl can witness a hypothetical filiation only on the condition of renouncing castration as well as her father, to make herself the representative of her mark in the Autre, on the Autre. How? By accepting to become an object delivered up to the risky vagaries of exchange and of adoption. This is a very strange state of acceptance. She has to accept to arrive in this place Autre, and to celebrate the power of this father on this real, his mark on this real, renounce castration – which assures filiation of her little friend, her little next-door-neighbour, or her brother – and even to renounce in a certain way to invoke her father's name. Because in this place Autre, her eventual recognition will find itself delivered up to a vagary – after all, there are laws of exchange – to know if she will be recognised, if she will or not be authenticated.

Therefore, the signifier "woman" is one of the names of the father, if it's true that he commemorates the taking of the real by phallic imaginary, in the phallic imaginary. We rarely see the real but, henceforth, it's not excessive to say that everything projected on this screen is to a certain extent marked by the feminine image. What we see, is reality as such projected on the veil of the phallic imaginary.

This is why I will go so far as to announce this evening, and I hope you will protest gently later, that if landscapes are capable of fascinating, of holding, of questioning us, or if they are objects of capture on paintings, it's perhaps because they will find themselves talking tirelessly about this feminine body, insofar as they come to be the foundation, not always visible of course, of this canvas which supports our reality.

There are circumstances where this fails and where the landscape may appear to us in its real crudeness. It's an experience which can be disagreeable but which sometimes is much sought after. You will then have a totally different perception of the landscape – it will become menacing, disquieting, peopled by what you do not know what, transforms itself, etc.

There is another proof of the capture of the real by phallic imaginary and therefore of its appropriation by sexual jouissance. It has to do with "woman" as one of the names of the father and therefore a testament to its civilising power. It is sufficient enough to have a little cultural or political sliding (I mean totally automatic manifestations, without the protagonists knowing about it) for a woman to find herself no longer recognised, identified by this mark about which I talked earlier, but on the contrary, denounced and humiliated as representing an object, an unnamed object, but in any case unlovable which has to be taken away or evacuated. For example, a situation of colonisation, or a total minority – political this time, finds itself Autrefied, vacillating on the side of the Autre. This could be enough to ensure that a woman is no longer the representative of the civilising mark, a name of the father but only the representative of the kind which hits all the representatives of this community.

Another demonstration of this is: if psychosis may have an effect of "push to the woman"[4] then it will bind the subject to an infinite chain where everything can be said, the chain which is properly constitutive of the Autre. Everything can be said and therefore nothing assures the significance, does not regulate the sense. But, what is produced in this case is that to sustain oneself in this place Autre, the subject will find himself irredeemably marked by a sign of infamy, which will be pointed as being of the order of the unnameable. This is totally classic which we see every day in psychosis, illustrating that if the consequences of the failure of this paternal nomination in the Autre are necessary, this is a failure which sends the subject, henceforth on to the enigma of the horrible object which he represents here. You know the way in which Schreber was cured, the change, that is to say, the substitution, from infamy to what he represents in this chain, of a feminine image which constitutes for him the entry into a possible normality. This is the only way in which he can maintain himself from a structural point of view, that is to say, insofar as he gets support from the Autre, the only possibility he has of maintaining himself in a tolerable way, is to stop to a large extent the hallucinations and to refind himself engaged with his fellows: to give himself a feminine image by way of the imaginary "I understood what was wanted of me, I could not understand it, I knew what was being looked for was an emasculation and I fought as best I could against these forces etc. but I understood". And it's therefore at the price of this identification that he won this kind of contentment.

We can also bring to mind, for those who were there, the case of a patient I saw recently on a Wednesday afternoon at St Anne. A totally charming man, an immigrant who presented in a very classic way, very banal, a delirium of persecution with auditory hallucinations. Everything played out obviously around this. On the one hand, he had renounced his own original coordinates, which were indeed his own and began to engage himself in the way of attachment towards his host country. And on the other hand, in this host country, he could only maintain himself in a position which supposed the renouncing of all pretension of mastery. In both cases, his subjectivity could be maintained only by a location in the Autre. This is an astonishing case, because of its simplicity and we see here at one and the same time, the mechanism of the beginning of his psychosis and the illustration of the clinical picture – he did not obviously dare to tell us how he was treated in offensive epithets and obviously these were of a sexual nature which offended him, even though, of course, he was not a homosexual in any way, etc.

So, I've reminded you of this setting to help us remember the constraints of structure into which we are in the process of placing ourselves. If what I'm telling you is right, we can see how the rapport a woman has with the symbolic is ambiguous. Firstly, her most obvious representative, S_1 imposes on her this kind of evacuation and assigns her to this place Autre, where it will be up to her own good will, by her effort and her devotion, which will be illustrated or not by the Name-of-the-father,[5] in the accomplishment of the capture on the real presentation of a woman. And this in a position which becomes even more ambiguous with regard to the symbolic order a woman would remain exposed to the risk, because of the very fact of this relocation which, she did not choose, of having to assume the responsibility for the failure of sexual rapport. Also, the question of *che vuoi?* What does he want of me? This question addressed to the father, remains central for a woman, is it not because this father, she thinks, does not say anything to her, because he has deprived her of the usage of S_1? From where can she exercise her word and give her authority, use her name, cannot be authorised apart from S_1 and the desire that this prescribes? From where can a woman give a place to what would be her word as a woman?

We can unfold the effects of this trajectory by returning to the formulae which we know, the formulae of sexuation.[6] If it is assigned to the woman by this S_1 raised from an order Autre of which it has to be underlined that it has no apparent genitor, if it has not assumed infinity from this order Autre, that is to say forever inaccessible, except in death, the only reference point proposed to her identity will be the procedure of the masquerade in order to take a place in the phantasy of a partner. From this we can draw this consequence, there really is no reason not to do: if she is not all phallic, she is always a little crazy. It's even what provides her charm, and we need to thank her, for this shadow which overwhelms her, which gives her enigma and the fact that precisely she doesn't have a friend – she is Autre.

Henceforth, we can see in terms of this journey which I hope will not seem to you to be too arduous, that the hysterical refusal to lend itself to the phallic imperative, that is to say to feminine masquerade – these false semblances, this masquerade imposed by the phantasy of the partner – or this will, no less hysterical, to make the woman valued as accomplished, perfect, detached from the constraints of castration, this refusal provokes a rupture with good sense. Good sense, orthodoxy, is never anything else but phallic economy. This refusal can at the same time be introduced into psychosis, and here not a simulated psychosis, but a clinically constituted psychosis of which it could be said also that it marks the realisation of The Woman. I'm saying exactly that – this is not a simulated psychosis.

Just the other day, Wednesday, at St Anne, I had the opportunity to meet a young woman who presented with a hallucinatory delirium. It was agreed at the examination that she was a hysteric and that her psychosis was perfectly simulated, the delirious elements hallucinatory etc., were not authentic and that was verified afterwards. On the contrary, the kind of mechanism I'm speaking about showed a perfectly constituted psychosis. So, what is the difference therefore between this and psychosis? Why is there sometimes a psychotic episode in hysteria?

There is firstly a really simple structural reason. If this entry into psychosis is an attempt to respond to the impasse, to the failure of sexual rapport, we can see quite clearly that this is a reaction to this implementation of place, operated by the Name-of-the-Father. But this implies that the Name-of the-Father should be recognised.[7] And if we stay with our Lacanian concepts from a theoretical viewpoint, it becomes difficult to talk about psychosis. Of course, this is a huge theoretical debate. This is also a clinical debate. Even in these cases of psychotic access, the esteem that a partner has for everything I'm speaking about here, is shown to be the most necessary. This should be developed within the problematic of identification, but it's as if the hysteric, to make herself be seen, heard, appreciated, admired, has need of this partner and by his esteem, by his intervention, her productions will take on a meaning for her. This mood can be rediscovered even at the very moment of a strictly psychotic episode.

There is yet another argument. If the milieu is in favour, to the extent that this episode is reactionary, an attempt, it will be transitory, it will get back in order fairly quickly and could only be an excursion, a little journey into psychosis.

We have other testimonies where the detachment from the phallic imperative is capable of provoking an oscillation in psychosis. This is not only reserved for hysteria.

In the same way, sensitive paranoia. You know that this is produced in very strongly moral people, generally isolated: and precisely this putting to one side of phallic economy, is totally within the observations of Kretschmer,[8] this often signals the entry into sensitive paranoia. Kretschmer had perfectly shown that sublimation was the most favourable method of evolution, of cure for this paranoia. It's certainly the same kind of detachment from the phallic imperative, but taken in an economy which justifies it, explains it and which, far from devaluing its representative gives it, on the contrary, a more elevated price. Religious sublimation, for example, understands this renunciation as a sacrifice. You see, there again, the power of the symbolic. It is not necessary to change economy. The same economy, passing from private and isolated renunciation to a collectively recognised sacrifice, can be translated clinically in a different way and is curative.

Another example, the "délire à deux". You know, it is organised on the principle of a perfect reciprocity, a perfect identification, a perfect love between two people. Every third factor, every third reference, in particular phallic love introducing divorce between these two people is excluded. This kind of couple are totally exposed to cultivate a delirium. And we can be sensitive to the fact that, it is in detaching, the putting of the phallic imperative to one side which may provoke this.

This is not all, there is still a way to give an account of these psychotic moments in a hysterical structure. This may happen when for accidental or other reasons, the phantasy holding this structure together, finds itself failing. In hysteria, this phantasy is constructed on the loss of an *objet*, the possession of which would permit the recognition by the father.

The hysterical phantasy maintains itself from these kinds of interpretations. We can think of situations where an accidental establishing of this phantasy is capable of provoking a psychotic episode. For example, it could be precisely a nomination. Someone could until then function very well with what would be a fault maintaining the phantasy, the failure of nomination. From the moment he is named – a nomination which could take on values, very different expressions – he reacts with such an attack.

Or indeed, these phenomena of post-partum which we don't individualise so well. We see clearly how it is this oscillation, the nomination on the side of mothers which provokes an access, before, more often than not, the patient finds her feet again.

In this way, in hysteria, the permanency of the phantasy is essential in maintaining the state and the implication of very diverse forms of this phantasy may provoke an access. But, you will say to me, up to now, we have learned that the implication of the phantasy provokes an attack of anxiety. Why, therefore, in this case does it finally provide a psychotic episode? It is not at all clear of course. The one thing we can say is that in the case of hysteria, it is necessary to take account of this privileged relationship with the Autre, of this support in the Autre and it is also possible it's from here that the putting into play of the phantasy is capable of having effects other than that of an anxiety attack.

This is how I wanted to take up again the question of the rapport with the father in hysteria. I could not avoid this detour to take account of the feminine position. But, even if I am a little bit advanced on what will be elaborated, it's the ways, the trajectories in place in the teaching of Lacan which we have to clarify properly, at the point where we now find ourselves.

QUESTION: I do not understand the status you give to these moments which you call psychotic. Voices are the only elements which Lacan takes up to distinguish psychosis in Seminar III, *The Psychoses*. Problems of language are first of all needed. But, I would prefer to say: a voyage to the land of the image of psychosis.

On the other hand, you say that for the hysteric, if the exterior milieu is favourable, it could all go well suddenly. What does that mean? Is there a possible taking up again of the symbolic? And in this case, how is this done, if it is not during an analysis?

CHARLES MELMAN: Language problems go without saying. If I speak about delirium and hallucinations it's to take account of the way in which, in classical psychiatry we hold on to massive elements as a testament to psychosis. I did not make a detailed picture as much as just go over an ordinary one. These few problems on this issue present themselves.

What I call the favourable attitude of the entourage, it's that this episode will not be taken as a psychosis. This presupposes being able to make a diagnosis about this episode as such, to not give it more weight than it merits, because the sanctions, the ways of recognising it will play a large role in the way it will play out. I wanted to give you the co-ordinates of structure, with this situation. This is how my lecture appears a little mechanical because structure, it's like that: once something finds itself displaced to such and such a place, this provokes consequences for something else.

QUESTION: In speaking about the image of psychosis, I meant to say that the hysteric identifies herself with the image, and will use the semiology of psychosis.

CHARLES MELMAN: No! precisely not! We must distinguish simulated psychosis from psychotic episodes.

QUESTION: I don't see what you call simulated forms.

CHARLES MELMAN: But it's not at all the same thing. You can have very diverse states of simulation in hysteria. Take all of Charcot's observations. Among his patients you can see that these are entirely simulated psychoses, copied from what is going on in the room. And then there are clinically authentic episodes. Simulation is another thing, it comes from a process of identification, from the effect of an "image".

I spoke about this patient who presented apparently with the clinical signs of a psychosis, who was followed up and treated for this for many years. And it could be shown at the examination that it was not hysterical psychosis but that it was a simulated psychosis by a hysteric. It's totally different.

QUESTION: Are the clinical criteria which you give socially tolerated?

CHARLES MELMAN: Yes, it's perhaps more frequent than we believe, but under a form which we spontaneously tolerate well. We are delighted when we bear that in such and such an African population certain kinds of expression are well tolerated, whereas that would mean isolation for us.

But we ourselves have it seems, a social, intuitive form of tolerance. There is a kind of consensus. We are prepared to accept a certain number of manifestations if a minimum compatible with social life is respected. We can cry and shout but we cannot annoy the neighbours, we can miss work, but not too much all the same. And I find that totally normal.

JEAN BERGÈS: What you said in the beginning about a phase which goes through the ear is very interesting, to the extent that it evokes a trauma. And then, there is the problem of mutism. There could be a mutism because nothing was listened to of these symbolic coordinates about which you spoke. Symbolic coordinates have a double sense, what is sent and what is received. And it is not impossible that, if this mutism, which is so often the object of questioning, whether that be hysteria or psychosis, it is exactly what happens when things are not heard.

CHARLES MELMAN: This is exactly a nodal point and from which arise a lot of situations which take up, again, the question of trauma.

From the fact that one's image is made on the model of alterity, on the model of the image of another and therefore, in this way, alterity finds itself introduced into the heart of identities looked for with oneself. In the same way there is a position from which the repression concluded by the Autre (that is to say from the minute the word comes to the subject from the Autre, this is his own message in an inverse form) is heard as marking no less than an alteration, a radical alterity. And it is all the more irreducible because it is no longer imaginary but of the order of the symbolic. To the extent that this kind of repression gives entry into a phallic order, over which the subject cannot prevail, to maintain his utterance. It's therefore a situation of strangeness, to hear one's own words as strange, that is to say, as imposed by another. It's here that are born images of breakout, of a closed mouth. It would be better to close the orifices, all the same, a breakout is produced which could be the place of his most secret, most true identity, regardless, perceived as unbreakable. And that is why trauma seems to be interpreted as linked to this mood.

On the question of mutism, it is obvious that from the moment I speak I find myself taken up in a commerce, whether I want to or not, what has also made a breakout and which really I blame. This has cost me a position I do not appreciate, a position I can rightly or wrongly think less favourably about than the other. But, if, from the moment I open my mouth to speak, I find myself embarked, on this kind of economy it can be seen that mutism is the part taken by another repression, that of the dead father, the imaginary father – but only insofar that this would be his silence. There is finally in mutism, a certain wisdom, even if we can think that it's not a bit satisfactory. What it does, on the other hand, is to double the wisdom of the psychoanalyst. But a mutism to the extent that nothing can be turned into a dialectic, shuts over on itself, does not permit any better elaborated return, able to be played differently. This last card, even if it is the most true, can only appear as an error if it stays alone, because it takes its price only in a game. If she is totally alone, her wisdom remains short. But, with hysterical mutism I think here we can consider a mode of repression which would be the good the true one to the extent that it will put into parenthesis all that is blah blah blah, into which we would like to carry the subject along at his expense.

QUESTION: But is this not true for both sexes?

CHARLES MELMAN: It has all the same a more frequent incidence if one of the sexes thinks that he is unfairly treated by the distribution. In this case, if you think that the rules of the game are not favourable to you can always take the position of refusing the game.

QUESTION: I do not see what presides at the entry to hysteria, or indeed to the choice of neurosis.

CHARLES MELMAN: No? So, perhaps you will understand it better with masculine hysteria. Perhaps you will understand it better from this side which makes the choice of neurosis and how this economy can be reversed. In what I said just now, the balance is interpreted as treating one of the sides unfairly. And from the moment we take on masculine hysteria we will see that the interpretation of hysterical economy is made in a totally different way.

After this lecture I will have to add, I was obliged to take account of the complicated and difficult ways through which sexual identities are put into place. And one of these may seem to be perilous, hazardous, difficult, and its more on this side that the question was asked about the journey, this journey which leads to sexual identity. This question is put more on the side of the woman and that is why hysteria is more often evoked from this side. For example, to assume the responsibility of the failure of sexual rapport, it will be the hysterical position which will question this insofar as her clinical expression will be a research into trying to solve that same failure. But, what has to be added immediately is that there is another way of talking about this same journey. A way that is no longer taken up in a hysterical device which is a proof that the difficulty is really there, on both sides, equal for the sexes. And if we can for one minute, abstract ourselves from the hysterical position, we will not be able to inscribe this failure to the debit of anyone. The partners have to make do, from one side or the other.

Now, there is a small point on which I would like to conclude. Lacan, in his implementation, does not mention our parental exchange systems. For us, it has not got to do with a restrained exchange, but with an "enlarged exchange", (this is according to Lévi-Strauss).[9] There were recently changes to the Civil Code, at the end of Giscard d'Estaing's rule, I think. There is no longer a head of the family, the woman is not obliged to follow her husband into his home, it was possible to give the names of the two families, even the name of one of them, to the children. There are changes which seem to be of little import, but which translate very important changes in our cultural references. Up to a time it was the boy who inherited the name. Even if it wasn't a question of heritage, of money, he transmitted his name, he had the obligation to perpetrate the generation, the family etc. The principle of general exchange which functions for us – it is strange that we don't speak much about these points – all the same now, a young girl has to detach herself from her generational tree to find a place eventually for another one. This kind of journey has consequences for subjective determinations. All these elements cannot be held as indifferent in the determination of values accorded to such and such a position and it is shown that these changes have results. But the way in which Lacan keeps that to one side is, I believe, a happy reminder of this: Conventions are able to move, to modify themselves without our fully appreciating what the consequences are, but we do not have to and I will emphasise this, mistake them for the structure itself.

8 March 1983

Notes

1 J. Lacan, "Seminar on 'The Purloined Letter'" in *Écrits* (trans. B. Fink). New York: W.W. Norton & Co., 2006.
2 S. Freud, "The Infantile Genital Organisation" in *The Ego and the Id and Other Works*, Vol. XIX, S.E. (1923–1925). London: The Hogarth Press, 1961.
3 S. Freud, *A Case of Hysteria, Three Essays on Sexuality and Other Works*, Vol. VII, S.E. (1901–1905). London: The Hogarth Press, 1953.
4 J. Lacan, *The Seminar of Jacques Lacan, Book III: The Psychoses, 1955–1956* (ed. J-A. Miller, trans. R. Grigg). London: Routledge, 1993.
5 Lacan, *Book III: The Psychoses*.
6 J. Lacan, *The Seminar of Jacques Lacan, Book XX: Encore, 1972–1973* (trans. C. Gallagher, unedited).
7 Lacan, *Book III: The Psychoses*.
8 E. Kretschmer, *Hysteria, Reflex and Instinct* (trans. V. Baskin and W. Baskin). New York: Philosophical Library, 1960.
9 C. Lévi-Strauss, *The Elementary Structures of Kinship*, rev. edn. (ed. R. Needham, trans. J.H. Bell, J.R. Von Sturmer and R. Needham). London: Eyre & Spottiswoode, 1969.

Chapter 17

The stage of abalility

Charles Melman

We are going to speak today about something which you know well and what is funny is that you don't know it because to know it you will have to go by the procedure which consists in naming it. This is called the stage of abalility.

Abalility is a French word. Some among you will know it because it has been part of scholastic speculation since Aristotle's time. But it is an original Latin word, *abalietas* formed from *ab* and from *alio* which has been translated as *abalility*. In scholastic tradition, abalility designates the property of creatures who are not from themselves, who do not owe their existence to themselves, but to another, *alio*. Creatures are distinguished by a *se*, from themselves and those properties are therefore aseity and then those who are *ab alio* are deemed to be inferior because they owe their existence to another. The creatures who owe nothing to anybody are obviously designated as superior. In particular, God – that is to say for Aristotle,[1] the first mover, immobile and insensitive – is from this aseity. But animated creatures who owe their genesis obviously to someone else and therefore imperfect, are from abalility.

This kind of distinction, which we no longer understand, had a huge importance in scholastic speculation, in allowing among other things, to distinguish essence from existence in animated creatures. Essence is not enough to confer an existence – I could say what the essence of a centaur is, but this does not guarantee in any way its existence. Existence is a quality which is given precisely by the Autre. Therefore, abalility orders the deliverance, or not, of existence. This is already something which should help.

Why am I speaking here about the stage of abalility and of what use will this be to us? I reminded you of the mirror stage the last time, the time of imaginary incidences of this abalility because is from an other that the speak-being is constituted. We can isolate this stage, perfectly well, it seems, that is to say, not according to a time but according to a place: we refer ourselves to the place where the symbolic and real co-ordinates of the foundational alienation of the speak-being is ordered, an alienation of which the mirror stage is a time.

The first advantage of this denomination of the stage of abalility is of course to situate, without any ambiguity, the properly alienating conditions, imaginary as well as real, also symbolic which determine the speak-being. Let

DOI: 10.4324/9781003167839-17

us remark therefore that this scholastic speculation continues most certainly to have resonances for our time.

We can consider the work of Lacan on the mirror stage[2] – or more exactly the mirror phase, because he later corrected it – as a putting into place of the prevalence accorded to the role of the form in the constitution of the creature. This prevalence had been confirmed apparently by authors who did not really know that all this came from Aristotle.

It must, immediately, be said that the implementation of the stage of ability is not in any way related to a denunciation of alienation in a kind of quest for our identity, for our authenticity. It is, in effect, totally clear to analysts that such a quest to realise one's being, has only one exit, one and only one realisation, death. This is really clear in Aristotle. If you give some attention to the specifications of Being for Aristotle, that is to say for him, the "first mover" you will find the following definition: Its immobility, its insensitivity, its impassability, its immutability, its perfection, a whole ensemble of traits where we are about to read the characteristics proper to an imaginary representation of death. With perhaps the consequences which the Greeks have for statues: the statue of such and such a personage, real or mythical, was the most just, the most loyal representation of what would represent one's being.

There is an example on which Lacan did not linger as if by chance.

For Greek speculation, what was the trait which characterised all men? The response given did not go without saying. All men – what is their being? Well, *all men are mortal*.[3] What are the more just consequences of the following assertion: *all men desire*. Because we can say that this trait distinguishes them from the animal, which, obviously knows only instinct. We see here all the trajectory, all the time that was necessary for this *all men are mortal* to turn with psychoanalysis into to *all men are desiring*.

What serves us only as a stop gap instead of a notification which is that of *desêtre*. This brings us to the question of ability because this desêtre, that is to say, what finds itself foundational of desire, because *all men are desiring*, this désêtre is caught in the Autre, it is from *ab alio*. There is here knotted the constitutive alienation of what specifies the speak-being, that is to say, what makes his desire, desire of the Autre.

What can we say about this message from this Autre, and which, is an inverse way, will make the I of the small speak-being? Because we repeat with Lacan, it's from the Autre that the subject finds his own message in an inverse way. It's a message with many voices and to advance in this specification of ability, we will this evening distinguish at least two.

The first of these voices is represented by what we can call the symbolic Autre: The symbolic Autre which, I recalled for you, finds itself ordered by the Name-of-the-Father and whose imperative, whose message thereby addressed to the small speak-being is "Enjoy" – a term which Lacan equivocates by saying that the small speak-being responds by saying "I enjoy" (or "I hear"). There is, then, on the side of the symbolic Autre, an essential message.

From the time the phallic object is the support of significance which he founds and assures, we can well see how the imperative of the chain is really that of jouissance. And without a doubt, we can recognise in this symbolic Autre thereby put forward what Lacan called, on another occasion, the "disque au courant".[4]

But, it is not obligatory that the phallic object should be the support of significance and this precision is not superfluous. In what could be its antecedent status, which we will qualify as "ante-paternal" the signifying chain does not function any less, but it is organised by another significance. Which one? This significance, which is clinically locatable, observable – these are not just points of view or artificial reconstructions – is debt. In this case, the metaphoric – metonymical game of the chain is essentially heard, as linked to the failure of the object in the Autre and what the subject will hear, what will be addressed to him at that moment and which he will assume at the level of the I, will not be "Enjoy" but "pay, it is necessary to pay". And, as we know, what he will have to offer in the long run will be his existence, the last thing which could remain open to him in this kind of attempt to make himself the pure object of this Autre.

What testifies to the fact that we do not lose our way is that this debt is part of what the symbolic Autre, regulated by the Name-of-the-Father, intimates to us – it is in fact an essential element, but is a payment, which as a general rule, is demanded one and for all, a symbolic payment. And this, in an economy of exchange because what is proposed, offered in exchange by the Autre for the price of this payment, of this acquitted debt, is precisely jouissance. It is in fact there that we can read a kind of pact linked to the father. The primordial pact, the symbolic pact, is indeed, this one.

Of course, it can happen – it's a scenario – that a certain form of elegance would be to give back to the father this jouissance, which he offers, and to make of it a sacrifice. It's these kinds of politeness which says, "But no, it's too much, thank you, but keep that for yourself". Because this jouissance, this phallic jouissance, it's precisely what comes to compensate for the failure of sexual rapport.

And it's here that we will hear the second voice of the message that the little speak-being receives from the Autre, this time not only the symbolic Autre but these real Autres, which constitute for him his parents. This message is itself organised as a response to the constraint which they (the parents) feel on the part of the symbolic father: he is himself taken up in a dialogue with the Autre: he is a mode of response to this constraint coming from the Autre, that is to say phallic jouissance itself substituted for this failure of sexual rapport. And this is how the little speak-being will find himself the receptor of messages which will come to be vectors of very contradictory imperatives, very diverse, which could vary from narcissistic happiness (narcissistic jouissance in the acceptance of this phallic jouissance constrained by the Autre) to punishment, from sacrifice to vindication, from protestation to disavowal, from encouragement to defence. No matter what, these messages that the little speak-being receives from these real Autres are always carriers of an already held position.

But, this held position is nearly always defensive with regard to this jouissance thereby constrained by this symbolic Autre. The question here is to know whether the message of one or other of the parents is neurotic or not.

What this little speak-being hears is always organised on the mode of engagement, and at the same time of a position held. And we cannot see how at any moment this would be a kind of holiday, a celebration assumed with regard to this phallic jouissance. There can be times for celebration, but these are times which are very limited in general.

To whom does this message, these messages coming from the Autre which are so different, address themselves? I'm simplifying of course, they address themselves to the little speak-being in so far as he himself is the proof of a failure. By his very presence, by his existence, he himself is the representative of this third presence which gathers together the couple, maintaining desire but also guarantees the failure of this couple, ensuring he will never be able to reunite, to make a rapport. And, this the child is in some way the proof: he is the evidence. What concerns him never misses to be marked by ambivalence, where, the general rule is that it is an excess of love which betrays the negative pole hatred, an aspect of affection, forming all part of the feelings which surround him.

This is what permits us to advance the question of abality: how will the little speak-being constitute himself from the Autre? If this message is addressed to the little speak-being as to a guilty one – because representing this phallus, cause of desire and at the same time the failure of its realisation – the task is also assigned to him to be the hero who will have to wait for reparation. That is how it will return to the child, to be sensitive to the kind of economy adopted by these real Autres who are his parents, to respond to the demands of the symbolic father, that is to say, to the evaluation which they make of the quality of the pact which they have concluded with this symbolic Autre. Is this a good or bad state of affairs? It's a pact, in any case, where jouissance does not in any way forget the failure of the object. But at the same time, he has to be sensitive to the demand, addressed to him to accomplish. He will have to be sensitive to the fact that these real Autres could also themselves fail: he is taken, held in a kind of vocation.

What evidence do we have for all this? They are multiple. For example, what happens for an adopted child? We see quite clearly these lines of forces which I'm in the process of mentioning. Most often, the child is received basically as a donation and not as a representative of this failure in the Autre, of this gap in the Autre which was the cause of the constitution of the couple. With as a consequence, their – inevitable – failings, which will no longer be absolved in advance, pardoned in advance, as being no more than the call of his participation in this original communal failure, but fairly often objectified, becoming those of a bold or incomprehensible child.

He himself will become objectified. You know, incidentally, that this could happen to a child of siblings, for reasons which I'm not going to develop. In the problems of adoption, we can locate the place, the role of representing the child and what is the value of this representation.

This separation between what I call the symbolic Autre and the real Autres illustrate themselves equally in a contemporary way. And that is how the child does not fail to put himself as a judge with regard to his own parents, of their economy which he is able to judge defective or dishonest, a betrayal, fraudulent, with regard to this symbolic Autre. And it's from this place of the symbolic Autre he judges them. It is not rare in adolescence. Sometimes there are families, family economies, where the child is totally put in this place, in this role of judge. In this way, it happens in cases where the parents are both psychotic, we are surprised to see that the child is not contaminated at all by the psychosis of the parents. On the contrary he/she becomes a kind of little precocious adult who lives in a position of vigilance, of spying on them, taking care of them, civilising them, giving them good advice. We cannot understand this except by finding this radical distinction between these real Autres (with their eventual abandonment with regard to the symbolic Autre) and the symbolic Autre to which the child, the little child has an access, I would say, no matter what these inevitable and full real Autres are.

Finally, another illustration of this kind of disassociation, the child will see himself proposing options in the choice of tasks to be done. In this way, he will sometimes be able to take the part of these real Autres who are his parents and for example, engage himself as he is called, to accomplish the vengeance of his parents if these live like despoiled people. This happens, there are some who are despoiled by the Autre – he could choose to receive what will happen to him as a message from these real Autres who are his parents and take up on his own account this kind of myth with which they constitute their economy. But he can also take the side of the symbolic father, if, for example he feels that the fraud committed by the parents, with regard to the symbolic father do not leave any other liberty for him as a child except to repair the damages or the imaginary damage which these ideal Autres have caused. This will, for example, be a frequent preoccupation in obsessional neurosis.

In this constitution of the subject from the messages he gets from the Autre in the putting into place of this abality, the principles of his economy will in this way, be put into place. The economy with the other, with one's fellow is an economy which is ordered by the kind of exchange which is knotted to the Autre. To give an immediate illustration, if the kleptomaniac is more specifically feminine and is produced in general without the slightest guilt, it's of course because a woman feels that the Autre, is in debt with regard to her. And all she is doing in a kind of way is a sort of retrieval. This could take us a long way! An economy organised by the principle of capitalisation of surplus value, like our own – I'm not judging, but locating how things happen –

is thinkable, is realisable, only in a society where it is supposed that there is in the Autre, someone who enjoys in a *surplus* way, who makes *surplus* jouissance of what we give up. This kind of capitalist economy is as a result of a limited sphere, it was not at all a universal economy. There have been cultures, civilisations which are, how shall I say it, obtuse, totally disarmed with regard to this kind of economy. They could not in any way understand what this might signify or represent. Here, I will ask you to read the way in which Lacan[5] underlines, *der Mehrwert*, surplus value, with *die Merhlust*, with surplus enjoyment, so that we can at least understand that the idea of capture for one's fellow, for the little other, of surplus value is thinkable only on the condition of supposing that what the Autre does, what we cede to it as a *surplus enjoyment*, that it is for him a *surplus enjoyment*. And why do we think that?

This kind of perspective always seems to me to justify my title, abality and always has to do with alienation, a foundational alienation. Therefore, in our exchanges, honesty – that is to say an exchange which would be founded on a fair price – is a very fragile given and we cannot, unfortunately, but qualify it as utopian.

There is nothing in the structure and in the economy of exchange which could say what justice could be! There is nothing which could teach us about a well-paid, well-calculated exchange, which would be something which we could leave to anyone, to either one of the "exchangers" without some after taste of remorse! To evaluate the accuracy or the justice of exchange, a symbolic sanction is necessary, that is to say a positive law which would say – the law does not say anything else – what is the fair part of jouissance which comes back to each one, that is to say what is the fair exchange at this time. Because laws vary enormously, and we do not have Roman law anymore. If honesty does not exist in this exchange, all you can do at the very best is to conform, to respect the law. You are not asked anything as to what your feelings are in this regard: all you are asked to do is not to commit an offence. But, if honesty does not exist, we have to remark that villainy exists. This is the paradox. You will see this fundamental asymmetry here. And what kind of villainy are we interested in, in this affair?

It's what consists in serving itself with this kind of knowledge which I'm in the process of speaking to you about – by giving you a chance of being able to make use of it – to engage in villainy – to increase the alienation of your fellows: the speak-being demands only to maintain the place where payment has to be made. Whether it's in the register of the political or in our modest analytic domain, what he wants is to be captured in the desire of the Autre. What better way to be captured in the desire of the Autre, than to pay for this? We know, I'm going to develop this a little bit, that the worst thing for him is that the Autre does not ask anything of him.

In this demonstration which should allow me to return to hysteria, we have to quickly remark that, if the little speak-being has to do with these real Autres who are his parents, the messages which come to him from them do not necessarily coincide. This is a banality! What arrives from one and the other in general, is not at all the same message. This is moreover, sufficient to show him that the idea of all is a strange thing, because they do not tell him the same thing. To the extent that the real father authorises himself from the symbolic father, where he gives support to his message by taking authority from the symbolic father, it would theoretically be this one who is supposed to have prevalence. But, it is not rare, for diverse reasons – perhaps because in his childish impotence, he identifies himself more from his own side – the child privileges the message which comes to him from his mother. Often, it's to do with accomplishing a revenge. And, we see, the range of choices which are proposed to the child and his freedom in the choice of message he would really like to receive from the Autre.

This brings us back to the question of feminine hysteria. Because from the two sides, paternal and maternal and for what concerns also the call of achieving the accomplishment of revenge, it will be in general the little girl – there are two exceptions – who will stay with the questioning of what the Autre will expect of her. Besides, she could traverse periods of mutism because the Autre says nothing to her, as if the Autre did not have a message for her. So, what could she say? From where could she take her orders, her will, her purpose, find her object? And this is without doubt what explains why often the little girl (I insist, we have to always introduce restrictions where we speak about a destiny which is perhaps easily the destiny of the hysteric) may be able to disinterest herself from her real family, to feel herself essentially concerned for this symbolic father, who calls her, if it is only at the level of maternity? There is here at least, a possible inscription in the desire of the Autre.

We have to remind ourselves of a large trait of hysterical identification, the interest for the real Autre, not parental this time but real, incarnate, which we find for example realised in a community in distress, a group in difficulty, carrying a demand to which she can sacrifice herself. Because to the extent that the Autre does not exercise demand with regard to her, she, the hysteric, feels herself as the vector of an excess. She feels guilty for this kind of super-fluousness which inhabits her and which should not be there, which is unjus-tifiably kept by her. That is what accounts for her very great sensitivity to everything which appears to her as demand, as if this demand were at the same time the imperative inviting her to sacrifice this excess of which she suffers, of which she tries to rid herself. Therefore, a major trait of hysterical identification will be to find herself concerned by the constitution of every group which serves as a realisation of this Autre, which substitutes for this Autre which did not ask anything of her and to which she can, in this way, sacrifice herself. Also, because of this failure of a security in the Autre, she finds herself highly vulnerable with regard to the word of her neighbour. She will be very sensitive to the demand underlying this word – there is no word without a demand underlying it – because she feels herself marked by this failure of accomplishment, by this failure of engagement in a trade with the Autre. Hence, this sensitivity, this particular faculty, this empathy for isolating what in the utterances of her neighbour is organised by demand, and which she will live from then on in a spontaneous fashion as an imperative which has to be satisfied. From where, when the circumstances lend themselves to taking a little bit of distance – sometimes, there isn't any – with the passage of time for example, the possibility of feeling this situation as an inexplicable constraint, even a machination, a manipulation to which she is led to cede every time. I will conclude therefore, on the consequence of this kind of disposition, this failure of the message received from the Autre, this failure of security in the Autre, and this kind of vulnerability with regard to the speech of her fellow.

It's a very strange thing, to be vulnerable to the speech of one's fellows. It does not at all go without saying. If, for example, you have a master and you tell him what you think of him "You, my dear man, you are an awful man, you are a crook, you are an idiot", this does not do anything at all to him. If he is really a master, this will not provoke the least bit of emotion. This is perfectly ok for him because it is he who nominates, it is he who uses signifiers; Signifiers have meaning, have weight when they come from him. But what is said to him has no relevance whatsoever.

I remember a seminar, in the last years, where Lacan[6] questioned this, this question of being, or not being, sensitive to the action of the signifier which falls, which make us circulate, the conditions under which it works, or the effect it has where it is from the word of one's fellow which takes on a virtue as if it were that of the Autre.

And I think we can here take note of the way in which there could be a corporal stigmata. If the word of one's fellow is always heard as an invitation to give up on this superfluous object, this object in excess, which the hysteric feels she has to deal with in a guilty fashion and moreover which remains for her enigmatic – also, her somatic symptoms are also erratic: she does not necessarily know where it will lodge, on top, or on the bottom, etc. – we can conceive how this word could have a translation which will bring along corporal manifestations, even if they are stigmata.

Does this word *abalility* please you? It's a word which says very well what it's about and which I truly believe has the advantage of breaking a certain number of phantasies, how will I say it, those full of goodwill, those which turn around understanding oneself, of realising oneself.

Where do these words come from? Very simply, from Aristotle! To search to realise one's being, to look to realise in oneself the maximum of being, the Aristotelian affirmation taken up by scholastic affirmation, and included in a religious speculation is nothing other than a pretension. It would be funny and instructive to locate the numerous clichés which fill own moral literature – because these are moral demands – and try to locate in a more precise way where this introduces itself, where it has come from, from where it was hooked up. And obviously take note of the *consequences*, because there are consequences.

I would like to finish on this before taking up next week the question of masculine hysteria, very different, and which will permit us in a strange way to throw light on feminine hysteria. So, this is how I wished to isolate, to situate the *stage of abalility*. This will permit us to recognise our general aspiration (or at least a circumstance where an exchange is made in this sense!) to alienation because this is our dearest wish, but equally to measure the effects of what passes, not any more for abalility but for aseity: with the embarrassment which accompanies the fact of being "for oneself", of not having found one's coordinates and one's message, and therefore our alienation in an Autre.

12 April 1983

Notes

1 Aristotle, *Metaphysics, Vol. I* (Books I–IX) (trans. H. Tredennick). Cambridge, MA: Harvard University Press, 1989.

2 J. Lacan, "The Mirror Stage as Formative of the *I* Function as Revealed in Psychoanalytic Experience" in *Écrits* (trans. B. Fink). New York: W.W Norton & Co., 2006.

3 Aristotle, *Prior Analytics* (trans. O.F. Owen) . London: H.G. Bohn, 1853.

4 J. Lacan, *The Seminar of J. Lacan, Book XX: Encore, 1972–1973* (trans. C. Gallagher, unedited).

5 J. Lacan, *The Seminar of Jacques Lacan, Book XVII: The Other Side of Psychoanalysis, 1969–1970* (trans. C. Gallagher, unedited).

6 This is Melman's way of reading the later Lacan.

Chapter 18

Masculine hysteria

Charles Melman

We will always have difficulty in orienting ourselves with regard to the question of hysteria, if we do not distinguish that the problem is not only the sex of the speaker but the place he occupies in the structure.

That is why we could begin to speak about masculine hysteria with a question. Why can we not hold the masculine position – yes – the masculine, position as being as hysterical as that which we have described for a woman? And why does it not arise from the same *"proton pseudos"*,[1] the same primordial lie because it is also inscribed in the category of the semblance?

We don't do this for a very simple reason. The word emitted from a masculine position, authorises itself, maintains itself from the place of a founding father from which it legitimately takes its value of truth. It proposes itself as truth because it emanates from this place founded in the Autre. By the same token, it sends the partner, this time the feminine one, to the lack of foundation in her speech that is to say to the *pseudos* character (whether it is *proton* or *deuteron* it doesn't matter), of her saying.

Let us put the question in another way. What makes us say that if a woman authorises herself from this masculine position, that is to say, identifies herself no less from this position in the Autre, and from the truth which from then on founds her speech, is she hysterical? In effect, why after all would it be anatomy which would decide her destiny, and not the deliberate choice of the speak-being? Well, we are not totally groundless in saying that it has to do with a hysterical displacement to the extent that we know that such an option, to be in the masculine position, is animated by a defence against castration.

That is to say, that from that moment this place will find itself invested by the woman for example, as a mission to be accomplished more than the realisation of a desire. Of a mission? This woman "who makes the man" as Lacan says in defining hysteria, will realise a kind of community, a new community where the dimension of alterity will be diminished, because the members of this community who are in this masculine position are fundamentally alike. They are alike because they each identify with the same place, with the same position, with the same reference in the Autre. And, no matter what their anatomical sex, they are not distinguishable except by their merits,

DOI: 10.4324/9781003167839-18

their classification in the realisation of this mission, which is to defend themselves against castration, to put an end to it. We can recognise a position, a manifestation, an hysterical expression, in this community, in the name of higher interests, to realise the true Man. Indeed, we have to recognise, today, in the organisation of our social life – our studies for example, of work – all this goes towards the realisation of such a community.

It's obviously something which is homogenous and synchronic with a kind of social appetite, or in any case, a social demand. Today this seems to go without saying.

We can immediately give a definition of masculine hysteria. By an effect of confusion and for the same reason a defence against castration, an anatomical man comes into a feminine position and tries to realise a community of fellows of which certain members distinguish themselves by pretending to be the True Woman. A certain number do this, especially, the male hysteric. In effect, from the feminine side, he who is delivered to this anatomical sign which is imaginary as a recognition by the father could at one and the same time be valued as a recognition of this total category. And, in this new category, the dimension of alterity is again unmade to the profit of a group of which the members no longer wish to distinguish themselves as in the preceding case, except by quantification: some show themselves to be more successful, better prototypes of the category than the others and, in particular, those who find themselves here marked by this anatomical sign, by this stamp of recognition supposed by the father.

Why do some arrive at this position? It is very clear that the Oedipal time[2] can be decisive in the determination of this transition, in the determination of this voyage. A little girl may want to make the man for the love of her father and with the concern to identify herself with those who appear by structure to be her legitimate representatives. By the same token we can say that in the Oedipus of the masculine hysteric, it's by a hatred of the father that the boy will refuse the identification which seems to him to be pre-formed, to which he seems to be pre-ordained, pre-invited, and to which he gives himself on the side of the Autre.

What could determine him in his choice is able to be redoubled also by the economy of a libidinal order, even more strict. I'm taking up again what was strongly remembered last Sunday with regard to the Seminar on *The Ego*,[3] the question of alienation which was brought up with regard to the psychosomatic. We can really see how to arrive at the position of the Autre, what is determining, is that a subject prefers to preserve what he is in his being. That is to say, that he has chosen to be what? It is never anything else but the phallus and that's what he chooses rather than consent to lose this quality concerning his being. By the same token, he finds himself, with regard to his subjective position oscillating, in a non-sense. Because it is really obvious that for us, this choice, always in the oedipal position, may be ordered by the future male hysteric, by this feeling that phallic realisation is much better assured, is much better guaranteed for him if he lines up on the side of the woman, that is to say, in making this option, this choice of being. With this feeling, ultimately being is far less hazardous than the attempt to have it. The attempt to have it engages, solicits the register of competition and opens the door to a risk, while the category of being is perfectly arbitrated with regard to the worry about competition: one is or one is not, but if one is, quantification is no longer necessary. And, then this choice may be determined also with this equal worry to preserve a jouissance which we know is exactly on the side of the Autre and also on the side of the slave. So how will we be able to recognise this male hysteric? On the whole he is a charmer, a seducer which is a testament to his concern about being recognised and above all – what gives us an explanation – to give himself value as a receiver of the *objet a* which, by his appearance he makes sparkle in this way. That is to say he gets caught in a feminine position.

The interesting thing is that it will be essentially from a woman that he will seek this recognition, a testament that it's really from this side that he situates the power. But it's not for him, in this hysterical position, to make himself recognised or to seduce by violence, by the arbitrary, by an imperative, without help, all of which are proper to S_1.

It has to do with making oneself recognised by a procedure of seduction in a duel confrontation. There again, we will find, not surprisingly, a dynamic because it's an essential time, a mechanism proper to the mirror stage.[4] One will be called, led to abdicate before the brilliance of the other, ready to recognise in this other also so brilliant, endowed with brilliance, his own image in so far as it is driven by an other. You know, this is a totally banal procedure and utterly frequent, that one can have one's ego driven in such a fashion that it should be assumed by an other. To put this in another way, in this attempt to make oneself recognised by a woman, it has to do, for the male hysteric, with proceeding as if he were, for this woman, her own image but her own image successfully and finally accomplished. And this would only be a revenge for the time where it was the feminine imago, ultimately the maternal one, who would exercise vis-à-vis him this killer-like fascination. Killer-like, because this will lead obviously to the abdication of one or the other, in order to recognise the image in the Autre.

We have to say here that this seduction suggests itself to a woman in this attempt at recognition not only at the level of having (at the level of what this image would be) but indeed at the level of the enigmatic being which would have supported her. This necessary, foundational indetermination is therefore sent to this enigmatic partner, which she, henceforth, shares with him.

In this arrangement where a man returns to a woman the question of being, sharing it with her and questioning himself at the same level as to what the Autre wants, to see this question sent back to her may have a troubling effect on the woman.

Therefore, it's apparently at the level of his being from the open question of what his being is about, that this image is proposed as seductive. But, if this imago affirms itself as more prevalent than the woman's, it's also because she finds herself marked by this penile insignia which henceforth, is supposed to deliver her the label of the "good form". That is to say that this imago is supposed to be loved by the Autre. In other words, what is thereby offered to a woman in this demand for recognition which operates by way of this seduction, is truly an image where she may recognise herself, even if this means that she has to eclipse herself, but where she can, nevertheless, recognise herself in a form which would assure the conjunction, an exceptional one, but this time successful, of being and having. In other words, to be a little bit crude, this is what realises the banal phantasy of the hermaphrodite.

It is in this way unique and outside competition that the male hysteric proposes himself to be, henceforth, made part of the feminine community, so that he will find himself near what could be a foundational position – because everyone, thanks to specular mirage, may find a possible accomplishment of his ego in this imago, which in this way has been proposed to him. And, if you wish, I will keep this trait which in masculine hysteria is a certain form of erotomania founded on this kind of bizarre certainty that he, in this position, will necessarily be loved, will be the one, preferred by women. That is to say, as if to the question of women, which he knows very well, what their being is and he will be well able to respond – "well indeed, here, I am".

It is true that in this procedure, this mirror system suggests to a woman an eclipse of what would be her own imago instead of what functions, henceforth, as an ideal. After all, a woman is able to consider this renunciation, as voluntary, it's she who will decide. As if this were her own sacrifice, as if it was her own leadership that operates this so called transformation, that topples over the *objet a*, which finds itself behind her (let us take this under an extremely imaged form, it's not important) for this male representative. As if it were her own renunciation of being which was responsible for this brilliance, as if this male in a position maintaining for himself this brilliance which she would also have yielded to him, was henceforth her product, her creation, even the child of her own selflessness.

I think that this point is not without some interest, because it allows us to decipher a mode of making men in an exclusively feminine way. A way which would escape castration and would operate by a process of donation, a donation made of a woman to a masculine imago which she would, henceforth, find having value as a masculine imago. It's indeed the imago which founds masculinity, founds being, founds the phallus.

I hope I will not shock you by telling you that this is a mode not rare in certain cultural zones and to name them – why not? – in particular the Mediterranean zones. With regard to these zones, we need to question ourselves as to the role of colonisation in the frequency, even the prevalence of this process which functions, as if in certain cases it was the only way out, when the reference to the real father, even to the symbolic father, finds itself impossible because of circumstances which would hold on, not to the specificity of the familial milieu, but to the specificity of the cultural milieu. In such and such historical circumstances, in such and such a zone, it may be difficult for a certain number of the populations to give value to the male child of what is in him of the real and the symbolic father: if, for example, he has to refer to a culture, not necessarily forbidden, but in any case presented as minor, even a serf.

From this we can reflect on certain characteristics. If the determination of this male hysteric is made from an oedipal entrapment of the little boy for example – to allow us to disengage from the cultural and historical conditions – this may ensure a resolute hatred of the father and a refusal to identify himself with this real father. Participation in the feminine community, the fact, of lining himself up in this position is therefore imprinted with the wish to take revenge on this real father. It has to do with constituting a man, but Autre this time who would escape castration and at the same time would permit the woman to escape this no less than he, that is to say, be no longer submitted to this disastrous economy of this pseudo-master, because it is not as a master that the male hysteric proposes himself to a woman.

This permits us to grasp why active homosexuality is not the rule in the case of masculine hysteria, so that we can ask, why, if he arrives at this feminine position, is this not a kind of invitation to a homosexual *passage à l'acte*?

But we find this is not the general rule. Why? Because if this hysterical process denies or disavows the father, it is to be able to surpass him and to exercise his own virility and to help save a woman from her condition. This is what can be called the myth of the male hysteric. If the *objet*, cause of his phantasy is truly essentially narcissistic – it is because it's really his own image, which for him maintains desire – it is nevertheless specific to the foundational myth of the male hysteric, that the feminine imago will function in the phantasy at the level of the substitute, the semblant of this narcissistic imago henceforth destroyed or in any case put between parentheses. In other words, if in the phantasy of the male hysteric the feminine imago is invested at the level of the semblant of oneself, it is always possible to make this self-re-appear, this marvellous object, this marvellous image which would constitute him. Here is, a kind of reversal of a position of being properly speaking the creator of this feminine imago, and may henceforth perfectly function as her product.

This image of oneself, this narcissistic image is the cause of the phantasy because it is there obviously to resurrect a time of childhood, where the little male was able to live invested at the level of the image of the object of the desire of his mother, to be for her the image representing the foundational object of her desire, that is to say the image representing the phallus.[5] This moment, it has to be said, has nothing exceptional about it in what constitutes a mother with her child, is this not right? But, if this moment finds itself retrospectively privileged, we can well see how this image of oneself, is a cause of phantasy and makes possible perverse *passages à l'acte*, of the homosexual type. I must stress, these, perverse *passages à l'acte* are not the rule. And what is decisive for a better heterosexual determination of male hysteria is that the feminine imago is primordially for him the cause of sexual attraction. This shows us very well what? It shows us that male hysteric is a secondary reactional elaboration with regard to the implementation of an initial phantasy which implies paternal castration.

Everything happens in male hysteria as if there were this intervention of paternal castration, making at the same time the feminine imago the support of desire of the feminine imago, but like a secondary elaboration, with regard to this first time, reorganising the phantasy in the way in which I've tried to situate for you. To love women, the male hysteric is without doubt hetero-sexual. But he produces something curious for himself which is from the position of the Autre, it's from the position of *heteros* that he loves them. That is to say, in realising this, we really have to say it like this, it is a strange form of homosexuality!

This gives to the *conjugo*, maintained in this way by the male hysteric, a small particularity. To want to think of oneself, to present oneself, to demand of oneself to be the support of the object cause of desire in the couple, it is obviously he who brings the right fuel to light the fire. In a certain way, we can also say that it is he who in the couple finds himself dressed in the most coloured, the most successful plumage. Henceforth, what seems a paradox and merits attention, is that sexual attraction by him can be upheld, not by the eruption of the conjoint but, on the contrary, by her failure, her insuffi-ciency, her lack, her demand duly expressed, which puts into relief for him his own excess and, henceforth, the generosity, the gift of which he will in some way make the alibi of his sexual activities. In other words, there is nothing here which is the effect of violence but on the contrary, what comes from gift, from love, even from nourishment, to compensate for this pretend asymmetry.

The approach of the partner may be regulated by the necessity to make himself recognised by her as the *real* man (not the pathetic one of the original foyer!) which is a phantasy I will allow myself to qualify as Stendhalian, if you wish and allows me to call the complex of Julien Sorel.[6] It's of course not an accident that Henri Beyle found this patronym *Sorel* for his hero Julien; You know the privileged attachment Stendhal had for his own sister and he even had relations which had the whiff of sulphur, but no matter. But, if there is a kind of phantasy which supports the different works of Stendhal and, I suppose give them this captivating and admirable side, we have nothing to regret – it's without doubt this matrix we see reproduced, every time.

Therefore, and I will finish on this, if for the male hysteric the approach of his partner is regulated by the necessity for her to be the true man, this part-ner will become Autre, which at the same time commands, directs his speech. Here, he is devoted to all the changes which, henceforth, the capriciousness of this real Autre can impose on him. From where the mythomania proper to masculine hysteria, which brings us to what I mentioned at the beginning: the question of non-sense: the non-sense from where his speech is articulated to the extent that he has chosen it. This male hysteric spontaneously, because of the fact that he finds himself lodged in the place of non-sense, the metaphysical vocation so willingly born in him, questions himself as to what would be the meaning of existence.

This is the point on which I will stop this evening. The next time, that is to say the 10th of May, I think there aren't any holidays, I will continue with this question of masculine hysteria, in particular with regard to the relation to the father, and with the economy proper to this disposition.

QUESTION: The phallic reference which appeared at the beginning of your lecture made me think of foreclusion. I found that in the end, the margin may not be perhaps too large between this particular loss, for the male hysteric and foreclusion. But, then you said that everything happens as if the paternal metaphor had functioned, all the same. What are we to think in terms of structure?

CHARLES MELMAN: In male hysteria we take account that there is an oedipal time, an oedipal invitation which was perfectly put in place. Male hysteria also has to do with castration as well as the Name-of-the-Father. He is a neurotic, a good neurotic, good like it should be, so there is no problem.

What happens after that – after that – I'm saying, he engages in a kind of chivalry, a kind of specific secret myth. He engages in a kind of attempt at achievement to resolve a double impossibility. On the one hand, identifying with his father, surpassing him – to such an extent that he doesn't resemble him in any way, yet, nevertheless realises him by putting him in this position of a non-castrated mythical father. On the other hand, putting himself in the group of the feminine community telling them in some way "I'm yours and I come to take you out of this place, and at the same time to resolve what the feminine impasse involves." We have to understand male hysteria as participating in a kind of history, organised in relation to original castration. This explains why, in general, a position of masculine hysteria is well established. As in every position, there can be difficulties, moments of wavering, moments of crisis but all the same it's something fundamentally solid in the structure.

QUESTION: From the clinic and precisely from the symptomatology, are these specific male hysterical somatisations?

CHARLES MELMAN: No, they are not specific. They are absolutely the same kind as somatisations of feminine hysteria. This is without doubt a point which we will have to take up again as it has to do with a disposition of structure, in this hysterical position indifferent to the anatomical sexes.

QUESTION: I'm asking myself about identifications in masculine hysteria. If the hatred of the father, this pathetic figure, as you've called him, orders this structure, this seems to me to locate certain identifications, for example with the paternal or maternal grandfather. Is there not a necessity in a hysterical structure to find masculine figures who are not so pathetic and who are not the father?

CHARLES MELMAN: It's possible but it's not necessary. Certainly, the grandfather seems to better escape this kind of destiny, because he is not taken up in an oedipal position. It's therefore a masculine image which can be invested in more easily. And it's also an image which participates more willingly in the familial myth, with an aura which puts him a little bit in the shade of the mediocrity of daily life.

QUESTION: Is there not a hatred of the father which does not depend on the real father?

CHARLES MELMAN: It surely has to do with the real father, to the extent that he is the representative, in a degraded way, of the symbolic father and it has to be said, in this case, one does not go without the other, that is to say, in the end, the one who puts the woman in a position of alterity.

QUESTION: I'm asking myself what is the specific racket which could be born from a *conjugo* between a male hysteric and a hysterical woman?

CHARLES MELMAN: Yes, but next time we have to see how the position of the analyst is not totally confused with that of masculine hysteria.

19 April 1983

Notes

1 Aristotle, *Prior Analytics*, Book II (trans. R. Smith. Indianapolis: Hackett Publishing Company, 1989. Ref. made in S. Freud, *Studies on Hysteria*, Vol. II, S.E. (1893–1895). London: Hogarth Press, 1955 and J. Lacan, *The Seminar of Jacques Lacan, Book VII: The Ethics of Psychoanalysis 1959–1960* (ed. J-A. Miller, trans. D. Porter). London: Routledge, 1992.

2 S. Freud, "Some Psychical Consequences of the Anatomical Distinction between the Sexes" in *The Ego and the Id and Other Works*, Vol. XIX, S.E. (1923–1925). London: The Hogarth Press, 1961.

3 J. Lacan, *The Seminar of Jacques Lacan, Book II: The Ego in Freud's Theory and in the Technique of Psychoanalysis, 1954–1955* (ed. J-A. Miller, trans. S. Tomaselli). Cambridge: Cambridge University Press, 1988.

4 J. Lacan, "The Mirror Stage as Formative of the Function of the *I* as Revealed in Psychoanalytic Experience" in *Écrits* (trans. B. Fink). New York: W.W. Norton & Co., 2006.

5 J. Lacan, "The Signification of the Phallus" in *Écrits*.

6 Stendhal, *The Red and The Black* (trans. B. Raffel, with an Introduction by D. Johnson). New York: Dover Publications, 2004.

Chapter 19

Paranoia

Charles Melman

It is strange to say that on the road to hysteria we are faced with a question which appears to be difficult to get around, just as much to advance about masculine hysteria as to respond to the question: *what is a woman?* This question, which arose for me in an unexpected way after our last meeting, is that of paranoia. It seems that we can now put into place what the structure of paranoia is and, at the same time, make considerable progress in our study of hysteria. We can now testify to the way in which hysteria is totally different – it has to do with something else completely – even if there are these famous pseudo forms, alongside, after or about paranoia, whatever you like to call it, which will sometimes make us speak about delusional hysteria.

With regard to this question, to begin with, what do we put into place? What founds the paranoid rapport of a subject with the Autre, the grand Autre, is that the subject, this supposed *subjectum*, is not so much the supposed as the underposed. In his relation to the Autre he finds himself determined by an infinite order, by a non-closed order.

This is what, immediately, cuts to the question of the neurotic who has a rapport with a signifying chain commanded by original repression. This repression introduces a limit and an unattainable limit because the repressed signifier finds itself fallen, separated, topologically cut off from the chain. We know for the neurotic that this *Uverdrängung* operates the closing and the vectorisation of the signifying chain.

What are the consequences for a *sub-jectum* of this rapport with an Autre which is in this way infinite? The first, surely the most dramatic, the most impressive, is that at the same time this *sub-jectum* no longer has any fixed place in the Autre. And this, no matter what the pact, he tries to give to this Autre with all the symbolic gifts he is able to propose, in which he will try to engage himself, all the offers he will try to make in order that this Autre, in accepting this gift, will recognise him. Therefore, there is this failure of a fixed place in the relationship to the Autre, because in the Autre, in the grand Autre, he finds himself deprived.

I could engage with this subject in an extremely rich clinic which I will call, for example, a clinic of domicile. It has to do with all the importance for the

DOI: 10.4324/9781003167839-19

subject of which the management of domicile is comprised, of this fixed place. This is something which is never not negligible – he could spend his life with this – managing his home. *A contrario*, when precisely such a mode of rapport finds itself put in place with an infinite Autre, it is not at all rare that banal symptoms are made manifest which are, at the same time, strongly explicit: a feeling of burglary in the home, intrusion into the home, or indeed that the place has already been taken. From an epistemological point of view, it's very interesting for us, to see how the modality of the rapport with the signifier, regulates perceptions for the subject. Because what is directly at stake is, properly speaking, projected here on to his sensible world, to his mode of perception. In his rapport with the Autre, with infinity, he will find himself deprived of every fixed domicile and will, henceforth, have the feeling that the place which for him will be the most intimate, the most closed, the most constrained, will find itself thereby exposed and open, despite all his precautions.

Another clinical element may help us to illustrate, with other forms of permutations totally well-known from this life of the home: all that may cause the trouble of jouissance at this home, for example, could be the noise made by neighbours. We see and we read about it every day, paranoid reactions properly experimental, produced by such manifestations. People, otherwise placid, likeable, not especially miserable, nor disturbed, can have paroxysms of sorts, sometimes even murderous ones, because of such noise of domiciliary jouissance, which is so common nowadays.

I will, with regard to this, go a little further. One can experimentally provoke a neurosis on oneself, nothing is easier. It is enough to order oneself a certain kind of prohibition, or a certain kind of repression to soon enough have a lapsus, or words which betray exactly what we would thereby like to defend. I had for a long time thought that one could not provoke a psychosis in an experimental way. I am no longer so sure. There is a circumstance which seems to me to be capable of provoking a psychotic episode in an experimental way; it's when the noise which upsets the jouissance of the home is represented by a foreign language. If anyone has the means or would like to amuse themselves by verifying this, insofar as this is necessary, it would be interesting to see how long a subject could resist such a situation. We can give the reason for this. In this situation where the jouissance of his own place, his domicile, finds himself thereby disturbed by a foreign language, the subject finds himself with the anxiety of the rekindling of an original situation, a hypothetical one but which we can, at the same time, say like this: this (situation) where the child finds himself in relation to a language which has ceased for him to be something foreign, which has become maternal only after the gifts of this language were accepted there. By the same token, his own value in so far as he is a subject, that is to say his phallic value, finds itself recognised. We can very well, if only in a mythical way, postulate this original situation.

I think I'm not extrapolating too much in saying to those who are interested in this manifestation, this always strange thing which is called racism or xenophobia, that is to this side that it is necessary to go looking. Why is it something which resurges so spontaneously, which reinvents itself like that so readily?

With regard to this, the famous "primitive scene"[1] whose traumatic character remains enigmatic – why is it that this story could very well be traumatic for a child? – and operates in much the same way? The child hears coming from his parents a secret language, I mean a series of noises, a series of sounds which remain for him for a certain period of time really enigmatic, a series in regard to which, as a child, he has nothing to offer and from which by the same token he finds himself obviously excluded.

This failure of a stable security in the Autre – because this Autre is infinite, and the subject cannot anchor himself – works in a devaluing way for the subject. The place from where he tries to authorise for himself, reveals itself to be fluctuating incessantly, always mobile, always inadequate because it's never the same, and at the same time he finds himself just as unjustified by the value, by which he tries to recommend himself.

So, as I remarked earlier, he can obviously engage himself in the offering of sacrifices to the Autre by hoping for some kind of adoption. We know these sacrifices: work, love, renunciation, sublimation. But these gifts will prove to be inefficacious because as a general rule – I will introduce an exception a little later on – they are unable to introduce a finite order into the Autre. This subject, in suffering, finds himself delivered up to a thing, that of the signifier, which pushes into him, which sweeps him along by the whim of a capriciousness which remains profoundly enigmatic, on a journey the destination of which he does not grasp and where the question of *what does he want of me?* – the question of *che vuoi,?* imposes itself on him without an answer. This suffering subject finds himself as a nomad in a real which is always moving, always displaced, transformed by the ebb and flow of the signifier and which, in a movement deprived of repetition, is therefore deprived of all regularity.

I would ask you to look at the marvellous experience which Schreber[2] has so very well described, I mean this kind of voyage, which has become a voyage because it's precisely a kind of exploration, because there is no repetition. Everything was presented endlessly in a kind of surprise, in a kind of newness, of originality, a flash and all this does not stop reappearing and just as quickly disappears without return.

It's from this that we can understand the extreme sensitivity for this subject; to grasp, to try and understand what is demanded of him, to interpret topics which have effectively the manipulative power to transform and to displace. There is the certainty that these utterances, like this, around him, promenade around him (it doesn't matter what; fragments of phrases heard in the street, something on the radio, a word in a corridor, it doesn't matter) the certainty of these utterances concern him. But, if his presence in being a virtual subject is never accepted in the Autre, because then he finds himself in a position of reject, it is inevitable, and it's always in this way that it happens: that by this very reject, the Autre wins, finds his significance. Why? We know that the signifying chain only acquires its significance from this rejected object, from the object from which it is cut off, from which it is separated. And, in such a situation the subject may have the conviction that everything articulated concerns him, to have himself put in a position of rejection, it is he who will thereby find himself upholding the significance of the chain.

Another remark: this situation where this *subjectum*, this subject in suffering finds himself endlessly without resources and dislodged from places where he tries to hold on in his relation to the Autre, depleted and dislodged at the whim of the capriciousness of this Autre, this situation gives him the feeling of being a creature without a shadow, without weight and therefore always exposed to the risk of being unveiled. This is what I will qualify as paranoid suffering, and this is regulated by the conditions of structure which we can perfectly well locate.

From this suffering is put into place what we can isolate as being the paranoiac solution, the kind of remedy which the subject will try to bring to this situation. I don't think it's excessive to say, that the destiny of the suffering subject will himself play on this rejection by what is signified to him by the Autre. To the repeated question of *che vuoi* (what does he want of me? What is it that he wants of me? What does he expect from me? What does all this mean? what does this signify?) he will conclude by admitting that what the Autre wants, it's his very own rejection because that is what is endlessly being signified to him. When he accepts this position of being the object of rejection he deprives the other of his quality of alterity, to assume it himself. It's he himself in this position of reject which becomes the Autre and from then on he occupies a place which we can qualify as properly feminine.

In other words, he makes his law of this reject and engages as if he himself had effectively become the foundational cause of a limit in the Autre. His rejection is the gift to which he finally consents: it will no longer be that of work, of love, of gifts, it's he himself who in some way will totally occupy this place. And it's as if, by the same token, he finds himself as founder, as a guarantee of this limit, thereby instituted as Autre. It has to be said that he can win this place in an easier way by being a rejected object rather than by being weak. This impossibility of being recognised, admitted by the Autre, can give him the feeling that his job is to please, to seduce. And in this he can be comforted by the fact that he finds himself in a position which from a structural point of view is a feminine position.

This helps us to understand why, as Lacan[3] remarked from the beginning, homosexuality is not the cause of paranoid manifestations which have to be interpreted as reactionary and defensive; but in the homosexual fear, the unease is linked to a disposition of structure, which is really paranoiac.

This subject, in all this adventure, manifests a certain courage – it's a trait for which he has to be admired – a courage which is rarely lacking. It has to be said that in general there is a battle by the subject to find some liveable stability in such a system. But, if paranoia is not a defensive modality against some kind of homosexuality, what we can recognise as defensive in his reaction, is the sublimation in which he will engage, to correct his status and the state of being an object of infamy, this state to which he is reduced when he accepts this rejection. Remember the injuries which accompanied Schreber, the President of the Court of Dresden, "You are only a slut", his voices said to him. He tries to correct his status as an object of infamy by sublimation, by a sublimation making him accede to being the object of supreme status. This procedure is not a simple change of sign, a negative which is enough to pass for a positive. It's a totally different thing. It's a procedure which involves the renunciation of this ex-sistence which seems to be so decried by the Autre to consent to make himself, of this Autre the pure object, the pure instrument. In other words, to the question of *che vuoi?* There is still the interpretation of what would be desire of the Autre. If the Autre cannot accept my ex-sistence, well then, I will renounce it and in this position of being a reject, I will make myself a pure object for him, a pure object arranged for his satisfaction, to satisfy him and also, I will make myself his instrument, his agent.

In such a situation where a renunciation of ex-sistence is carried out, this sublimation is not only seen in paranoia but also in other procedures which concern sublimation. This is nothing exceptional. Religious sublimation also goes by way of the sacrifice of ex-sistence. It is in a certain way too the renunciation of ex-sistence and the gift of the Autre of what would be the dearest thing, because it comes from the Autre and where this Autre is ordered by a father, it's a way, isn't it, of giving back to him that which would be the most precious gift?

But it ends up with this, in a system where such a renunciation operates, the signifier loses its function of representation, to explore and give up what the speak-being is about, which finds itself entirely submitted to its imperative. Of course, we are all sensitive in a certain way to the signifiers which fall on us: kind words, or words of calumny, this could have consequences, that could send you running for help. We smell something in the gut, neuro-vegetative manifestations, unease or, on the other hand, feeling well, but all the same, we resist. What is it that makes us, in the end, hold up under this torrent? It is because the subjective position is maintained in a real, which I will remind you is normally refractory, in the shadow of the movement of the signifier. So that in the case where the gift of ex-sistence is given to the Autre, we can very well see that for such a speak-being, the signifier loses its function of representation, because what it could represent is in some way, evacuated. Henceforth, this signifier becomes an imperative and no longer the representative of a subject but the *being* itself of this ex-subject.

This ends of course with the constitution of a new community. A community of pure semblants because this procedure ends up in some kind of way abolishing the category of the Autre when the subject is renounced, is evacuated from the chain. Everyone is at this moment perfectly identical, one signifier is the same as the next. And there is in this community an exception to the rule in every ensemble. It is now the paranoiac himself who is this exception insofar as he would have been totally successful in renouncing this subjective position: with the aim of an ideal, an accomplished ideal, he holds himself in this position of exception.

We end up here in an organisation with a rather special dynamic, quite a new one. If from his place of exception the paranoiac now gives value to the community to which he belongs (which could be a random community, it could be a family community, it could be a social community, it doesn't matter), if he makes it known that as a general law that what would have been addressed to him in a personal way, that is to say, to have to renounce ex-sistence, it will end up that he will stay in a place, that of the reject. This place of exception, he will have a right to it, because he will have perfectly accomplished this renunciation.

The others, the members of the community, if they are invited to proceed there, are also invited never to succeed because if they are successful they would put the place they occupy into danger. Here there is something totally banal, occurring frequently and perfectly contradictory in this kind of wish: that the others engage themselves, on the condition that above all, they will never be successful. But, in a reversal which interests us, if this place of exception validates itself by the fact that the subject has precisely renounced his position as subject, to make himself a pure object and a pure instrument of the Autre, he reclaims at the same time – it's here that the reversal is curious, precise, understandable – the right to ex-sistence, it will be that only now, and thanks to him, this limit operates in the Autre. He retrieves this and it's now an ex-sistence which henceforth will be one of pure capriciousness, insofar as there is nothing which could reign it in or control it.

This is what I have undertaken for you under the rubric of the paranoid solution: how, at the price of an acceptance of what is heard and accepted as the wish of the Autre, the paranoiac gains a status, a stable place and a putting into order, in attributing, what's more to himself, the paternity of this chain and by a reversal, he reclaims the right to a kind of ex-sistence, limited to pure capriciousness which nothing can rein in.

It's from this establishment of the major traits of the clinic of paranoia and the way in which French psychiatry isolated it which has enabled it to be understood. As you know, these major traits are the delusion of grandeur, the delusion of jealousy and the delusion of revenge.

- The delusion of grandeur. He who occupies this place of exception, can only have the conviction of being a considerable personage and nothing nor nobody can imitate him, because its effectively the place which escapes castration: the place of the at-least-one. We understand therefore that, in a really legitimate way, he can only find himself in a delusion of grandeur. He cannot do otherwise.

- The delusion of jealousy. Jealousy comes from many different processes, but this delusion of jealousy can be very well justified by the care that all loving respect should be reserved for this place. After all, that God should be jealous is something which has been explicitly articulated. He demands that all this respect should be given to his representations or to his person.
- With regard to the delusion of revenge, it is true that this place demands in some way, tributes and gifts. It's the place of the at-least-one which exercises itself, for whoever, with what's more the feeling of debt never perfectly paid, this invitation to contribute to this imaginary treasure of the Autre. It's really from this place that the demand is felt.

There is an extremely simple step which has yet to be made. These demands – to be recognised in one's grandeur, to be the exclusive object of the love of his subjects, to be equally the source of appeal of gifts and of donations – we are compelled to recognise, that we give these to God, when we call him Father. All the same, we have to immediately say that this Father, whom we recognise as having such demands, has a major trait which distinguishes Him from paranoiac demands. This Father, this God marked as Father (this is not the God of the philosophers but of religion), there is something which He does not ask of his creatures, it's to renounce ex-sistence. If certain people believe that they are rendering homage to Him, by giving Him the gift of their ex-sistence, in consecrating their life in a monastery for example, if certain people engage in this, it is their affair. But He, as a Father, recognises this existence as good and pleasant. It's really in this that there is a major hiatus between the God of religion, of revealed religions and this kind of paranoiac demand. I remember a discussion a long time ago now, in trying to understand what could be said about the experience of Schreber[4] which was not the same as a religious experience. I think we have the exact response here. Schreber could well have pushed all that in a very lucid fashion, the farthest away possible, to try and forge this private religion. This is an essential difference between this and revealed religion.

So, you will say to me, yes, but why? Why this difference and what holds it together? Because you always make reference to the structure, what is it about the structure which means that the Father such as religion reveals, does not institute what the paranoiac tries to foment, even if it is putting Him in his place?

It seems to me that all this is fairly compact, fairly dense. To respond to the question without making this evening too heavy, I will immediately come to the conclusion in jumping to the third time of my exposé. After, the "suffering" after the "solution", it is called "the paranoical logic" – a very interesting logic which I will eventually speak about before the end of the year.

Why is it different? Well, we can, I think, prove what Lacan[5] tried to specify about paranoia when he spoke about the Borromean knot. He used to tell us that in paranoia the Borromean knot had this particularity that the real, the symbolic and the imaginary found themselves in continuity. You will remember that. This is a formulation which at first glance is rather enigmatic.

But, in the exposé which I've just given you, we see how the real and the symbolic are effectively in continuity, because, we have to do here with a real which finds itself continuously displaced and reorganised, modified according to the flux of the symbolic due to the very fact of this failure of a limit in the Autre, because all operates as if there was no cut between them.

But, how do we understand the fact of the imaginary being equally in continuity with the real and the symbolic? We could think that with putting the knot straight that it passes from R_3 and R_2, from a space with three dimensions to a space with two dimensions. There is no more crossing over. The knot is strictly maintained according to a Euclidian plan, R_2, which we love so much, in which we spontaneously think. You know that it was necessary that the researchers had to think in three dimensions, one dimension more, then simply write their formulae on the board to organise them in space to discover the double helix chromosome. We can ask ourselves if this Euclidian space, to which we aspire, this space to which we have grown accustomed is not a paranoiac ideal? It's like as if in this putting into place of this ideal, we should be spontaneously more at ease ...

But it's not enough to respond to the question as to what the putting into continuity of the imaginary, with the real and the symbolic means. So, we can perhaps note this: in the end, this position of exception, this position of rejection, this position therefore Autre, which the paranoiac here takes on, is held up essentially from an imaginary representation which he gives it and is not a fact of structure, a real cut which would effectively put into place this real, this Autre. This position of exception would have to find itself endlessly validated, demonstrated, produced by exceptional characters, which the paranoiac has to endlessly show, sacrificing himself in order to hold on to the fiction of this place, of this dimension. And, that is why the paranoiac God, despite traits the similarity of which I've already noted, is essentially different to the God of revealed religions, which is put into place by a cut and therefore never attainable, and that is why it is not a question of rejoining Him, nor are we ever able to contemplate His face.

It's therefore in this way that we can hear, it seems to me, this formulation of Lacan when he says that in paranoia the three categories find themselves in continuity. We can also understand why the paranoiac finds himself limited by this work, by this force of labour which constantly consists in his devoting himself in giving value in an imaginary way to this category of the real without which this imaginary representation would cease to exist. This is how Schreber finished, in this kind of obligation, constrained to live his life in front of the mirror, dressing himself in women's clothes. It is because he is destined for the permanent jouissance of his gods and to produce endlessly, in some way, but under an essentially imaginary mode, manifestations of the presence of their alterity – which he will be able to renounce if there is something of the symbolic sanction of his feminine position. As you know, this symbolic sanction is positioned on the horizon because he has begun to feel it in his stomach, the movement of first embryos which are going to populate, are going to repopulate the world. There was here a beginning of maternity which would be the hoped-for symbolic sanction, giving peace and comfort to all this trajectory.

This detour via paranoia will permit us, I believe, to grasp in the best way possible what is in the relationship of the male hysteric to the father. Hysterical paranoiac reactions are pseudo-paranoiac modalities, even if the pictures and closely linked longings can be held together. And, from these we will slide easily, and I will try to make you sensitive to this the next time about the question of what a woman is: why is the hysterical position not confused with the feminine position, why she is not the attribute of it, it's inevitable condition?

We will take up these positions next Tuesday, the second last seminar of this year. And, on the 14th of June, I will deal with the question of hysterical resistance, the mode of hysterical resistance to psychoanalysis.

We have to, all the same, consider with regard to paranoia, that we have two things with Lacan. On the one hand, all his work begins with his thesis, the mirror stage,[6] that is to say on the putting into place of the imaginary conditions of paranoia, how the imaginary itself has this dimension, this paranoiac quality. All his texts nourished by this position, for example, a proposal on "Psychical Causality",[7] or his texts on Criminality,[8] on "Aggressivity in Psychoanalysis"[9] are texts which are always current and always amazing. Then we have, "On a Question Preliminary,"[10] which takes on in a far more general way what the psychoses are about. And, then we have at the very end, the Borromean knot, three lines and a drawing to say: there it is, the paranoiac Borromean knot.[11] I imagine that you like me, or some among you, can be a little moved, a little distracted in front of this graffiti. What is this kind of procedure that he could put into our hands like that? A key, a formula, a representation? I know that as far as I'm concerned I received with this a certain reticence. This is an under-statement to say the least.

Well, by the detour which I've just made this evening, the conditions which are strictly speaking symbolic of the determination of paranoia, it seems to me that in taking up this question via this link we arrive at what is of a teaching value of this formula, this final Lacanian formula. What would be the interest of repeating the formulae even if they are Lacanian, for their elegance, for their arbitrariness or for their beauty? Obviously, this looks "chic", but in the end, it's not going to satisfy us. It should be an instrument in our work, that is what Lacan wanted, he did not wish it to distract us. It seems to me that by the detour which I've done for you, here, this evening and what you can verify in your own time, we begin, to know what this drawing of Lacan allows us to grasp, which would otherwise stay obscure in the clinic of paranoia.

I did not artificially construct this investigation into the way in which the imaginary could find itself in continuity with the real and the symbolic. It's something which appears to me as not resolved. The continuity of the real and the symbolic seems to me to speak for itself and to be very rich. For the rest I have run out of ideas. They are perhaps more than likely the constraints of elaboration, which demands that we work something out which led me to this last feeling which does not appear to me to be either forced or inexact and which allows us to understand a lot of things, a lot of traits in this wonderful clinic.

QUESTION: On the side of the man, the push to the woman; on the side of the woman, erotomania. Is this one and the same question?

CHARLES MELMAN: It is totally clear to the extent that psychosis operates as a vector of a rejected signified to the subject that it is a push-to-the-woman. If the subject finishes by consenting to it, he recognises his place in a position of alterity, and from then on also in a feminine position. But it's not for all that, that this femininity will find itself confused with that which is normally or physiologically – if I may express myself metaphorically, an establishing of a symbolic determination.

This symbolic determination implies the cut which isolates a place Autre, and therefore, gives it its status. Even if those who, if I may say so, are going to populate this place and maintain this status, staying in a certain enigma, a certain investigation as to what is owed to the father, if he does or does not intervene. Nevertheless, from the moment that the paternal function operates this kind of cut, which manages, which gives its guarantee to this place Autre, those (men and women) who populate this place can lay claim to a femininity, marked by the agreement of this father. They are not in the end there as strangers, they are there in a place which he has managed and which guarantees them. So, the situation of push-to-the-woman of psychosis does not find itself guaranteed by any cut and is maintained only by manifestations of the imaginary register. It is not from this place that one could conclude that a woman is mad and if they are, it's not at all for the same reasons, it's not from this place in any case that this is deduced. I evoked erotomania in relation to masculine hysteria, which I mentioned comprises a paranoiac dimension and I believe that we will have to take it up to show the proof of the structures I'm speaking about.

I have to say that since the beginning of my studies in psychiatry, I have been amazed by this kind of consistency that I perceived in the forms of paranoiac delusions: the delusion of revenge, the delusion of grandeur, and the delusion of jealousy which have been so well individualised and late enough, by the French clinic. I had the occasion to see, with my own eyes, a delusion of revenge transform itself. He was a very courageous fellow. He was stopped in front of the Elysée where he wanted to seek an allowance for his son who had a handicap. He therefore arrived in the clinic with a delusion of revenge. With the helpful psychotherapist and with this kindness and attention and interest, he consented to abandon his delusion of revenge. It was, after all a great result. But, at the same time, as he abandoned his delusion of revenge, he began to say "Listen, doctor it's strange, but it's been a few days since I received a letter from my wife, I'm wondering what has happened". There again, in an experimental way, a delusion of jealousy has come to take the place of the preceding one, and which, in spite of the anecdote, has at least the merit of illustrating that it really has to do with the same structure, which are the differing expressions of a position which is obviously one.

Good, so until next Tuesday.
10 May 1983

Notes

1 S. Freud, "The Wolfman Case" in *An Infantile Neurosis and Other Works*, Vol. XVII, S.E. (1917–1919). London: The Hogarth Press, 1955.
2 S. Freud, *The Case of Schreber, Papers on Technique and Other Works*, Vol. XII, S.E. (1911–1913). London: The Hogarth Press, 1958.
3 J. Lacan, *The Seminar of Jacques Lacan, Book III: The Psychoses, 1955–1956* (ed. J-A. Miller, trans. R. Grigg). London: Routledge, 1993.
4 Freud, *The Case of Schreber*.
5 J. Lacan, *The Seminar of Jacques Lacan, Book XXII· R.S.I., 1974–1975* (trans. C. Gallagher, unedited).
6 J. Lacan, "The Mirror Stage as Formative of the *I* Function as Revealed in Psychoanalytic Experience" in *Écrits* (personal translation).
7 J. Lacan, "Presentation on Psychical Causality" in *Écrits* (trans. B. Fink). New York: W.W. Norton & Co., 2006.
8 J. Lacan, "A Theoretical Introduction to the Functions of Psychoanalysis in Criminology" in *Écrits*.
9 J. Lacan, "Aggressivity in Psychoanalysis" in *Écrits*.
10 J. Lacan, "On a Question Prior to Any Possible Treatment of Psychosis" in *Écrits*.
11 Lacan, *Book XXII: R.S.I.*

Chapter 20

Another approach to masculine hysteria

Charles Melman

We saw the last time what the failure of domicile is in the Autre for the subject in paranoia. The word domicile is just right, because, as you know, *domus* has the most fine link with *dominus*. In paranoia, therefore, for the subject there is no place which is fixed in the Autre. Therefore, he is forced to manifest himself in a stable way in the real, at the price only of an endless imaginary usage. It's without doubt what gives to the paranoiac this kind of permanence, the famous paranoiac rigidity, that is to say this petrification, but also this vigour, of not allowing himself any mobility with regard to this constraint.

What could possibly intrigue us, is this failure of a fixed place in the Autre is also found in hysteria. But, instead of a petrified kind of deployment for the hysteric we have a sort of versatility of representation which he gives, something unforeseen, or indeed what is called his mythomania, an inconsistency of his representation. How is the same failure of a fixed place in the Autre, how is this to be translated by such contradictory pictures?

Hysteria rules itself by a phantasy but, and here lies its particularity and its richness, it is a phantasy attributed to the Autre. It's a phantasy the satisfaction for which will impose itself like a duty. We can immediately say that it's a phantasy organised by a look, and a look which will have the duty to satisfy, which will have the duty to assure jouissance.

Is this not near enough the Schreber[1] position, this look in the Autre, of which the subject would have to assure his jouissance under the form of an imperative, under the form of a constraint? There is an essential difference between them and we will show on the way with another clinical remark how the hysteric has to take a place in the phantasy, to invest, to maintain and not, as in the case of Schreber, to guarantee it by this taking up of a position. This goes back to what I told you the other evening, in specifying the difference in the real, proper to paranoia. This dimension will only be supported in some way, will only be maintained by the imaginary representation to which the paranoiac devotes himself, whereas in hysteria it has to do with a real which find itself perfectly in place, which holds, and for which the hysteric feels himself called simply to play his role in some way.

DOI: 10.4324/9781003167839-20

The question which we now ask and which is difficult, is to know why in hysteria there is this dominance of a look in the Autre? Why, for him as well as for her, the permanence of always feeling the need to give oneself over to be looked at? The easiest way is to begin with the mirror stage, to this moment which I have mentioned many times: when the hysteric abdicates and gives to the other, the small other, the master position. Something plays in the field of the scopic, in this kind of renunciation of representing this master figure. But, the imaginary is not enough. We are about to give symbolic determination to what is produced in the imaginary. Because, this abdication, this renunciation is commanded by symbolic coordinates, which ensure the sharing between the masculine and the feminine positions. These symbolic coordinates introduce *hétéros*.

What interests us, always with regard to male hysteria[2] is all these who for reasons which belong to the difference of sex but not only that, all the speak-beings who are not able or who do not want to give assent to symbolic recognition by the father are arranged on the side of hétéros. That is to say all these speak-beings who do not want or who cannot witness their castration guaranteed. The male hysteric is ranged from the side of hétéros because he refuses this membership of the lineage which would necessitate a symbolic recognition by the father. What makes the richness of this Lacanian conceptualisation, is that on the side of *hétéros*, on the side of the Autre, will be ranged all those who, no matter what their sex, cannot, for very diverse reasons be recognised symbolically by the father – for example simply by the fact that he belongs to a different lineage – or those who are determined by the fact of the difference of sex, or indeed those who do not wish because of the way in which they have taken up the oedipal position, something like this "Well, you will never have me, I will leave the place you assign me and the function you give me".

To arrive also at this place of *hétéros*, two consequences produce itself of the order of the imaginary, which concerns the image, the imago.

One, I have already largely dealt with, it's an uncertainty of the form, from then on dedicated to a malaise, and which seems fragile, exposed to dislocation. This badly worked out form, enigmatic, is necessary for he who is the carrier, to endlessly unite it, or what is even easier, to make it recognised by his fellow, as the title of fellow exactly: to engage in a kind of commerce where the subject is able to verify, by the address which will be sent to him, that he is indeed a fellow and indeed shares this form. There is here in hysteria a kind of "social" necessity, social, if I may say so, which is easily spotted.

A second trait is maybe for us more interesting and more enigmatic. It seems as if who is in this position of *hétéros* who puts a stain on the landscape, that he is excessive there and therefore, the feeling that there is nothing paranoiac which is proper to hysteria, to be exposed, to be seen, to have been looked at, to attract the eye. To make a stain on the picture, is finally to represent the look itself – that's what, the stain on the picture means. Why by making a stain on the picture, being an obscure point on the picture, and representing the look itself, will this in return give the feeling of being seen? This could be a paradox, but is resolved very easily. We find it quite easy in the clinic to verify these two modalities and their consequences.

That the hysteric may be a voyeur is a situation totally confirmed, totally patent because the position *hétéros* where he is, gives him a kind of eternal glance of the eye. He has an eye on the world, a kind of perception, a kind of analysis which testifies well, to simplify, that he is E.T., is a certain way out-side things. And, in his type of analysis, in his kind of critique, in his kind of analysis of the thing, he carries out a kind of reversal of the system: it's the world which becomes for him in some way strange, *hétéros*. In this visual quest, what he is looking for is his being itself. To give a simplified image, it's a look which slows down in front of the shop window in looking for the quality of what is exposed there and in what attracts the eye. All this, I'm emphasising, in the quest for his own being.

On the other hand, no matter how much of a voyeur he is, however impregnated with the feeling of being seen, there is nothing strange in this if we recall the functioning of the drive. Or, indeed, what Lacan[3] talks about somewhere in his little narrative, which was taken from Sartre, on the voyeur, surprised in watching through, the keyhole the shame that is produced at the moment where he is seen, at the moment this look revealed to him what his being was about.

We don't therefore have to think that there is something of a paradox in the fact of finding oneself projected as a stain on the picture. To find oneself in the position of the look, also organises voyeurism as well as the feeling of being endlessly seen, that is to say unveiled, revealed in one's being.

No matter what, to find oneself in a position of *hétéros* because of a con-flict with the father (or else by the fact of having been rejected by him or not having been recognised by him as one of his own) means that there is a part played which will engage the hysteric with this father. This consists, among other things, in a competition, with the ordinary representative of this father, because he has recognised him as being his own. It has to do with showing to this father that his true son is no longer where he believes: the true one: his worthy representative, is he who wants to escape castration and to arrive in this position of *hétéros*, who will be up to the measure of cojoining being with having. But, it has to be said, it will also in the end arrive at the same posi-tion as this imaginary father. Because simply, hétéros is the position of the imaginary father.

In other words, this look, in the last resort in order for the hysteric to assure jouissance, is indeed the look of the father. It's like as if, there is a duty to transfigure this stain on the landscape, to rehabilitate it by giving it the best representation, the representation which is the most dignified and the most seductive of all. Here we will refind the problem of the mirror, and it's like as if here the castrated son, (the recognised son) constituted a menace for the imaginary father. In recognising him in his castrated representative, he risks finding himself castrated and therefore destroyed. He has to be defended, protecting him by offering him the spectacle of a creature finally perfectly fulfilled. Moreover, in taking care to guarantee his jouissance, as if it had to do with the fact of ensuring that he would not go astray, that his look would not abandon the earth, would stay attached to the earth.

For those among you for whom this is sensitive, I will comment that the very important and decisive discussions which took place on the dogma of the Trinity, were essentially, about this. Can it be said, for example, that the Son is equal to the Father, and does not it risk in this way in bringing about a revalorisation, a fall of this Father? Schisms have been produced in the Church, and in particular within the Eastern Churches, on this point of the interpretation of the Trinity.[4] One group maintaining, in some way, the equality of the Father and the Son, the other side thinking that there cannot be a leap, a difference in level, a hiatus between the Father and the Son. In other words, to say that *two* is not equal to *One*. For those of you who are really interested in this, I will note that these little things, apparently about nothing at all, byzantine (it has to be said) have indeed shaken the best formed souls and spirits. There have been the most precious consequences for what could be the social organisation and for the relationship to authority, for example, the most sensational regarding the world of the father and power.

Therefore, it's really for the father that this rivality, this competition is played out. To the extent where it would seem to be abusive, to give his love and confidence to his legitimate pretend representatives, to his sons, it has to do with testifying to him that from the other side, the side of *hétéros*, they could be his best children, his best sons and for diverse procedures like sublimation, engage themselves in all the exploits characterising those who are in this position of *hétéros*.

But there is the endless question of *che vuoi*? In finding himself at this place – without having wanted it, he may have chosen it but without knowing it, without having foreseen the consequences. The subject is brought to re-question the desire of the Autre, in finding himself. And, we can see well how he does it, the consequences of his position, of his duties: the fact of rediscover himself here like a stain in the picture, he will interpret these unexpected consequences as so many duties dictated by this Autre which as a result he will have to accomplish.

We find once again, in the oedipal position of the male hysteric, what I pointed out to you the last time as being hatred for the symbolic father: the father who orders, who commands the privation of the mother, and who engages his children in a competition, lost in advance in the quest for the good object. Because it's ultimately this, the oedipal invitation: firstly, you will not have her; secondly, run after her, and thirdly, run forever! This is it, this is the programme. So, we can see how hatred of the symbolic father and of the programme which is here prescribed, this hatred turns round into a love for the father, imaginary this time, from the position of *hétéros* and from the place itself where this imaginary father maintains himself. It now has to do with making of himself the faithful representative. That is how the stain in the painting, which the hetéros thereby presents – I do not say represents, but presents because it has to do with his being – this stain in the picture will be interpreted by him as the scopic object of the desire of the Autre, of this desire therefore attributed to the Autre. It has to do with satisfying it and trying to hold on to it, in taking the best forms, the best representations capable of success.

It's here that we can, it seems to me, locate the frame of the phantasy, of this phantasy put into place in the Autre. In this phantasy, the male hysteric will be able to displace himself, transform himself, take very diverse forms to satisfy this look in the Autre. He is not held by a precise form, but doesn't risk losing his way because all these changes accomplish themselves for the jouissance of this father: They all accomplish themselves in the window, in the spectacle of this phantasy, and for the ever greater glory of this imaginary father. So in this way, we can say that the ethics of hysteria will in effect be, an aesthetic. What will command in some way his conduct, his morality, what will be his wisdom, will subsume itself under this aesthetic constraint.

After this putting into place the phantasy which orders and which makes the hysteric work, in a new kind of way, we can more easily analyse what happens for the male hysteric in his encounter with his male fellow and then with a woman.

With his male counterpart, we understand immediately that the hysteric has a complex task. It has to do with making himself recognised as a fellow: he is also a creature of this father, but superior. That is to say that he will have to make this mysterious object shiny, to maintain his image, by the fact of his position of *hétéros*. But just for a moment, the time for an eclipse, because he renounces this object in giving a gift to the Autre. What is extremely odd and interesting, is that finally he respects the established order: he wishes to show himself, to make himself superior his partner, he all the same respects him, does not wish his destruction, his disappearance. On the other hand, if he makes a mistake, he is not able to make himself recognised any more. It has to do with letting him vacillate for a minute, and then immediately, resuscitating him.

The male hysteric finds himself here engaged in a process where it always has to do with showing how much he could do if – if what? That's indeed the question. He does not do all he could. It's here that is inscribed what we can call the ordinary failure of hysteria and its impossibility. If, eventually he arrives at that place of his fellow, by the same token he loses all his subjective bearings, finds himself deprived of his phantasy and plunged into anxiety. He shows all his virtual talents but in general he tries not to fulfil them. Because for him there is only one way to accomplish them: no longer in a competition, but in a position which would be outside the competitive zone and not letting him out of his original place of his position, hétéros.

In his relationship with his fellow male and in an attempt to make himself recognised, and, therefore to make himself loved, the hysteric always changes at the whim of his interlocuteur and wishes for him to ensure a reply of a rather particular kind. What kind? Every meeting decides alterity, irreducibly separating the two interlocuters, but it has to do with, in this kind of response of the male hysteric, lifting this impossible, to be a witness to the fact that the other could be the same. In the final analysis, in this meeting a co-opting of the two partners could be made possible which would be perfect between them: they would be twins.

An ideal of fraternity is situated here, its source is located here: a rapport with ones fellow which will definitely abolish the dimension of alterity and sign the greater glory of the father. Because, if the dimension of the Autre finds itself abolished, nothing will any longer testify to a castration in the Autre because all will be regarded as identical, under the same look. There is, therefore, at the direction of one's fellow, an invitation to put oneself under the empire of this look in the Autre. We can very easily see here the origin of the ideas of fraternity, these ideas, it has to be said, which are *nice* and which may of course also be a social ideal.

But, in the meeting with a woman, there again, because of this *hétéros* position, the male hysteric can only engage with her as a depositary of the object cause of desire. In other words, in the most beautiful affair – it's him. This is a situation which has nothing exceptional about it and I won't press you to follow up on all the literary examples. For example, in the loves between Musset[5] and George Sand[6] largely retold by their novels as by their own letters, it is possible to see a representation of this kind. Let us remark that this situation for the male hysteric, frequently encounters the complicity of the partner, who is therefore comforted, in not having to assume the role, because it's he who is in charge. But, and because there is always a but, she will also have to pay with a devalorisation of herself, a devalorisation which is necessary for love to be realised. In effect, if it's he who makes this object brilliant, makes it shiny, holds it, represents it, she cannot at the same time, enter into this affair, except, in a devalorised position. The problem is that he loves himself because of her. And, in this situation she is no longer at his level, he will find that he will never be in love nor be loved as he should.

He will never meet a beloved one, because it's enough in some way to believe that he has met her but as soon as the game of this elementary mechanism has begun she will find herself out of favour.

That is why there is always without doubt, in this kind of system, a pre-ference, a kind of predilection, properly hysterical so that the amorous exchange will stay at the level of the look. That is to say just the reciprocal equivocation of what could have been, but it has to do above all in not accomplishing when one knows in some way the true killing which is from then on exercised on the partner. And these are things which one explicitly finds in all the literature, in particular romantic literature. It has to do with preserving, doesn't it, the partner, of not sacrificing him in what would be a *passage a'l'acte*?

It is curious that from the fact of this *hétéros* position, the hysteric finds himself the guardian of an order, where, it has to be said, everything can be accomplished. Because only the extraordinary merits the attention and the look of the Autre, of the father. All this will be in the greatest sacrifice as well as in a huge perversion; one and the other can alternate.

What interests us most of all in this new order of which the hysteric is the representative, is that the pleasure principle does not apply here anymore, let us say, in a standard way. It is not any more about finding one's pleasure, in the resolution of tension at the most basic level, but on the contrary maintaining oneself permanently at the most heightened level of tension, in order always to be a witness to being this lovable figure for the Autre, whereas the lessening of this tension is, in general, on the contrary, synonymous with depression.

Of course, an image imposes itself. It has to be given because it is true, it is not a gratuitous image. It has to do with the most beautiful representation in the phantasy and – it's that of a phallus in erection. There never has been a representation which could be better than that for the imaginary. And, to the extent that it has to do with always assuming, permanently, the highest level of tension, we can well understand how this in turn, links to this imaginary representation. We see how, through the imaginary, the desire of the hysteric is a desire which has to be unsatisfied, why is it a desire of dissatisfaction? Because it has more to do with coming to terms with oneself in an erection – as if it were the end of this essentially imaginary operation. It has to do more with coming to terms with a representation in erection than to accomplish an act which we will immediately see how it brings with it a dissatisfaction. Otherwise, worth would be given to this dissatisfaction, which is on the verge of being quasi physiological and which is well known, noted for a long time, which is the kind of deception always inherit in the realisation of the failure of sexual rapport.

In any case, in this position of *hétéros*, the hysteric presents himself as the possessor of a knowledge, which, by being commanded by the Autre and vowing himself to the maintenance of the father, offers himself willingly as wisdom. When one maintains oneself in the position of *hétéros* we are not looking for the wise ones, for the good behaviours. It's from this side that this originates, if I may dare say so. In this wisdom, the hysteric will have to realise the triumph of the father by the exhibition of a phallus which would be perfectly mastered.

In fact, Lacan[7] says somewhere, this is the father accomplished: he who would be master of his desire, able to command to the real, the phallus, in so far as it is imaginary is its most legitimate representative.

He would be in a position to ensure this representative would obey him with finger and eye – to the eye, it has to be said: I speak only of this.

It's exactly what the hysteric tries to realise: to be such a representative for this phallus which would never stop obeying the eye. This is the reason, obviously for all the tension, all the effort and the trembling in the fear of failure always possible for this hysteric.

This is also the reason for his own division with regard to this task, obviously he is not completely there. And, a little bit tired because of this constraint, this guard always there, it happens that he will question what he is doing there and engage himself in these moments of – "I've had enough" – and he goes on strike. With this idea that the Autre – it's here that we can refind the relative homogeneity with the paranoical position – that the world will flow from the minute he will stop being there, his weapon at his foot, that everything will fall again.

He is obviously surprised to notice, that in general, things will continue to work around him, because that could obviously have repercussions for the immediate entourage. With this disposition linking the problem of the psychical economy with the pleasure principle, in this brutal lowering of tension, we find a sort of vacillation, the kind of alternative the hysteric attempts.

Psychoanalysis by the fact that it comes to the place of the Autre, by the fact equally that it finds itself willingly invested with the *objet a*, or at least flirting with it, psychoanalysis can find itself willingly confused with the hysteric especially when the hysteric himself does not believe that his place – is indeed a hysteric one, this confusion can then happen. Before the putting into place of the four discourses it was, I find, very difficult to make the distinction, and for many theorists of analysis – and among the best – the distinction of places was absolutely not done. That is why hysteria could always appear as the best possible condition to occupy this place of the analyst, as if there were a kind of predestination and affinity between them.

And yet, there is an essential difference: if the place of the analyst is confused with the hysterical position, the relationship with the object, with the causal object, will stay suspended in an eternal quest, until there is finally a renunciation by mutual fatigue. That is why moreover, that the desire of the hysteric is to be unsatisfied, in the "it's not that", in denunciation and in the quest for what could eventually come to light.

If this kind of coalescence, of confusion is not worked out, we could imagine that the treatment could – this is never guaranteed – finish, no longer in an incessant search, but by the recognition of the object, the simple *objet* which supports the desire of the subject. We could imagine that at the same time the analyst would not resist the invitation to demean himself. Resistance, Lacan says, is first of all with the analyst. This is not to be heard in a general and polyvalent way, but in a precise and localised fashion.

What is also at play in this distinction, it's obviously the problem of the end, possible or not, of an analysis – of analysis "terminable and interminable". Each one of us is summoned by this question, can ask themselves about it, even if, for the moment the procedures of the pass are not active, are not current. That is why next week, I will finish this seminar on hysteria by evoking the way in which the hysterical position produces a resistance to analysis, and again it seems to me this evening that I have put the central themes in place.

QUESTION: This dimension of spectacle which you have highlighted with the notion of achievement, does this not also pose the frontier with obsessional neurosis?

CHARLES MELMAN: Hysterical achievement can be also in the accomplishment of sacrifice, in the accomplishment of castration, it will be the one who says, "You see, I give more, I sacrifice more than you". The obsessional will not surely engage in a competition where it would have to do with giving more than the other!

QUESTION: It happens that subjects whose apparent symptomatology is obsessional reveal themselves responding to the plan of structure as you have described.

CHARLES MELMAN: Masculine hysteria, I don't know why, is not very well regarded. It's more chic to be an obsessional. All the same, it has to do with satisfying what it is about the scopic, we could put a lot more trust in the hysteric. ... It has got nothing to do with generalising foolishly about artists but if an artistic vocation no matter what – and certain realisations of existence are by themselves works of art, it's very beautiful – we can only but admire and be grateful. In other words, let us rehabilitate masculine hysteria!

QUESTION: You spoke rather belatedly about the distinction between the analytic position and that of the hysteric.

CHARLES MELMAN: Of course, it is sure that there is an affinity from both sides, that's the problem. It's not that long ago, I heard an excellent colleague saying that the hysterical position was identifiable with the analytic position. I think it's very interesting for the analysis and for analysts to state that they are not absolutely identifiable, even if it could seem to play in this way, as if the analyst could more easily comfort the enigma of his desire in so far as he is an analyst by leaning on the hysterical position. During one of the study days, about 10 years ago, Lacan said that the hysterical position was that of *not yet*. In other words, "one more effort", is a position which does not lack a certain dynamism, a certain force. But, we will have difficulty in concluding on that, and it's not because we will not conclude on that, that we will have to lower our arms and say to ourselves that because things are like that, that all we have to do is keep ourselves quiet in our corner and cultivate our garden.

What is admirable in the position of he whose teaching we have followed, it's that on the one hand he was totally clear that he was not in the position of *not yet* and yet all the same, this did not stop him from being animated by an energy, by an effort, by a tension which showed very well that he did not have the need for this kind of illusion or this kind of alienation, to work, to function.

QUESTION: You said that the hysteric could engage in an ideal of fraternity. Can one extrapolate, to say that the militants on the left would have more than the others ...

CHARLES MELMAN: I don't think that's the important issue or we should say such things. But, it has to do finally with pointing, at the moment where it is possible, that there could be ideas which maintain themselves with such dispositions. That does not mean that we are going to analyse this. But the structure is totally rebellious to such ideas. An ideal of fraternity can only conclude by the expulsion of those who would be from then on in a position, no longer of others, but of foreigners. The society of brothers has always concluded on the expulsion of the foreigner. It cannot function in any other way. There is no fraternity which could be the least of the universal world. Very dignified, courageous efforts have been done, which in general have not turned out very well. We can historically say how cunning was reintroduced into the affair and how that went in the direction of a resuscitation of the dimension of masters. In any case, analysts can refer to the impossibilities of structure and not envisage for themselves an ideal of fraternity. That's it!

17 May 1983

Notes

1 S. Freud, *The Case of Schreber, Papers on Technique and Other Works.* Vol. XII, S. E. (1911–1913). London: The Hogarth Press, 1958.
2 Lacan, J. *The Seminar of Jacques Lacan, Book XVII: The Other Side of Psychoanalysis, 1969–1970* (trans. C. Gallagher, unedited).
3 J. Lacan, *The Seminar of Jacques Lacan, Book II: The Ego in Freud's Theory and in the Technique of Psychoanalysis, 1954–1955* (ed. J-A. Miller, trans. S. Tomaselli). Cambridge: Cambridge University Press, 2007.
4 B. Whalen, "Rethinking the Schism of 1054 – Authority Heresy and The Latin Rite", *Traditio* 67 (2007), pp. 1–24.
5 A. de Musset, *The Confession of a Child of the Century.* (trans. D. Coward). London: Penguin Books, 2012.
6 G. Sand, *L'édition complète des oeuvres de George Sand.* Caen: Presses Universitaires de Caen, 2017.
7 J. Lacan, "The Subversion of the Subject and the Dialectic of Desire in the Freudian Unconscious" in *Écrits* (ed. J-A. Miller, trans. B. Fink). New York: W.W. Norton & Co., 2002.

Chapter 21

Resistance to psychoanalysis

Charles Melman

The ethic of hysteria is commanded by the guilt of being Autre with regard to the father. Autre, because they do not apparently share the same approach. This causes a limitation on the empire of this ethic. And, as I mentioned the last time, this translates at the level of the form which will be lived as a stain on the picture and therefore will have to be anthropomorphised, rectified, to be made recognised in the image of one's fellow by humanising it in some way. And, we will indeed see how, in this place, the ethic of hysteria engenders the taste of a beauty which is good in itself.

Let us remark that the famous *kalos kagathos*,[1] the famous moral on the beautiful and the good, could only be a moral of the slave, could only be engendered from a slave's position in that it came to infiltrate a society of masters. What is most instructive for us, the master does not give a damn whether or not he is handsome: this does not feature in his concerns, this is in some way an acquired privilege. As far as being good is concerned, let us even not speak about it!

Therefore, this guilt with regard to the father translates at the level of concern for the form and obviously also for the phallic validation of this form. The hysteric is profoundly divided. On the one hand, her representation and her speech are taken up in a dialogue lived as essentially alienating, in an alternating way, because called by social dialogue she engages in a worldly participation, in an earthly, invited participation. On the other hand, there is this subjectivity from where she watches herself and from where in a certain way, she admires herself. We can therefore, of course, highlight this division between the movement of social participation in which the hysteric feels herself having a role, a task to be carried out and on the other hand the distance she keeps with this subjective position, a distance which could be qualified, why not, as celestial – which could remind us of the traditional divisions, the top and the bottom for example, or indeed the earth and the sky.

After all, this division, this splitting, properly speaking, is subjective division and all I am trying to do is rely on what belongs to the division proper to each subject. But, the specificity of the hysteric is to make of this subjective division, the cause, to bring this subjective division to the place of the cause.

DOI: 10.4324/9781003167839-21

We see here the power, the richness of the four discourses.[2] The position of the hysteric, is to bring this division into the four discourses, on top and to the left, to the place which makes cause and also to what commands. Now, by this procedure, it is this division which becomes the failure responsible for organising the world. And it is this splitting, this division which will induce and nourish this eminently hysterical aspiration at the beginning of the world, to the final realisation of a community where all of us would be together. It's from this division, put into the position of cause, with which this hysterical aspiration is engaged in the accomplishment of a universality.

Let us return to this meeting with a "partner", let us call it that, a social partner, whatever it may be. As I have introduced it from the beginning, it is this meeting which engages the hysteric in the worry of making herself known in this mundanity which registers this dimension of splitting. And indeed, this meeting with a social partner perfectly illustrates, and I will make use of it for a little while, the positions which Schema L.[3] puts into place.

The axis $a - \grave{a}$ of egotistical confrontation finds itself here organised by a mimetism which calls for reciprocity – this is precisely an attempt to resolve the splitting, and at the same time there is this Autre dimension which I posed as at fault, a cause of guilt. In this aspiration to mimetism the hysteric finds herself completely captivated at this very moment.

In organising this imaginary axis, there is no less this ex-sistent place of $ from where the subject contemplates himself in this realisation, this anthropomorphisation which he is in some way trying to accomplish, this place from where he admires himself.

But, for the jouissance of the fourth term, the Autre, about which it's satisfying the look – because it is not so much finally the partner as the look of this Autre which assures jouissance. If we start again with the introduction of guilt because of this faulty dimension of the Autre, with regard to the father, we can see how this feeling of work to be accomplished is engaged: to assure the jouissance of this Autre which the hysteric would find herself capable of ensuring it fails, it lacks.

The difficulty is that in this egotistical confrontation, this concern to give oneself value can operate only by brief eclipses. It supposes a certain voyeurism loaned to the Autre. As if it had to do with the gaps of the eyelids which fall away just at the time of batting the same eyelids; to use an even more crude image, the coat of the exhibitionist opening and closing. In any case, this jouissance of the Autre can proceed only by eclipses, by subtle apparitions, destined very soon to die out.

Thus, in order to preserve this fellow engaged in the dialogue even if he appears sad and a little bit clumsy, he has to be preserved, this fellow who could have been chosen and could not find himself on the side of the Autre. So let us – we keep in mind this schema with its axis $a - a^{1}$ and this kind of transivitism in which the hysteric engages – in a concern over fusion, of perfect collusion in order to efface this dimension of alterity which weighs, has to do with being one or even the other, because from the minute the relationship is specularisable she gives herself over to a movement of interchangeability, to be one or the other.

For example, this interchangeability extends: either man or woman, or one and the other, even if it is at the same time in the same relationship, to arrive at the place of the man and at the same time at the place of the woman. Because this attempt means that it has to do with accomplishing the interim, being the one who serves, who would permit the annihilation of alterity, whose guilt the hysteric tolerates. And, all this to realise sexual rapport, which, by virtue of ranging herself in the category of the Autre, the hysteric accuses herself that this Autre will be able to fail.

So, that in the mirror, in this one or other, we can read the S_1 and the S_2, we can give them these symbolic coordinates. And, even to read this S_1 and S_2 in the way which Lacan emphasised in all his last seminars, in particular, at the beginning of *RSI*,[4] by distinguishing the signifier One of the symbolic and the signifier One of meaning. This is an heuristic distinction which you will easily understand. The One, the signifier One of the symbolic is the signifier which puts the real into place. The signifier One of meaning, is the one by which God would have proceeded to the nomination of objects, animals, persons who people this real, what Lacan called *naming*.[5] We will see later on how these emphasise their difference.

But in any case, in this egotistical confrontation, one or the other and one and the other – we can immediately distinguish them, emphasise them in their differing valences by isolating two poles.

- The One of the symbolic, the S_1.
- The One of meaning, to be put on the side of S_2.

The problem, and here we advance a little, is that in truth the hysteric will not recognise herself at the level of S_1, nor at the level of S_2. Both positions are assumed at the level of facticity.

The One of the symbolic is prohibited, because its allocation is precisely this place Autre. It is something about which we cannot jest because it is the kind of allocation which may be without remedy (and this is something that can easily be verified in a treatment), the kind of allocation which may be very difficult to disentangle.

And, the One of meaning, S_2, why is it that the hysteric rushes to assume this position? The One of meaning takes its meaning from a finitude which is, strictly speaking, phallic. The One of meaning, does not mean anything else other than representing phallic finitude – this she can accomplish, one can imagine, with this One of meaning. But, for the hysteric, this phallic finitude is in reality incompatible with the infinitude she feels, insofar as she participates in this place Autre and at every attempt to catch it, every attempt at *Begriff*, at catching the concept, she can only reply "It is very pretty all this but I'm to the side, but continue, keep going".

We have to point out a paradox here. If the hysteric suffers from the fact that there is no universe – because there is this Autre dimension and therefore there is no universal father – by the same token she supports the symptom and makes herself the representative of what is not working. She finds herself in this way on the side of this Autre which denies power, which I will permit myself here to call the catholic power of this father (catholic as understood in its etymological sense) that is to say, the universalising power of the father.

But, the paradox is, if the hysteric is in this Autre position, she finds herself by the same token on the side of this imaginary father, that is to say from this original $, *urverdrängt* from which the $ of the hysteric authorises herself. What is marvellous is that a male or a female hysteric never authorises from himself or herself. It is only ever authorised from the fact, that in the Autre there is precisely this *Urverdrängt*, there is an $. Therefore, to arrive in this place Autre, the hysteric, relying on this $, will arrive at the very place of this imaginary father. And the mutation which operates, it is he or she who will be the loudspeaker, the voice carrier of this imaginary father. Henceforth, she will say, on her father's behalf, that there is something which is not working, which is wrong.

If we wish to grasp what makes an obstacle to the treatment of the hysteric, and it's what I hope to conclude these talks on this year's theme, we have to envisage that there is an essential solidarity between the $ of the speak-being and he who finds himself *Urverdrängt*, repressed. And, I will go as far as using this image, a complicity of the reunion in this common tomb. And, this is how the hysteric finds herself, in part, caught and attached to what could really be called the God of religion. She cannot subsist without Him, that is to say without this *Urverdrängt* in the Autre, but she has the certitude that He also cannot subsist without her. And there is here, if you like, a very rudimentary dialectical type: for example, so that there can be children, there has to be a father but on the other hand, and inversely, it is necessary to have children for a father to assert himself.

We can grasp the validity of this speculation in this complicity: the $ of the subject when he is an expression of it, when it founds his authority, when he puts it in this master position which gives value to the discourse of the hysteric, this $ gets its voice only by referring to an original $. This reference will go a long way and engages an essential solidarity because the hysterical subject willingly gets involved in making himself the *porte-parole*, the carrier, the missionary in some way of he who would be dead in the Autre, and by this death will rejoin him, thereby permitting him to resuscitate his voice. We can bring together here two great forms of hysterical expression:

• Sometimes it is the representation by One of meaning even if it is badly accepted. The signifier One of meaning implies a phallic representation to celebrate the power of this father, his vital manifestation, his power to generate. The acceptance of this place where the hysteric is represented by

S_2, by the One of meaning, is the inauguration, why not call it like this, of carnival, of sexual celebration.

- And, then also as well, there is this place $, which is the most essential place where the hysteric always makes of herself the representative of the father, no longer this father who can generate and who is powerful, with the phallic image, but the representative of the dead father in so far as ultimate power and last truth: the truth even of the real, precisely beyond this phallic imaginary. What makes the acceptance of this place $, of this representation of the dead father, it is that contrary to the representation by One of meaning the representation by $ is, open to infinity. This is totally consistent with the organisation of hysteria.

We could here, talk about countries not that far away, where women's dress, their ordinary clothes are black, a reminder of a never-ending mourning for this dead father, and at the same time the necessity to have to pursue this work of mourning which is never ending. This never ends when it interprets itself from the position of the Autre. Why? Because you can sacrifice to him all you want, this will not stop the fact that the position of the Autre, the place of the Autre, maintains itself as such, you will never exhaust the place of the Autre. This type of permanent mourning, supported in a cultural context by women, seems to be a reminder of having to sacrifice sexual jouissance to this dead father. After all, what is the work of mourning except to have to renounce sexual jouissance for a supposedly decent period of time? We can see how, to keep oneself in this Autre position this work of mourning intends never to be completed.

So, I think we will end here, with the isolating of these two positions which give this apparently contradictory appearance to the clinic of hysteria. On the one hand, the phallic image; on the other hand, the evocation, the presentation of this dead father to whom sexual jouissance will have to be sacrificed. We understand that they are both in the same place. And I do not run the least risk of offending you by telling you that these two positions marry in the end, these two positions are associated, or disassociated in time, or within the hysterical ambit. In this way, maternity will celebrate the One of meaning, this vigorous father; and then the necessity of virginity will pay homage to the dead father.

The religious myth barely feels the difficulties in conjoining these positions of maternity and virginity in a way which appears to everyone as perfectly acceptable and rightly so, because this myth goes before unconscious truths which can be registered only in this way. Otherwise, we cannot see how this could be socially shared, is not this true? This "meeting" of maternity and virginity associated in this way will perhaps remind us that the marriage of the hysteric is not essentially knotted with her partner, the genitor of her children but, more essentially with this dead father also present in the Autre. It is he who is the true partner, the master look is his, the dominant one.

This specificity permits us to understand one of the difficulties of the treatment – let us pass regarding the clinical pictures. Hysterical resistance to the treatment is linked to what we have to consider really as being the force of this Autre position. It is an extremely strong position, why?

Firstly, let us note, it is an absolutely unsinkable position: you can go anywhere you want with this position, you will always be sure to find yourself at home, you obviously can recreate it, you will find your slippers again without worrying about the concrete demands of the situation, all the positive languages you have to deal with, you do not give a damn, you are at ease all over the place. And, I will dare say it like this, it is good that a woman is able to pass to the level of an object of exchange, is it not? That is also why a woman will always have a rather special relationship – a rather particular one, with regard to engagements (national) etc. Do you see the force of this position, in its permanence, its indifference to every symbolic arrangement, to the specificity of every symbolic arrangement, no matter what?

On the other hand, something else interesting, this Autre position, is transmitted in a direct way, that is to say without passing via castration. Once the yoke has been understood, this is passed on to the children who wish to be inspired by it. This is transmitted without this painful work of a gift to the Autre, of recognition by him, nothing of that at all! It passes like this, a legacy like this, from hand to hand.

To occupy this place is a very strong position, because the jouissance attached seems to conjoin jouissance and death in a single place: the body. This does not go without saying; the body as a support of jouissance and death. If we make the Borromean knot intervene here, we will have a tendency to say at the same place the three orders will be conjoined. *That of the body (symbolic) that of jouissance (imaginary) and that of death (real). That of the body to the symbolic, that of jouissance to the imaginary and that of death to the real.*

Moreover, we have a very obvious clinical illustration, because the old authors had perfectly located the erotic expression of hysterical pain. They had certainty understood this expression as at least a little bit strange, but they did better: they saw in these hysterical pains the clear expression of an excess of corporal jouissance, a kind of *plus-de-jouir* of oneself. And I will use a Freudian term here of an affect, *eingeklemmt* (Translated as "caught"). There is, here, the kind of expression in the body of an excess which is not able to let itself flow. The old authors read perfectly well here the call to a salutary phallic intervention, that of the father himself, preferably. As a result of which we have the traditional kinds of therapy traversing the ages. Some advise marriage and others pregnancy, a little pregnancy, like that, *en passant*, to arrange matters.

But, were these pains themselves the expression of a *plus-de-jouir* evocative of an excess calling on phallic intervention and already homogenous with this phallic intervention? Or were they capable of evoking, of making this death heard in this way at the horizon? We can understand here how hysterical symptoms present themselves with this ambiguity, and are the expression of this collusion between jouissance and death.

So, if in this case, real, symbolic and imaginary are able to conjoin in a single place, that is to say, in this body which is at the same time the representative of the Autre, because a mental place is always a surface, we can perhaps understand that the collusion of the three orders in one place, a unique but same surface, may perhaps necessitate the intervention of a fourth which is what knots them. This has to be seen, and I propose it for your reflection.

But, this approach, in any case does not seem totally free. Because the representative of this Autre, the hysteric, sees herself as a depository of a fundamental knowledge, of a knowledge which she knows or which she thinks is linked, let us not be afraid of words, to the order of the world. From the minute she is representative of the Autre with her body, she supposes this knowledge which inhabits her to be inevitably a subject and a subject in which she fervently believes. This happens immediately, in some way, from the fourth ring, that is to say, from of the Name-of-the-Father.

What is really amazing is that ordinarily the hysteric resists apprenticeship. She participates in the best cases in a certain number of knowledges, refined, elaborated, sophisticated, but will never implicate the knowledge of which she finds herself the depository and to whom she thereby attributes a subject. No question, if I may dare say, that this enters. Some, moreover, complain about difficulties in apprenticeship.

There is here an effect of resistance. The problem is that the belief given to this subject attributed to knowledge, of which she is the depositor, takes account of the aptitude for transference. The hysteric can only wish to see this subject incarnate itself and in this way be ready for her knowledge.

But – what a weird, strange thing when this subject finds himself incarnated by an analyst, we find here the risk of a fundamental misunderstanding. Because engagement from a hysterical position in analysis is made from a legitimate wish to be cured ... this to be heard as an accomplishment of this knowledge, of which the hysteric in this way finds herself the depositor: that this knowledge would finally be successful at what? To succeed, precisely to lift this impossibility of sexual rapport and to be cured in this way once and for all. This aspiration for the realisation of this knowledge turns in certain cases of analyses towards positions which belong in a certain way to voca-tions of prophecy, for example, or to generalised therapy – the expression of a knowledge which in the end would be witness to a true, authentic guide to life, a guide to a successful life.

This misunderstanding can occur if, instead of contributing or encouraging this disposition which we can perfectly understand, an analyst finds himself looking for a process which does not go in the direction of an encouragement, of a sublimation of this knowledge. This misunderstanding is further enhanced if an analyst insists on the putting into place of an unconscious knowledge as being a simple way of warding off the failure of sexual rapport. Finally, this can happen if an analyst tries to get out of the game while the going is good thereby adapting himself to a possible jouissance. Because unconscious knowledge is nothing more than a way of dealing with castration and trying to make do with it. If the analyst engages himself in a kind of prompting for an implication – it has to be said – of this unconscious knowledge, we can see how his presumption is felt as a putting into place of the order of the very world itself, that is to say as something, in the end, fairly exorbitant. And, really one could, with the hysteric, ask the question: what will remain, if because of this implicating she is no longer able to enjoy her knowledge? Or again, to question what she enjoys, what better can we promise her?

We can here, very gently and politely conclude on the following few remarks. If the hysterical position arises from a subversion, that of the $ subversion of the subject, this does not all the same make it as subversive as all that. On the contrary, we can qualify the hysterical position with a perfectly justifiable term here as conservative, including its political connotations. She is conservative to the extent that she remains attached to the father insofar as it's his knowledge which for her guides the world. That's why the hysterical position fundamentally watches over respect for castration and therefore, it has to be said, respect for neurosis even when she finds herself at certain times exalting phallic celebration. We cannot get out of this celebration of the paternal function because it is at the same time the celebration of the symptom. That is to say that things are not going so well and she has to get on with it. If, in all this, the hysteric still finds herself tolerating the symptom – that is to say representing what does not work, what could not work – this is not in any way to subvert it, but instead to try and accomplish it: to try and lift what is interpreted as the limitation of the power of the father. So that on the contrary, he can be realised in all his glory, splendour and his arrival is finally, truly accomplished.

In situating this kind of difference of language between the hysteric and the analyst we can more easily grasp what is the "rock" of castration, it is the word which comes to me, this "rock" of castration which Freud pointed as being unsurpassable. Obviously, the subject complains about castration, in other words he makes symptoms of it. But, on the other hand, he enjoys it and it's even this he enjoys. On the question of presence of the economy of forces, on the question of knowing who will take him away from his complaining or his jouissance, we can surely conclude that he finds so astutely and so well the way to make his complaint, his jouissance – that in the end, he can gain from both sides, which is no longer that bad!

In a certain way, the problems happily find themselves in suspense and call on analysts of our generation, of your generation, to see if it is possible or not to get over this difficulty. Because if one trusts in the economy of forces at present, we do not really see how we will get out of this in a subjective economy. Therefore, the question has to be asked, where will we get the energy to get out of this? Here we have an embryonic response. It will of course be at the insistence of the analyst. The analyst is not satisfied, he begins again, he has the appearance of finding that ...

This is it, the desire of the analyst, the famous desire of the analyst. Because he could in some way link up with a certain state of affairs, with his analysand, saying "There you go, we have done a good bit of the road together and we have seen a little ... but, we have to do more, let us not dramatise"! But, the analyst, because he is implicated, should be able to get over that and not conclude on a knowledge arrived at from his own symptom: in the place where it costs, to make it so that it will be fruitful, that it will be beneficial. On this, Lacan was unique, believing that analysis, if it makes any sense, should go through all this, go the whole journey.

It is here that the desire of the analyst enters. There is obviously the risk from this moment that there is something at play which we saw with Lacan: the side, how will I say it, not only unsettling, we can see this very well, but strictly speaking intrusive, of his vow. In other words, who authorises you? To which Lacan could only respond "In his wish, the analyst can authorise only from himself".[6] Obviously, for him there is no father in the Autre who authorises him because it is precisely by his vow that he finds himself the analyst, by his own small vow. And in this dimension he finds himself implicated.

I think I have been relatively faithful and pretty much prudent without running the risk of execrating myself too much in speaking. And, I hope to have made you sensitive to a question, which is never-ending for every analysand and every analyst. It is also this which will oblige groups of analysts, whether they want to or not, re-interest themselves in the question of the pass, no matter how difficult it is. The question will resurge again in the real as long as we continue to treat it as foreclosed, is that not so? That should give us a little cause for concern.

Therefore, it is on this matter that I will conclude this year. Next year, I will propose another theme for you, in the same line in a certain way because it has to do with the Psychoses. We will continue to work "On a Question Preliminary to any Possible Treatment of Psychosis",[7] which is exactly thirty years ago since Lacan introduced it. Are we still at the preliminary question? I think this question of psychosis is directly linked to the conclusion which I've just given you about hysteria.

QUESTION: We speak about the work of mourning. But we also meet the contrary of the privation of jouissance: for example, a "merry widow" or an erotic reactivation.

CHARLES MELMAN: You mention what is called in the clinic, maniacal mourning. The ceremonies of mourning which belongs to festivities, are a way of entry into an analysis of this.

This means very simply that it is well perceived that the death of the father – which we hear as a symbolic death, even if the real death of a father will remind us of this symbolic death – is for us at one and the same time generative of our access to sexual jouissance. At the same time, this is only at the price of a sacrifice of which mourning is in general the commemoration. The "work of mourning" is a good term, it implies that suffering has to be undergone and produced for the jouissance of the Autre. In certain regions we find funeral meals more gargantuan than the meals of baptism or marriage which reminds us that this time may conjoin both these aspects. Let us remark that it is an expression which has the particularity of not registering itself in myth (sadness, contemplation, remembering) but is a counterpoint. This possibly maniacal time will remind us of this strange condition: our jouissance goes by what Lacan used to call in *R.S.I.* with regard to the Freud's work, *enmoïsement*.[8] [This is a pun on Moses, the ego and putting on.] The love for the father is equally present in the manifestations you've mentioned. These mournings are expressions of love: we thank him for having loved us now that he is dead. He really wanted to do that out of love for us, he went as far as that!

QUESTION: In sacrifice, there is a compensation, there is all the same, a benefit.

CHARLES MELMAN: Of course. And without a doubt we suffer in no longer having rites as good as this. We surely suffer from the delinquency of our rites. For example, we could have rites of passage between puberty and adult age. Those among us who take care of adolescents would have nothing more to do.

If we leave it to the young people to invent rituals, they will break their bodies on motorcycles. Formerly, military service played its role, but nowadays it is not done so well. Moreover, ethnologists never miss giving us evidence that the so called primitive peoples benefit from these rites, that they do well with them. Afterwards, they can obviously hide themselves in the forests with the girls, in all serenity, they are content: it is prescribed. Margaret Mead[9] went into ecstasy with this kind of wisdom.

Are you in agreement with all I've told you? So – happy holidays!
14 June 1983

Notes

1 P. Davies, '"Kalos Kagathos" and Scholarly Perceptions of Spartan Society', *Zeitschrift Für Alte Geschichte* 62, no. 3 (2013). 'Kalos Kagathos' is referred to by J. Lacan in *The Seminar of Jacques Lacan, Book VII: The Ethics of Psychoanalysis, 1959–1960*. Paris: Editions du Seuil, 1986.
2 J. Lacan, *The Seminar of Jacques Lacan, Book XVII: The Other Side of Psychoanalysis, 1969–1970* (trans. C. Gallagher, unedited).
3 J. Lacan, "The Purloined Letter" in *Écrits* (Personal translation).

4 J. Lacan, *The Seminar of Jacques Lacan, Book XXII: R.S.I., 1974–1975* (trans. C. Gallagher, unedited).

5 J. Lacan, *The Seminar of Jacques Lacan, Book XII: Crucial Problems for Psychoanalysis, 1964–1965* (trans. C. Gallagher, unedited).

6 J. Lacan, *The Seminar of Jacques Lacan, Book XXI, Part 1: Les non-dupes errent, 1973–1974* (trans.C. Gallagher, unedited).

7 J. Lacan, "On a Question Prior to any Possible Treatment of Psychosis" in *Écrits* (trans. B. Fink). New York: W.W. Norton & Co., 2006.

8 Lacan, *Book XXII: R.S.I.*

9 M. Mead, *Continuities in Cultural Evolution.* New Brunswick, NJ: Transaction Publishers, 1999.

Appendix

Report on the study days on hysteria at the Freudian School of Paris, 24 June 1973[1]

With regard to the question which hysteria poses for us, I will firstly make a few comments on the history of our ideas. The first thing which surprises us is that hysteria is mentioned in our very first written documents (Medical Papyrus, 2000 and 1600 years B.C.) and written in a surprisingly modern form. Its versatility, its polymorphism, does not in any way distract from its ability to be recognised. *Hysteria* is identified as feminine, but with a patho-logical aetiology not too far from our own. This is very interesting because it has to do with the unstable and migratory character of the uterus in the feminine body. Hippocrates[2] adopted the theory of the wandering uterus which coincided with the Aristotelian theory of the proper place (*oikeoin topos*) "for everything, its natural place."[3]

Unfortunately, or otherwise, for the woman, her sex wanders. We can recall the platonic conception of the Idea and of matter (taken up by Aristotle as form and matter) in so far as the Idea imposes itself on matter, holding it, mastering it, impregnating it.

This is about the workings of the master signifier. In any case, we can compare it to Galen's[4] theory on hysteria: what the hysteric demands is to be impregnated: she suffers if she is not impregnated.

With St Augustine,[5] in the name of the Christian God, we arrive at the division of the soul with the body, the spirit with matter, which results in placing the hysteric on the side of evil, of that which escapes divine power.

What strikes us with Charcot[6] is the phantasy aspect of hysteria: with its representation as an illustration of a half-saying, with these hysterical mani-festations, with these half bodily paralyses (which go from left to right, from top to bottom). In any case what astounds us is this metal gadget with a screw and a plug to constrict the ovary – a wonderful attempt at mastery!

The problem Freud introduces us to is the concept of conversion, of somatic compliance. But Freud entered into this field of division without criticism. And so, the second topology[7] implicates an economy of the psychical apparatus founded on the pleasure principle and the reduction to the lowest level.

With the beyond of the pleasure principle, the principle of somatic conver-sion has to be looked at again: the energy not flowing, on its way to being converted, endlessly demands to express itself. What is striking, is that from 1910 onwards and right up to the end, Freud says nothing about hysteria. In the last article from 1910, "Some General Remarks on Hysterical Attacks,"[8] Freud analyses attacks as grammatical sentences. It seems to me that what interested him with hysterics was not to see them but to hear them, that there is an impossibility with the word, as a result of a traumatic origin. Here, is the anchoring point. This formed for him the phantasy that psychoanalysis would one day bring to light a word transparent to itself. In 1910, in "The Future Prospects of Psycho-Analytic Therapy"[9] Freud outlines a luminous future: when psychoanalysis will be widespread in the community, playing a hygienic role, neurotics will no longer have to use defence mechanisms, because this will be immediately understood and interpreted. It's very touching! If like as if at a dinner party the etiquette requires that "When the ladies wish to retire to the powder room, all they have to say is I'm going to gather some flowers." Now as everyone understands they will have no more need for metaphor and need only say: "I'm going to the powder room."

To return to our subject matter. I shall begin with the easiest assertion: the hysteric speaks with her body. Does it not have to be said that it's usual for the speaking being to appeal to his body as evidence of the truth of his discourse? This can be observed in mimicry as an agreement with the Autre, or again as the signs of affect as the excess of my body (tears, blushing, etc.) bearing witness to my involuntary capture by the Autre. Parade is linked to the human imaginary as an appeal to the Autre and especially in love and war where my body is witness to the truth of my engagement with the Autre. Clinically, we know that the failure of this engagement is problematic. (See Freud's interest in the War Neuroses).[10]

I propose that the hysteric makes of her body a gift, she makes of it a servant of the Autre, so that the Autre can be her master, her body becoming a place of sheer enjoyment according to the order of sacrifice and love. As evidence of what this gift could be: the cervical feature, serving as a limit and function to be re-found in the symptom: a lump in the throat, choking, dyspnoea, aphonia, even the scar which our techniques of resuscitation leave after a suicide attempt. If the hysteric perceives that her existence is tenable only from the lack in the Autre which it gives as a gift, and if she considers herself to be responsible for this castration of the Autre, we understand that she for her part, commits herself to compensatory activity. Herein lies a paradox, as her aim is that this activity will not succeed to the extent that this success would achieve the death of the Autre and in this way the loss of her position. That is why she lives her love as quarrelsome. She hears every word as a demand and she commits herself to a sacrificial activism, in order to satisfy the enjoined imploration. Look at Bertha Pappenheim[11] and her militant feminism: worker for Jewish culture, social worker, mother of orphans, anti-Zionist, caught up in a passion for German, later Nazi, culture. Tragically divided in this compensatory activity.

The impossible, guaranteed by the violence and the arbitrary nature of the legislator is understood as impotence, side-lining her existence. Because of this she makes of herself a therapeutic object, fearing the miracle which might be produced. Her facile attachment to the idealised figure of the priest or the doctor, the former for knowledge of her body, the latter for her soul [...] each will know their male opposite number. There is an everlasting appeal to the coming of a master who will totally and finally enjoy her, thus permitting her in her turn to totally enjoy.

These particularities are able to account for the drama of the division of jouissance with sexuality, of her anxiety with regard to a debt which is never settled. There is division because she has to ensure the jouissance of the Autre as a demand of the superego: she has to work in the scopic field to ensure the perfection of the image to be offered for the jouissance of the Autre. Within the domain of the voice, she has to ensure satisfaction of what is heard, as a demand, the prevalence of orality. There is an attempt at sublimation, in both these registers (to be a sheer look, sheer capture, sheer voice) to lead her to sexuality, to make of herself in this way, Mother, or The Woman: all the women for a man. Confronted with the man to whom she has given a gift of her own impotence, faced with the sudden appearance of the phallic sign which represents her own body as a return of the sexual object, for which she had retreated for the Autre, disgusts functions as a barrier. In the same vein, her castrating activity, in the guise of a moral imperative for everybody around her, yet always fearing that her wish will be realised because she would then lose all her bearings with regard to her desire.

Another aspect of division: a persecutory kind of over-sensitivity, pseudo-paranoical, in the face of manifestations of love, for which she meanwhile appeals (See what Freud says on violation by the father).[12] This is accompanied by a pseudo-perverse activity in the pursuit of a forever fatal relationship.

There is indeed, a double personality, in the division between, on the one hand, the multiplicity of masks she wears to function as an object of desire, to be found in every word addressed to her (empathy, finesse, signs of a worldly life), and on the other hand, the unique character of fidelity, to be the one for the Autre. The relationship she has to mothering represents love finally purified: to make a master, to make a real man. All this is around the fundamental phantasy: a homosexual temptation in so far as it has to do with an attempt to take – herself, to enjoy herself – she at least would know how to handle him with regard to making love. There is a demand for equality and for the interchangeability of partners, as if $\frac{1}{2} + \frac{1}{2} = 1$, repressing the zero.

To conclude, let us return to the symptoms of mutism. If the hysteric stops speaking, we see there, without a doubt, the return to the Autre of this silence which manipulates and for which she yearns, but also her repugnance for a word which engages her in such servitude. Thus, there is hope for a supposedly natural communication, archaic, intuitive, to be understood without speaking, furtive looks in mutual silence: something may indeed happen there. Can we not understand this silence on the position of agent in her discourse, as the presence of the sheer subject, as a sign of the omnipotence of the Autre in so far as it is barred?

LAURENCE BATAILLE BASCH: Did you say to be a sheer look, a sheer voice?

CHARLES MELMAN: There is a kind of pressure to make a spectacle, to make a scene in the register of the look. She is weighed down by all of this, she is exhausted at the end of the day. With regard to the voice, there is an attempt to be witness to sheer silence. A patient once said "when I speak, I have the impression that I'm playing at comedy. I am only real when I keep quiet." We only have to believe her!

ERIC LAURENT: And masculine hysteria?

CHARLES MELMAN: That's a relevant question. It is no less frequent and would have to be taken up with other coordinates. But, as for the essential, from the matricial point of view, it's consistent.

JEAN ALLOUCH: There are two things which must be interpreted differently: after 1910 it is no longer a question of hysteria, and Freud would have linked certain signs in attaching hysteria to trauma. We can understand this in a different way.

For Freud, trauma has a different meaning to that of the medical discourse of the time, where it is seen as something privative: the hysteric is suggestible because there is weakness there at the beginning, so that there is no obstacle to suggestion. Freud generalises the concept of trauma and in so doing destroys it. It has not got to do with a weakness, but a surplus of energy. Trauma is already the sign of what would later be defined in "Beyond the Pleasure Principle." It is already shown that the excess energy is not capable of being taken up by the ego.

CHARLES MELMAN: With the second topology, Freud freed himself totally from a message which would have come from the Autre, in this case, the hysteric. Freud believed that there was an accident in nature, either too early or too late. He hoped that there was only the accidental, the contingent. He began to engage, from 1910 onwards with the dream theory which was enough to interpret to lift the symptom. This archaic dream was indeed something to be enthusiastic about! The second topology is a re-examination. If the death drive is difficult to accept, it's because it is preferable not to know anything about it in an economy maintaining the concept of somatic conversion.

CLAUDE CONTÉ: You speak about the castrating activity of the hysteric with regard to her entourage and a fear that her wish will come to pass. It seems to me that this does not take account of the castrating machine: for example, the hysteric wants to make a show and exhausts herself in so doing. Why not link this to seduction? In this way she arouses the desire of the masculine Autre on whom she depends. But which desire does she want in so doing? From the moment this desire reveals itself as sexual, something goes wrong for her, so she evades something. Who is the hysteric in this evasion?

CHARLES MELMAN: I tried to make some formulae intelligible. That being said, I adhere to what I said. We can make links between this "making a scene" and the intended castrating effect: After the seduction, there is nothing to see. Contrary to what is believed the hysteric holds a certain restraint, which preserves her phantasy. Ah, the day she will let it be seen, we will see what we will see!

COLETTE MISRAHI: And what she can show, or make seen, is the child. In analysis it's often the child who she makes appear, instead of anxiety. And sometimes the child may even be called Flower!

CHARLES MELMAN: Yes, indeed I've tried to show how the relationship with the child could be conflictual.

JACQUES LACAN: It is obviously striking that with the second topology Freud did not in some way translate the discourse of the hysteric and that he did not translate it in a condensed way in these terms: there is no sexual rapport. Because if there is someone, a typical example, that is to say who pays the price with her skin, that which I postulate as real, it's the hysteric. Because it is clear that on the other hand, all the same, in the detail, that's what Freud said. Trauma, it's the encounter with something which for her is the sign of sexual rapport, but as to precisely what, it's here that she does not respond to any degree. If it is the real, which is what I'm saying, that there is no sexual rapport, it opens up a question, a question which I will not develop now, but which is this: that if we can have any hope of the real, it's to the extent that as speaking beings, and linked to this existence as speaking beings, linked by a coherence which is not yet elucidated, linked to this, to this real, I would say the possibility of acceding to it as to this impossible, like this constituted impossible, it's linked to that which the speaking being, in being put forward as a speaking being, there is hope of having access to the real for him. So what specifies the relationship of the hysteric, of whom we cannot say she is nothing on this road to the real? She knows the way but it has to be said that she keeps a good distance, that's the least that can be said. Because it cannot be said that the hysteric circumscribes in a military way this road to the real, although all the same things turn around, even if it is only in this emergence of the analytic discourse.

What then constitutes the discourse of the hysteric? It is, I believe, and with this I wish to bring witness of my response, in what Melman has said. It's this: to this real that there is no sexual rapport (that sexual rapport cannot in any way be registered that is to say, to take sense) to this real, this other formula is substituted. I think you will see one of the motivations for the title of my seminar of this year: "There is *as yet* no sexual rapport". And all her behaviour is determined by it. I note, but I cannot anymore remember who, someone who was the very definition of "seduction". Seduction means that she knows, and Melman has well emphasised that she has pinpointed that to be the object of the man, she has to support herself from *a* and on this condition that this will not entail any jouissance. And what I already wrote on the board, to give the two terms to help support the woman, with her partner, these two terms have to double up, precisely by this *a* by which the woman is the object of seduction, and with this which is the narrow rapport with her jouissance, by which I will write. S (A). That is to say, the question which I asked in my seminar this year, if a woman ever knows and because of that can ever say what her jouissance is about. She is divided by this, and this is the central point, the point of conflict by which the hysteric supports herself, she is there between the two: seduction on one hand, militant love on the other. Ultimately, that's what guided Bertha Pappenheim towards the end of her life. Militarism, with regard to which a question was asked earlier, it's love, love of humanity.

Therefore, to give my response to what such a substantial discourse suggests to me, precisely with regard to the clinic, with what Melman has brought to us, all holds together not in this "pas" (not) but in the mirage of this "not yet".

JEAN CLAVREUL: It is said and it's true that hysteria changes, that the hysterics are no longer the same. Some people even say we do not see real hysterics anymore, or that we don't have anything to learn from them nowadays. And yet I think that nobody doubts that it's not so much that hysterics have changed but a certain discourse which we hold and if they no longer have anything to teach us its perhaps to the extent that we hardly listen to them, that appears to me to be significant. In any case is to point out that during the great era of hysteria I'm talking about that of the Salpêtrière, of the time of Charcot,[13] that which followed immediately on the great era of medicine, that's when medicine during the 19th century acquired its scientific status, an era in which in any case medicine could think it had acquired an aptitude for producing a rigorous nosology. I would say there is a succession, like two explosive breakthroughs which succeed each other. And, I think we can say something analogous every time something of the order of hysteria is found. That is to say that it's a great time of something which may be within the scientific approach. But also within the history of thought perhaps in particular that of religious thought, to the extent that witchcraft, demonic possession, mysticism, all these manifestations where we quite readily see hysterical manifestations, all these have surely not come about accidentally. There is something here which seems to me to be very important to point out and which, I believe can be located by referring ourselves as to what could be the dependence of the discourse of hysteria with regard to the apparition, the blossoming, the development of the discourse of the master.

In focussing therefore on the interest which the discourse of hysteria holds for us, that at the same time diverts our attention from something which we could say is its blindness or fascination (reciprocal, by the way) which is inevitably produced when the attention is fixed on the symptomology, or when, in one way or another we let ourselves be taken in by the seduction of the hysteric. It seems to me therefore that it's in this aftermath of the Freudian contribution that Lacan situates when he speaks of the discourse of the hysteric between the discourse of the master (I said earlier just after it) and before the discourse of the analyst.[14]

It's never without anxiety that this situation where the hysteric is basically the initiator of a certain type of relation, it's never without anxiety that hysterics discover that they are in some way the indispensable support and even the agent of the desire of the father, or to say things differently, that they look to establish someone in his place who would be a master. But precisely what they have to discover, is that the master, he, or the father, fades away to the extent that one looks for him; and he pathetically, and with difficulty holds the place which she gives him, which is this same place which should be the support of the discourse of the master. Psychoanalysis certainly does not and especially the psychoanalyst must not attempt to play this role with his well-honed knowledge with regard to the desire of the hysteric. When an analysand discovers that it is necessary to have an analysand for there to be an analyst, it's always felt by him as the discovery of the absence of the discourse of the master.

But it's not there that the analyst takes risks. What is carried out in analysis is something else altogether […] For psychoanalysis, something else happens, it's the possibility of taking into account not only the hysteric as such, but her discourse, that is to say to accept her as a speaking being, that is to say in fact, as a speaking subject of her phantasy, speaking of her rapport with object *a* if you wish. The risk that we run, it's certainly not to put too much emphasis on the importance of the object *a* or the game of desire and of jouissance but to use it to constitute of it a new discourse of mastery. This would end up with the reconstitution of a sort of nosology where the vagaries of the organisation of desire would be listed in the same way that the doctor studies and lists the normal or the pathological.

JACQUES ADAM: In a more fundamental way is homosexuality not linked to the homosexuality of the father of the hysteric? I'm saying this following a session where a person had heard that the hysteric is homosexual, "O. K. but my father wanted a son and not a girl. I am a homosexual but I've got it from someone."

JEAN CLAVREUL: Perhaps you are making reference to the allusion made by the hysteric to the castration of the father, always a difficult problem for her to confront?

FRANÇOISE DOLTO: It is said that Freud no longer concerned himself with hysteria. I wonder if the rapport between Anna O.[15] and Breuer did not make him phobic? And then there was Groddeck. It was he who gave the word *Ça* to Freud. Freud took this up in his topology and Groddeck[16] helped him with hysterical conversion in children's troubles brought to the doctor. Groddeck was the first to speak so well of the hysterical familial symptoms in the trio of the father – mother – child. This is a trap for parents who wish to understand their child, instead of living and allowing them to live. We cannot understand anything at all of the desire of these adults. Hysterics are people, men and women staying in the illusory belief that the value of sexuality, is for a woman to produce, for a man to have a hard-on for himself and the other, a mirror of oneself. This continues in the ego ideal of adults. Children then are in an impossibility of assuming their desire, and so they make a conversion in their own bodies. They are stupid, someone says. There are children, who through their Oedipal phase have become hysterics by an identification with their own sex through the behaviour of a domestic animal. The father for the girl, the mother for the boy, give this animal as an example with regard to their narcissistic emotional relationship. A trapped child, he will become even more trapped with the so-called instruction in sexuality at school.

MOUSTAPHA SAFOUAN: At the risk of appearing a little excessive, I will say that psychoanalysis began with hysteria, and psychoanalytic knowledge will always be worth only what our knowledge of this structure is worth.

By this I mean we can do our work, and well, without knowing what the transference is. We can obtain appreciable modifications in the treatment of an obsessional neurosis without being able to say exactly how we have obtained them. But it is out of the question to introduce significant modifications in a case of hysteria without knowing ... I'm about to launch a nasty word here. Let us backpedal a bit and let us say: without ridding ourselves of all knowledge But, it's hardly believable.

So let us take up this sentence, which we often hear from hysterics, in different forms, depending on style and temperament: For example, "The positive transference, it will never happen!" or: "It's incredible how you leave me indifferent," to which sometimes she adds "It is beginning to worry me" or again "It's impossible for me to love you".

At first sight, this is a negative sentence. But, by dint of having heard it repeated with this insistence, we are obliged to tell ourselves that because it's about an intellectual negation that there is therefore a denegation in question. From this time onwards there will be no doubt about the truth, easy to find: all we have to do is deny the negation, which gives: I was going to say; this is impossible; let us rather say: as I did not give her, the analysand, any particular reasons to love me, this can only be an appearance of love. Not even that! For where has this appearance come? So, it can only be a reappearance of love: a repetition.

Let us suppose now that we have this little strength called patience, which does not mean that we are going to resign ourselves to routine habits; let us suppose that we suspend a received knowledge, even if it is well founded, then we end up by learning, sooner or later, that it has to do with a sentence which has nothing particularly negative about it. By this I mean that its impact lies not in the form of the negation, but that it's a sentence, like many others, which is in fact only a half-sentence: the other half is repressed. If this were restored, it would give very different results. For example, "It is impossible to love you ... because it is impossible to love shit." At this moment we begin to know.

To clarify the oscillation with which I began, let me say this: it is impossible to analyse a hysteric without knowing. Besides, this is a known fact, but one that we cover with a prudish silence, I don't know why. Some of our colleagues are incontestably competent with all kinds of analyses, but when it comes to displacing a hysterical structure by one inch, there is no doubt about it, they do not know.

Let us now enter into the heart of the matter. To get straight to the point, I will point out: the form of the law, presented as a demand or command, is the source of a lure, which consists in the law's appearing to be born out of the mouth of the one who proffers it. In other words, it is a law that the will of the Autre imposes or wants to impose and not as a law to which the other submits herself. Besides, does she submit herself to it? Here is the snag.

But, in the meantime we see the possibility of a wish to be the lawmaker. A little bit of reflection will be enough to convince us that if there is the blindest of wishes, that is to say a wish that has no possibility of being fulfilled except in the sharing of this wish with its object that is to say in this lure: An author of the law exists.

What I have just said can be summarised in a formula: there would be no reason to believe in God if it were not for the role that was expressly assigned to Him in the beginning: as the creator of eternal verities for which you would not need to be an analyst to understand the impact and even the justice of it.

Let us now suppose a subject who settles himself into this belief, sacred or profane. We see, first, that this movement is not without a reciprocal division: that is to say his or one's own. Secondly, we can translate this confidently into our language by saying that the subject in question demands the symbolic father, and will not be happy with anything less. Thirdly, we can conceive of the possibility that, by an obscure pathway but not impossible to trace, is precisely that of a questioning of the paternity of this divine, this symbolic father, something may result which I will call, 'knowing too much about maternity'. Because it is a fact that the hysteric ignores nothing that concerns the ways of motherhood.

We will keep present in our minds this constellation, this package of premises, and we ask what consequences it has with these few coordinates for the subject we have just defined.

So that you are able to appreciate fully the response, it is essential that I recall here Lacan's thesis on the function of beauty.[17] Lacan defined beauty as this brilliance which dazzles us and is interposed between us and the second death. Now, what is this? What is this second death?

Hegel[18] says "the life of children is the death of parents". This is doubtful. Most often we observe the contrary. What is not doubtful, but only analytic experience permits us to affirm this, is that the subject comes to be a parent only to the extent that he rids himself of the phantasy which Hegel describes, without knowing that it is a phantasy, which is to say, Hegel takes it for reality.

Knowledge is the second death. It is precisely because all tools fail him, which would permit him to accede to this knowledge, that the one we call psychotic is sometimes pushed to fulfil the second death in a real, physical death. And the first? If there is a second, there is also a first.

The first is that of narcissistic birth, of the narcissistic birth of this image which is also the model, par excellence, of every corpse. A poignant citation from Maurice Blanchot,[19] has recently reminded us of this.

Now, let us remember the moving moment when Dora[20] spent two hours contemplating the *Sistine Madonna* of Raphael in the museum of Dresden. I, for my part will not turn my nose up at Raphael. It's a fact that his *Sistine Madonna* is indeed one of the images of beauty before which desire experiences itself in its intimate tenor of nostalgia and regret while at the same time its pain and sickness are veiled. But in any case, this is not a reason for us in our turn to remain mute before it.

Let us imagine that the stomach of the Madonna if I may say so, begins to inflate, to round out, advancing into real space, and imagine the effect this would produce on the one contemplating it. This gives us an idea of the strange convulsions that every time her discourse, and not her vain curiosity, puts her closer to the *reality* of maternity and that finally this body not yet, not a dispossessed body in the imaginary or the real, as would be the case with a neurotic or psychotic, but a unique condition of the hysteric, a possessed body: a body that spits, vomits, bleeds, grows fat, and develops symptoms: all this leaving her without any understanding.

There is nothing surprising in this: because in this "too much" she knows too much about maternity and therein resides, not the distance, but the formal hiatus between this knowledge and the truth. And what is this truth? There are many formulate. I will choose the following one:

Only the law makes jouissance condescend to desire. But the hysteric does not hear it this way. She wants, it would be better to say that she dreams, for this can only be a dream she dreams, then, of a desire which would be born of love: and this in turn can only sharpen the antinomy between love and desire.

Let understand this because in a certain way, such an antinomy does not exist. What I mean by this is that desire always brings along with it a certain amount of love; a little or a lot, repressed or not, it is not important.

But what of love? The inverse is not true: despite all the praise that has been addressed to the little god of love, it has remained completely incapable of engendering the least little bit of desire.

But what is love, if not the fibres of being tending toward an object? And all this lack would be void of desire? Ah yes, for there are lacks and there are lacks.[...]

With regard to lack, philosophers have defined the concept as privation, as a real lack. Analytic experience has brought forth, to the point where it is impossible to misconstrue it, another kind of lack, which is distinguished from the first in that the recovery of the missing object (or called as such) brings no plenitude, no satisfaction; this is frustration. Love is this frustration. Let us understand by this I mean pure love, like as we say pure oxygen, that is to say that it is never seen or ever so concretely except in some socially institutionalised forms, the most exemplary example of which is courtly love, or else in poetry, specifically, in the English metaphysics or in certain Arab mystics. Therefore, I'm saying that love in this sense is frustration because at the root of love there is abolition and abandonment, to say nothing of the betrayal by the object. Of this object one retains only a sign, a look, salutation, simple presence, I was going to say a picture, why not a photo? This affinity between love and object loss or mourning has been noted by many analysts beginning with Freud himself. They never dreamed of finding the lost object in the object itself; the object of the aim of love.

Desire belongs to another order, one to which I referred earlier in talking about Lacan's formula because I think that it's always his formula and about which I've have said that the hysteric consents to it with difficulty. But then what does she do?

Take a child and tell him the story of the stork that nips a mother or future mother on the leg. If this child has strong dispositions toward obsessional neurosis, he will begin to limp. This is a symptom founded on the following reasoning: "The stork nipped me, thus I have a baby in my belly." The obsessional is in fact a naïf; that is why we can work with him more or less well. But if the child's dispositions bear towards hysteria, he will also limp; there will be the same symptom, but not the same reasoning: he will say: "The stork nipped me, however I do not have a baby in my belly, you are lying!" We have to ask ourselves, why does the hysteric hold onto this, "you lie"? Does she have to pose the other as a liar? The reason is that it is precisely in this lie of the Autre that her faith, or her little faith, in the phallus resides. [...]

She wants the phallus to go walk-about, for it to be a wanderer. And this is why, wherever she goes, she brings war with her, ideological war, war of prestige, which we know has no object, but of which she meanwhile makes herself the focus.

It is only when she renounces what is at stake, but we will have to precede her there, it's only at that moment that she will be ready to conquer the real truth. This is to say that she has never demanded anything other than to be loved for her imperfections, those imperfections with which she has always been reproached. It is at this very moment, then that we learn from her, from this mother in sufferance, that there is only one trauma; which endures, and it's the trauma of birth.

SERGE LECLAIRE: When the reference to the phallus arrives as the ultimate signifier, as the significant signifier, this signifier which replaces our belief in mythology or in science, this place of an ultimate signifier, it could indeed make one or other of us say that psychoanalysis is really a phallocentric theory on the same model as the doctrines or theocentric religious. I have the feeling that something of this phallus escapes us. Not least when we mention the phallus as a part of the body, that is to say something which would be nearer the side of the object.

The question is therefore: Is the phallus a signifier? Is it this pure signifier, this original signifier once again? Is the phallus the object? And I don't think that last Sunday, you missed hearing what I had to say concerning the phallic drive, as an attempt, more or less blind by the way, of reintroducing something of the order of the phallus as object, even as a partial object. For me, it's a question of the phallus, when something of castration as such is envisaged. This is castration not in any way to be understood from a more or less representable perspective, but strictly, from a structural point of view or even from a structuring one. By this I mean this point as this double reference through which something of the irreducible difference of the signifier and of the object may be ensured. The phallus is neither a signifier, nor an object, it is at one and the same time signifier and object.

MOUSTAPHA SAFOUAN: You have used two formulae "neither signifier, nor object", because "one and the other." So, in fact there is one and the other, but this excludes the first formula. I agree more with "one and the other." Indeed, it's an object, but as it is an object which has to be used from time to time, it's only in psychoanalysis that it is noticed that this is not done all alone, but that it raises a certain problematic where this same phallus intervenes again but this time as a signifier [...].

As we are having these study days with an eye to what the I.P.A. is organising around the same time, it's the right time to remember that indeed in analytic theory, in analytic conceptualisation, a certain slope is followed according to which the advent of sexuality ... Here, without taking things into account, are two points of view which exclude each other, expanding this idea of maturation and at the same of gift of accomplished oblativity. It's one or the other. Indeed, we can read the most recent publications, where we see the proximity of these two points of view, up to this very day.

The phallic question arises and tends to be elaborated in the School as Leclaire mentioned earlier. It's not for nothing, because, indeed in sharing things, in leaving to one side biological science, or the support one could take from maturation (which in any case, would entail no conflict because they are connected by nature). If one puts to one side this reference, we will see that far from functioning as a gift – which is evidence itself, that it's not a detachable object – the phallus, therefore, as a signifier, functions, au contraire as the sign of a threshold, in other words as a sign that there is a threshold beyond which satisfaction is not obtained by way of the gift. It is the signifier which indicates the limit the gift is able to bring as satisfaction.

Notes

1 This chapter was produced from notes taken by Philippe Julien, Monique Chollet and Philippe Kuypers.
2 Hippocrates, *The Corpus: The Hippocratic Writings, Vol. I* (trans. A.F. Adams). Loeb Classical Library, Cambridge, MA: Harvard University Press, 1989.
3 Aristotle, *On Rhetoric: A Theory of Civil Discourse* (trans. A Kennedy). Oxford: Oxford University Press, 1991.
4 G. Galen, *Method of Medicine, Vol I* (trans. I. Johnston and G.H.R. Horsley). Cambridge, MA: Harvard University Press.
5 St Augustine, *On Christian Teaching* (trans. P.P.H. Green). Oxford: Oxford University Press, 2010.
6 J-M. Charcot, *Lectures on the Diseases of the Nervous System* (trans. G. Sigerson). London: The Sydenham Society, 1877.
7 S. Freud, *Beyond The Pleasure Principle, Group Psychology and Other Works*, Vol. XVIII, S.E. (1920–1922). London: The Hogarth Press, 1955.
8 S. Freud, "Some General Remarks on Hysterical Attacks", in *Jensen's "Gradiva" and Other Works*. Vol. IX, S.E. (1906–1908). London: The Hogarth Press, 1959.
9 S. Freud, "The Future Prospects of Psycho-Analytic Therapy" in *Five Lectures on Psychoanalysis. Leonardo Da Vinci and Other Works*, Vol. XI, S.E. (1910). London: The Hogarth Press, 1957.
10 S. Freud, *Introductory Lectures on Psychoanalysis*, Part III. Vol. XVI, S.E. (1916–1917). London: The Hogarth Press, 1963. See also, Freud, *Beyond The Pleasure Principle*.
11 S. Freud, *Studies on Hysteria*, Vol. II, S.E. (1893–1895). London: The Hogarth Press, 1955.
12 S. Freud, *Studies on Hysteria*.
13 J-M. Charcot, *Lectures on the Diseases of the Nervous System* (trans. G. Sigerson). London: The Sydenham Society, 1877.
14 J. Lacan, *The Seminar of Jacques Lacan, Book XVII: The Other Side of Psychoanalysis, 1969–1970* (trans. C. Gallagher, unedited).
15 S. Freud, *Studies on Hysteria*, Vol. II, S.E. (1893–1895). London: The Hogarth Press, 1955.

16 G. Groddeck, *The Book of the It* (trans. P.G. Christensen). Madison, WI: University of Wisconsin Press, 1993.
17 Lacan, J. *The Ethics of Psychoanalysis.*
18 G.W.F. Hegel, *The Phenomenology of Spirit* (trans. A.V. Miller). Oxford: Oxford University Press, 1976.
19 M. Blanchot, *Infinite Conversation* (trans. S. Hanson). Minneapolis: University of Minnesota Press. 1992.
20 S. Freud, "The Dora Case" in *A Case of Hysteria, Three Essays on Sexuality and Other Works*, Vol. VII, S.E. (1901–1905). London: The Hogarth Press.

Bibliography

Works by Freud

Freud, S. "Draft – G. Melancholia" in *Pre-Psycho-Analytic Publications and Unpublished Drafts*, Vol. I (1886–1899). S.E. London: The Hogarth Press, 1966.

Freud, S. "Hysteria" in *Pre-Psycho-Analytic Publications and Unpublished Drafts*.

Freud, S. "Points for a Comparative Study of Organic and Hysterical Motor Paralysis" in *Pre-Psycho-Analytic Publications and Unpublished Drafts*.

Freud, S. "Project for A Scientific Psychology" in *Pre-Psycho-Analytic Publications and Unpublished Drafts*.

Freud, S. *Studies on Hysteria*, Vol. II, S.E. (1893–1899). London: The Hogarth Press, 1955.

Freud, S. "On the Psychical Mechanism of Hysterical Phenomena: Preliminary Communication" in *Studies on Hysteria*.

Freud, S. "Neuro-Psychoses of Defence" in *Early Psycho-Analytic Publications*, Vol. III, S.E. (1893–1899). London: The Hogarth Press, 1962.

Freud, S. *The Interpretation of Dreams*, Vol. IV, S.E. (1900). London: The Hogarth Press, 1953.

Freud, S. *The Interpretation of Dreams (Second Part) and On Dreams*, Vol. V, S.E. (1900–1901). London: The Hogarth Press, 1953.

Freud, S. "The Dora Case" in *A Case of Hysteria, Three Essays on Sexuality and Other Works*, Vol. VII, S.E. (1901–1905). London: The Hogarth Press, 1953.

Freud, S. "Fragment of a Case of Hysteria" in *A Case of Hysteria, Three Essays on Sexuality and Other Works*.

Freud, S. *Jensen's Gravida and Other Works*, Vol. IX, S.E. (1906–1909). London: The Hogarth Press, 1959.

Freud, S. "Some General Remarks on Hysterical Attacks", in *Jensen's "Gradiva" and Other Works*.

Freud, S. "'Civilised' Sexual Morality and Nervous Illness" in *Jensen's Gravida and Other Works*.

Freud, S. "The Future Prospects of Psycho-Analytic Therapy" in *Five Lectures on Psychoanalysis. Leonardo Da Vinci and Other Works*, Vol. XI, S.E. (1910). London: The Hogarth Press, 1957.

Freud, S. *The Case of Schreber, Papers on Technique and Other Works*, Vol. XII, S.E. (1911–1913). London: The Hogarth Press, 1958.

Freud, S. "The Unconscious" in *The Case of Schreber, Papers on Technique and Other Works*.

Freud, S. *Totem and Taboo and Other Works*, Vol. XIII, S.E. (1913–1914). London: The Hogarth Press, 1955.

Freud, S. "Instincts and their Vicissitudes" in *On the History of the Psycho-Analytic Movement, Papers on Metapsychology and Other Works*, Vol. XIV (1914–1916). S. E. London: The Hogarth Press, 1957.

Freud, S. "Narcissism" in *On the History of the Psychoanalytic Movement, Papers on Metapsychology and Other Works*.

Freud, S. "Repression" in *On the History of the Psychoanalytic Movement, Papers on Metapsychology and Other Works*.

Freud, S. *Introductory Lectures on Psycho-Analysis*, Part III, Vol. XVI, S.E. (1916–1917). London: The Hogarth Press, 1963.

Freud, S. *An Infantile Neurosis and Other Works*, Vol. XVI, S.E. (1917–1918). London: The Hogarth Press, 1955.

Freud, J. "The Wolfman Case" in *An Infantile Neurosis and Other Works*, Vol. XVII, S.E. (1917–1919). London: The Hogarth Press, 1955.

Freud, S. *Beyond the Pleasure Principle, Group Psychology and Other Works*, Vol. XVIII, S.E. (1920–1922). London: The Hogarth Press, 1955.

Freud, S. "Beyond the Pleasure Principle" in *Beyond the Pleasure Principle, Group Psychology and Other Works*.

Freud, S. "Identification" in *Beyond the Pleasure Principle, Group Psychology and Other Works*.

Freud, S. "The Psychogenesis of a Case of Homosexuality in a Woman" in *Beyond the Pleasure Principle and Other Works*.

Freud, S. "Dissolution of the Oedipus Complex" in *The Ego and the Id and Other Works*, Vol. XIX, S.E. (1923–1925). London: The Hogarth Press, 1961.

Freud, S. "The Infantile Genital Organisation" in *The Ego and the Id and Other Works*.

Freud, S. "Negation" in *The Ego and the Id and Other Works*.

Freud, S. "Some Psychical Consequences of the Anatomical Distinction between the Sexes" in *The Ego and the Id and Other Works*.

Freud, S. "Verneinung" in *The Ego and the Id and Other Works*.

Freud, S. "Civilisation and its Discontents" in *The Future of an Illusion, Civilisation and its Discontents and Other Works*, Vol. XXI, S.E. (1927–1931). London: The Hogarth Press.

Freud, S. "Fetishism" in *The Future of an Illusion, Civilisation and its Discontents and Other Works*.

Freud, S. "Femininity" in *New Introductory Lectures on Psycho-Analysis and Other Works*, Vol. XXII, S.E. (1932–1936). London: The Hogarth Press, 1964.

Freud, S. *"The Question of aNew Introductory Lectures on Psycho-Analysis and Other Works*.

Works by Lacan

Lacan, J. "Family Complexes in the Formation of the Individual" in *Encyclopédie Française*, Vol. 8. (edited by A. de Monzie). Paris, 1938 (translated by C. Gallagher, unedited).

Lacan, J. *The Seminar of Jacques Lacan, Book II: The Ego in Freud's Theory and in the Technique of Psychoanalysis, 1954–1955* (edited by J-A. Miller, translated by S. Tomaselli). Cambridge: Cambridge University Press, 1988.

Lacan, J. *The Seminar of Jacques Lacan, Book III: The Psychoses, 1955–1956* (edited by J-A. Miller, translated by R. Grigg). London: Routledge, 1993.

Lacan, J. *Dialogue avec les Philosophes Français.* Société Française de Philosophie, 23 February 1957.

Lacan, J. *The Seminar of Jacques Lacan, Book IV: The Object Relation* (edited by J-A. Miller, translated by A.R. Price). Cambridge: Polity Press, 2020.

Lacan, J. *The Seminar of Jacques Lacan, Book V: The Formations of the Unconscious, 1957–1958.* (translated by C. Gallagher, unedited).

Lacan, J. *The Seminar of Jacques Lacan, Book VII: The Ethics of Psychoanalysis, 1959–1960* (edited by J-A. Miller, translated by D. Porter). London: Routledge, 1992.

Lacan, J. *The Seminar of Jacques Lacan, Book VIII: Transference, 1960–1961* (translated by C. Gallagher, unedited).

Lacan, J. *The Founding Act*, June 1964 (translated by C. Gallagher, unedited).

Lacan, J. *Proposal on the Psychoanalyst of the School, 1967* (translated by C. Gallagher, unedited).

Lacan, J. *The Four Fundamental Concepts of Psychoanalysis* (edited by J-A. Miller, translated by A. Sheridan). Paris: Éditions Seuil, 1978.

Lacan, J. *The Seminar of Jacques Lacan, Book XII: Crucial Problems for Psychoanalysis, 1964–1965* (translated by C. Gallagher, unedited).

Lacan, J. *The Seminar of Jacques Lacan, Book XIII: The Object of Psychoanalysis, 1965–1966* (translated by C. Gallagher, unedited).

Lacan, J. *The Seminar of Jacques Lacan, Book XIV: The Logic of Phantasy, 1966–1977* (translated by C. Gallagher, unedited).

Lacan, J. *The Seminar of Jacques Lacan, Book XVI: From an Other to the Other, 1968–1969* (translated by C. Gallagher, unedited).

Lacan, J. *The Seminar of Jacques Lacan, Book XVII: The Other Side of Psychoanalysis, 1969–1970* (translated by C. Gallagher, unedited).

Lacan, J. *The Seminar of Jacques Lacan, Book XVIII: On a Discourse that might not be a Semblance, 1970–1971* (translated by C. Gallagher, unedited).

Lacan, J. *The Knowledge of the Psychoanalyst, 1971–1972* (translated by C. Gallagher, unedited).

Lacan, J. *L'Étourdit*, Lacan 1972 (translated by C. Gallagher, unedited), unpublished.

Lacan, J. *The Seminar of Jacques Lacan, Book XX: Encore, 1972–1973* (translated by C. Gallagher, unedited).

Lacan, J. *The Seminar of Jacques Lacan, Book XXI, Part 1: Les non-dupes errent, 1973–1974* (translated by C. Gallagher, unedited).

Lacan, J. *La Troisième.* VII Congress of the Freudian School of Paris, Rome, November 1974.

Lacan, J. *The Seminar of Jacques Lacan, Book XXII: R.S.I., 1974–1975* (translated by C. Gallagher, unedited).

Lacan, J. *The Seminar of Jacques Lacan, Book XXII: Joyce and the Sinthome Part 2 (1975–1976)* (translated by C. Gallagher, unedited).

Lacan, J. "The Function and Field of Speech and Language in Psychoanalysis" in *Écrits* (translated by B. Fink). New York: W.W. Norton & Co., 2006.

Lacan, J. "Kant with Sade" in *Écrits*.

Lacan, J. "On a Question Preliminary to any Possible Treatment of Psychosis" in *Écrits*.

Lacan, J. *"The Mirror Stage as Formative of the Écrits*.

Lacan, J. "Science and Truth" in *Écrits*.

Lacan, J. "Seminar on 'The Purloined Letter'" in *Écrits*.

Lacan, J. "Presentation on Psychical Causality" in *Écrits*.

Lacan, J. "Aggressivity in Psychoanalysis" in *Écrits*.

Lacan, J. "On a Question Prior to Any Possible Treatment of Psychosis" in *Écrits*.

Lacan, J. "The Signification of the Phallus" in *Écrits*.

Lacan, J. "The Subversion of the Subject and the Dialectic of Desire in the Freudian Unconscious" in *Écrits*.

Lacan, J. *"Response to Jean Hippolyte's Commentary on Freud'sÉcrits*.

Lacan, J. "A Theoretical Introduction to the Functions of Psychoanalysis in Criminology" in *Écrits*.

Lacan, J. "Variations on the Standard Treatment" in *Écrits*.

Lacan, J. *The Proposition of the School* (translated by C. Gallagher, unedited), 1967.

Other sources

Abbé de Choisy, *The Transvestite Memoirs* (translated by R.H.F. Scott). London: Peter Owen Publishers, 1973.

Abraham, K."A Short Study of the Development of the Libido", in K. Abraham, *Selected Papers on Psychoanalysis*. London: Routledge, 1988.

AncientEgyptian Medicine: *ThePapyrus Ebers* (translated by C.P. Bryan). London and Chicago: Ares Publishers, 1930.

Aquinas, T. *Summa Theologica* (translated by A.J. Freddoso). South Bend, IN: St. Augustine's Press, 2010.

Aretaeus, *Consisting of Eight Books on the Causes, Symptoms, and Cure of Acute and Chronic Diseases* (1785) (translated by J. Moffat). Farmington, MI: Gale Ecco, 2018.

Aristotle, *On Rhetoric: A Theory of Civil Discourse* (translated by A Kennedy). Oxford: Oxford University Press, 1991.

Aristotle, *Metaphysics, Vol.* I (Books I–IX) (translated by H. Tredennick). Cambridge, MA: Harvard University Press, 1989.

Aristotle, *Organon* (translated by O.F. Owen). Vol. II. London: H.G. Bohn, 1853.

Aristotle, *Prior Analytics* (translated by O.F. Owen). London: H.G. Bohn, 1853.

Aristotle, *Prior Analytics*, Book II (translated by R. Smith. Indianapolis: Hackett Publishing Company, 1989.

Athenaeus of Naucratis, *The Learned Banqueters* (translated by D. Olson). Vol. I. Loeb Classical Library. Cambridge, MA: Harvard University Press, 2010.

Augustine. *The Confessions* (translated by H. Chadwick). Oxford: Oxford University Press, 2008.

Augustine. *On Christian Teaching* (translated by R.P.H. Green). Oxford: Oxford University Press, 2008.

Babinski, J. *Hysteria or Pithiatism* (translated by J.D. Rollerston, edited by E. Farquhar Buzzard). London: University of London Press, 1918.

Bernheim, H. *Hypnotisme, Suggestion, Psychotherapie*. Paris: Fayard, 1995.

Bichat, X. *Physiological Researches Upon Life and Death* (translated by T Watkins). Philadelphia: Longman, Hurst, Rees and Browne, 1816.

Blanchot, B. *Infinite Conversation* (translated by S. Hanson). Minneapolis: University of Minnesota Press. 1992.

Breasted, J.H. *The Edwin Smith Surgical Papyrus* (translation and commentary). The Papyrus Ebers. Vol. I. University of Chicago, Oriental Institute Publications, 1930.

Canguilhem, G. *On the Normal and the Pathological* (translated by C.R. Fawcett). New York: Zone Books, 1991.

Charcot, J.M. *Lectures on the Diseases of the Nervous System* (translated by G. Sigerson). London: The Sydenham Society, 1877.

Charcot, J-M. *Oeuvres complètes de J-M. Charcot*. Sydney: Wentworth Press, 2018.

Clastres, P. *Society Against the State: Essays in Political Anthropology* (translated by R. Hurley). New York: Zone Books, 1990.

Daumezon, G. "Essai historique critique de l'appareil d'assistance aux maladies mentaux dans le department de la Seine depuis le début du XIX Siècle", in *L'information psychiatrique* vol. 36, 1960.

Davies, P. "'KalosKagathos" and Scholarly Perceptions of Spartan Society', *Zeitschrift Für Alte Geschichte* 62, no. 3 (2013).

Descartes, R. *Discourse On Method* (translated by D.A. Cress). Indianapolis/Cambridge: Hackett Classics, 1998.

Descartes, R. *Meditations on First Philosophy with Selections from the Objections and Replies* (translated by M. Moriarty). Oxford: Oxford University Press, 2008.

DiagnosticandStatistical ManualofMentalDisorders (DSM–5), 5th edn. Washington, DC: American Psychiatric Association, 2013.

Ey, H. *Manuel de Psychiatrie*. Paris: Masson, 1960.

Falret, J.P. *Des Maladies Mentales et des Asiles d'Aliénés*. Sydney: Wentworth Press, 2018.

Foucault, M. *The Birth of the Clinic: An Archaeology of Medical Perception* (translated by A.S. Smith). New York: Panther Books, 1973.

Freud, S. *Selected Letters of Sigmund Freud to Martha Bernays* (compiled by A. Patel and A. Mehta). North Charleston, SC: CreateSpace Inc.

Freud, S. *The Complete Letters of Sigmund Freud to Wilhelm Fliess* (edited and translated by J.M. Masson). Cambridge, MA and London: Harvard University Press, 1985.

Galen, G. *Method of Medicine*, Vol I (translated by I. Johnston and G.H.R. Horsley). Cambridge, MA: Harvard University Press.

Galien, *De La Formation Des Enfans Au Ventre De La Mere Et De L'Enfantement A Sept Mois (1556)* (translated by G. Christian). Whitefish, MT: Kessinger Publishing, 2010.

Gide, A. *The Immoralist* (translated by D. Watson). London: Penguin Classics, 2008.

Groddeck, G. *The Book of the It* (translated by P.G. Christensen). Madison, WI: University of Wisconsin Press, 1993.

Herbermann, C. (ed) *Ancient Diocese of Mâcon*, Catholic Encyclopedia. New York: Robert Appleton Company, 1913.

Hegel, G.W.F. *Phenomenology of Spirit* (translated by A.V. Miller). New York: Oxford University Press, 1979.

Hippocrates, *On Ancient Medicine*. Vol. I. (translated by A.F. Adams), Vol. I. Loeb Classical Library. Cambridge, MA: Harvard University Press, 1989.

Hippocrates, *The Corpus: The Hippocratic Writings, Vol. I* (translated by A.F. Adams). Loeb Classical Library, Cambridge, MA: Harvard University Press, 1989.

Hughlings Jackson, J. *Evolution and Dissolution of the Nervous System (1881–1887)*. London: Thoemmes Continuum, 1998.

Israel, L. *L'Hysterique, Le Sexe, et le Medicin*. Paris: Masson, 1997.

Janet, P. *The Major Symptoms of Hysteria: Fifteen Lectures Given in the Medical School of Harvard University*. Whitefish, MT: Kessinger Publishing, 2007.

Jorden, E. *A Briefe Discourse of a Disease called the Suffocation of the Mother*. London, 1603.

Kretschmer, E. *Hysteria, Reflex and Instinct* (translated by V. Baskin and W. Baskin). New York: Philosophical Library, 1960.

Leriche, R. *The Philosophy of Surgery*. Bibliothèque de Philosophie Scientifique. Paris: Flammarion, 1951.

Lévi-Strauss, C. *The Elementary Structures of Kinship*, revised edition. (edited by R. Needham, translated by J.H. Bell, J.R. Von Sturmer and R. Needham). London: Eyre & Spottiswoode, 1969.

Liébeault, A.A. *Sleep and its Analogous States considered from the perspective of the action of the mind upon the body*. Paris: Masson, 1866.

Locke, J. *An Essay Concerning Human Understanding* edited by P.H. Nidditch). Oxford: Clarendon Press, 1979.

M. Mead, *Continuities in Cultural Evolution*. New Brunswick, NJ: Transaction Publishers, 1999.

De Musset, A. *The Confession of a Child of the Century* (translated by D. Coward). London: Penguin Books, 2012.

Pabst, G.W. *Secrets of a Soul*. Berlin, 1926 (A Psychoanalytic Film), viewed 24–25 April 1982, Study Days on Psychoanalytic Discourse, École Normale Supérieure, Paris.

Paracelsus, T. von Hohenheim, *The Hermetic and Alchemical Writings*. Vols I and II (translated by A.E. Waite). Eastford, CT: Martino Fine Books, 2009.

Paré, A.*Oeuvres*. Lyon: Editions du Fleuve, 1962.

Pinel, D., C. Caille and L. Ravier, *Traité Médico-Philosophique sur l'aliénation mentale, ou la manie*. Paris: Richard, Caille et Ravier, an IX, 1801.

Plato, *Gorgias* (translated by R. Waterfield). Oxford: Oxford University Press, 2008.

Plato, *The Symposium* (translated by C. Gill). London: Penguin Classics, 2003.

Plato, *Timaeus* (translated by P. Kalkavage). Hackett Classics, 1955.

Plato, *Laws* (translated by T.L. Pangle). Chicago: University of Chicago Press, 2016.

Le Pois, C. *Selectiorum observationum et consiliorum de praetervisis hactenus morbis affectibusque praeter naturam*. University of Lausanne. E. Typographeo. F. Hackii, 1768.

Proust, M. *In Search of Lost Time* (translated by A. Mayor, revised by G.J. Enright). New York: Random House Inc., 2014.

Rabelais, F. *The Life of Gargantua and Pantagruel* (translated by T. Urquhart and P.A. Motteux). New York: Penguin Random House, 1994.

Rank, O. *The Trauma of Birth* (edited by E.J. Lieberman). New York: Dover Publications, 1993.

Reich, W. *The Function of the Orgasm*. New York: Touchstone Books, 1974.

Russell, B. *Logic and Knowledge*. Nottingham, UK: Spokesman Books, 2012.

Sand, G. *L'édition complète des oeuvres de George Sand*. Caen: Presses Universitaires de Caen, 2017.

Sartre, J-P. *Being and Nothingness: An Essay in Phenomenological Ontology* (translated by S. Richmond). Abingdon: Routledge, 2018.

Sophocles, *The Three Theban Plays: Oedipus Rex, Oedipus at Colonus, Antigone* (translated by R. Fagles). New York: Penguin Classics, 1984.

Spencer, H. *On Social Evolution*. Chicago: University of Chicago Press, 1975.

Stendhal [Marie-Henri Beyle], *The Red and The Black* (translated by B. Raffel, with an Introduction by D. Johnson). New York: Dover Publications, 2004.

Sydenham, T. *The Works of Thomas Sydenham. M.D.* London: The Sydenham Society, 1850.

Thomas à Kempis, *The Imitation of Christ* (translated by R. Challoner). Gastonia, NC: TAN Classics, 1991.

Whalen, B. "Rethinking the Schism of 1054 – Authority Heresy and The Latin Rite", *Traditio* 67 (2007), pp. 1–24.

Winnicott, D. *Playing and Reality.* Foreword by F.R. Rodham. New York: Routledge, 2005.

Index

Note: Page numbers with italic *f* denote Figures

For Product Safety Concerns and Information please contact our EU
representative GPSR@taylorandfrancis.com
Taylor & Francis Verlag GmbH, Kaufingerstraße 24, 80331 München, Germany

www.ingramcontent.com/pod-product-compliance
Ingram Content Group UK Ltd.
Pitfield, Milton Keynes, MK11 3LW, UK
UKHW021451080625
459435UK00012B/461